ORTHOPAEDIC RADIOLOGY

PATTERN RECOGNITION AND DIFFERENTIAL DIAGNOSIS

To my late father,
Alfred Reichenbaum

ORTHOPAEDIC RADIOLOGY

PATTERN RECOGNITION AND DIFFERENTIAL DIAGNOSIS

Second Edition

Peter Renton FRCR, DMRD

Consultant Radiologist
Royal National Orthopaedic Hospital, London and Stanmore
and University College London Hospitals
Honorary Senior Lecturer,
Institute of Orthopaedics,
University College London

with the editorial assistance of

Veronika Aurens BA

MARTIN DUNITZ

© Peter Renton 1990, 1998

First published in the United Kingdom in 1990 by
Martin Dunitz Ltd
The Livery House
7–9 Pratt Street
London NW1 0AE

Second Edition 1998

A CIP catalogue record for this book is available from the British Library.

ISBN 1-85317-434-3

Distributed in the United States by:
Blackwell Science Inc.
Commerce Place, 350 Main Street
Malden, MA 02148, USA
Tel: 1-800-215-1000

Distributed in Canada by:
Login Brothers Book Company
324 Salteaux Crescent
Winnipeg, Manitoba, R3J 3T2
Canada
Tel: 204-224-4068

Distributed in Brazil by:
Ernesto Reichmann Distribuidora de Livros, Ltda
Rua Coronel Marques 335, Tatuape 03440-000
Sao Paulo,
Brazil

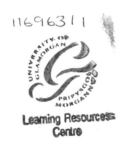
Composition by Scribe Design, Gillingham, Kent, United Kingdom
Printed and bound in Hong Kong by Imago

Contents

Preface to the First Edition

The aim of this short text is to provide an easy to read system of orthopaedic radiology for trainees in both orthopaedics and radiology. The approach is based on pattern recognition, first popularized by that great teacher Dr George Simon in his book *Principles of Bone X-ray Diagnosis**, which is now out of print. Diseases are described according to their predominant radiological features, rather than their pathological groups. These features form the basis of individual chapters. Using this method of instruction, it is inevitable that some conditions are described in more than one chapter. This is desirable as it reinforces information and also reduces the need for cross-referencing. The emphasis of each chapter, however, alters the way in which each disease is described.

The author hopes that the text will provide an understanding of radiological change and differential diagnosis, comprehensive lists of which are interspersed throughout. Suggestions for further reading are given at the end of the book.

*Simon G (1960) *Principles of Bone X-ray Diagnosis.* Butterworths, London

Preface to the Second Edition

The aim of this book remains to introduce trainees in radiology, orthopaedic surgery and rheumatology, as well as general radiologists, to the broad spectrum of radiological imaging.

Since the first edition, magnetic resonance imaging has become readily available and it would therefore have been impossible to write an orthopaedic textbook without taking this into account. The basis of this book and its method remains the plain film and the differential diagnosis obtained from it but, wherever necessary, corresponding MR images have been included, as well as CT and radioisotope scans, and to some extent ultrasound scans. New chapters have also been added on imaging of joints and on the spine and soft tissues. A brief chapter on methods of investigation in orthopaedic radiology has also been included.

List of Tables

Acknowledgements

This book was written at the suggestion of Professor Leslie Klenerman, formerly of Liverpool University and of Northwick Park Hospital. I am grateful for his encouragement.

Many of the illustrations have been taken from the files of the Radiology Museum of the Institute of Orthopaedics, London, with permission. I am conscious of my debt to my colleagues and indeed, to all those who have sent us films over the years. The illustrations have been provided by the Medical Photographic Department of the Institute of Orthopaedics and I am especially grateful to Mr Dirk de Camp for the care he has taken over them. Mr Fred Chambers was responsible for the computer-generated images of the human body; the statistics relating to tumours came from *Dahlin's Bone Tumours**, with permission from the author, publisher and the Mayo Foundation.

I am also most grateful to my colleagues Dr Sarah Burnett and Dr Asif Saifuddin for their help and advice. Dr Hugues Brat of the Catholic University of Louvain (Brussels) read the completed manuscript and made many helpful suggestions.

This book could not have been undertaken without the constant help of the Radiology Museum secretary, Veronika Aurens, BA, who also typed and arranged the manuscript. I am most grateful to her and to Messrs. Alan Burgess and Clive Lawson of the publishers, Martin Dunitz Ltd.

Peter Renton 1998

*Unni KK (1996) *Dahlin's Bone Tumours*, 5th edn. Lippincott-Raven, Philadelphia.

Chapter 1 Decrease in bone density

Loss of bone density may be:

1 generalized;
2 regional, affecting many but not all bones, often in continuity, for example, a whole limb;
3 focal. Focal lesions may be multiple and separated by normal bone.

A bone which shows a decrease in density can be described as osteopenic. This term does not imply a particular pathology and avoids labelling a patient with a specific disease entity which may not be present. It is used to describe a subjective radiological appearance of bone which may be due to different causes and is also subject to observer variation. Osteopenia may also be mimicked by faulty radiographic technique, especially by the use of a high kV.

Normal bone consists of cortex and medulla, which vary in thickness at different sites. Typically, the cortex is thick in the midshaft of the femur and thin at the distal femoral metaphysis. Medullary trabeculae often reflect local stresses, which are well demonstrated in the femoral neck and vertebral bodies. The overall radiographic image of a bone is largely due to the anterior and posterior cortices overlain. At the margin, particularly of a round bone, the curved cortex has sufficient depth to be radiologically visible end on. Cortical bone loss is the most significant factor in the reduction of bone density.

The major causes of generalized osteopenia are:

1 Osteoporosis
2 Osteomalacia
3 Hyperparathyroidism
4 Marrow infiltrative disorders and diffuse malignant disease

OSTEOPOROSIS

Most osteopenic patients are osteoporotic; however, the terms are not interchangeable. Osteoporosis may be defined as an absolute quantitative deficiency of bone substance. The bone which remains is qualitatively normal. Therefore, there is a decrease in bone mass per unit volume.

METHODS OF ASSESSING OSTEOPOROSIS

Visual assessment

Radiologically visualized bone density is the result of a balance between osteoblastic and osteoclastic activity, between bone formation and resorption. Therefore, if osteolysis exceeds osteogenesis, a loss of total bone mass occurs. Radiologically, osteoporosis becomes visible when approximately 50% of bone mass is lost. Bone loss is seen at the cortex and the medulla.

Radiographic photodensitometry

Comparison is made between the subject's metacarpal and a normal metacarpal embedded in perspex and radiographed on the same film, or an aluminium step wedge. This is an adequate, simple and fairly reproducible technique which requires an accurate light densitometer. The technique is now obsolete.

Radiological quantitative morphometry

Using a standard radiographic technique, the thicknesses of the midshaft and medulla of the second, or second, third and fourth metacarpals are assessed at right angles to their midpoints. The measurements made with Vernier calipers can be used for various calculations to assess cortico-medullary ratios. There may be difficulties in visualizing the inner cortical margin, and, if the cortices are not homogeneous (as in hyperparathyroidism), the cortical width does not represent cortical bone mass. This technique is also now obsolete.

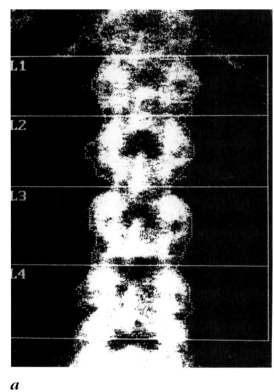

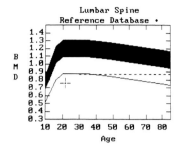

	Lumbar Spine Reference Database ◆			TOTAL BMD CV FOR L1 - L4 1.0%		

C.F.	1.001	1.046	1.000

Region	Area (cm²)	BMC (grams)	BMD (gms/cm²)
L1	10.92	7.52	0.688
L2	12.36	9.43	0.763
L3	13.78	10.12	0.734
L4	14.82	11.84	0.799
TOTAL	51.88	38.92	0.750

BMD(L1-L4) = 0.750 g/cm²

Region	BMD	T(30.0)		Z	
L1	0.688	-2.91	68%	-2.91	68%
L2	0.763	-3.01	70%	-3.01	70%
L3	0.734	-3.35	67%	-3.35	67%
L4	0.799	-3.14	70%	-3.14	70%
L1-L4	0.750	-3.10	69%	-3.10	69%

◆ Age and sex matched

a

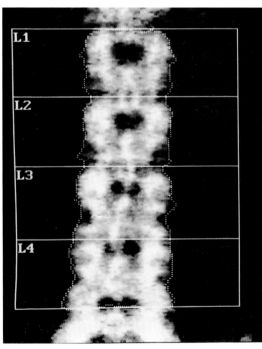

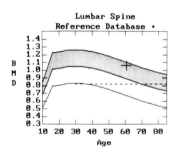

	Lumbar Spine Reference Database ◆			TOTAL BMD CV FOR L1 - L4 1.0%		

C.F.	1.005	1.044	1.000

Region	Area (cm²)	BMC (grams)	BMD (gms/cm²)
L1	13.06	12.46	0.954
L2	13.91	14.86	1.069
L3	15.86	17.12	1.079
L4	16.79	18.33	1.092
TOTAL	59.61	62.77	1.053

BMD(L1-L4) = 1.053 g/cm²

Region	BMD	T(30.0)		Z	
L1	0.954	+0.27	103%	+1.56	122%
L2	1.069	+0.37	104%	+1.81	123%
L3	1.079	-0.04	100%	+1.47	118%
L4	1.092	-0.22	98%	+1.35	116%
L1-L4	1.053	+0.05	101%	+1.52	119%

◆ Age and sex matched
T = peak bone mass
Z = age matched

b

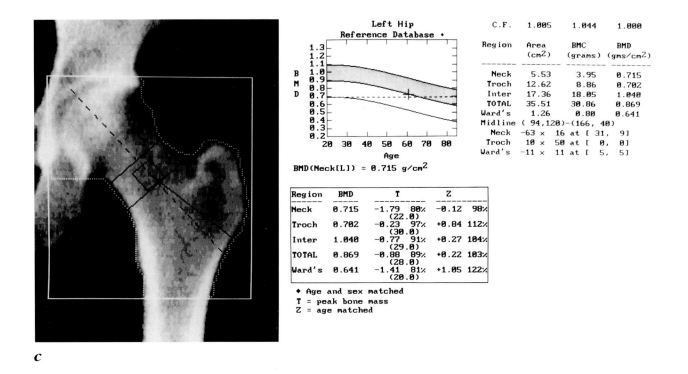

c

Figure 1.1 *Dual energy X-ray absorptiometry (DEXA) scanning. Accurate measurements are most commonly taken from the lumbar spine and proximal femur; results are usually expressed in terms of the number of standard deviations above and below the mean of an age-related control population (Z-score) or of a young healthy adult population (T-score). (**a**) This 21-year-old patient has osteogenesis imperfecta type I-A and shows marked decrease in density in the lumbar spine, equivalent to the lowest normal bone density in a 75-year-old. (By courtesy of Dr H Brat.) (**b**) This scan shows an increase in density in the lumbar spine above the expected norm for this age, but this is probably because of the presence of osteophytes in degenerative disease. (**c**) Further imaging of the femur shows the patient to lie exactly on the predicted value for bone density at her age.*

Photodensitometry

Single photon absorptiometry (SPA) uses a single radio-iodine source and a detector. The apparatus is portable. Measurements are obtained at sites of thick cortices, such as the midshaft radius, but also calcaneus and distal radius. There is an accuracy error of 4–6%, but the extremity needs to be placed in water to keep soft tissue absorption constant.

Dual photon absorptiometry (DPA). The use of a multi-energy isotope of gadolinium-155 permits scanning of thicker parts, such as the spine and hip. The isotope, and hence the scan, are relatively expensive and the test slower than SPA.

Dual energy X-ray absorptiometry (DEXA). The machine uses an X-ray source and integrated data interpretation (Figure 1.1). Scanning time and radiation dose are low and accuracy high (error 4%). Lateral scanning of the vertebral bodies allows more accurate measurements of spinal bone density to be made without inclusion of aortic calcification, vertebral osteophytosis or the posterior vertebral elements that would occur on an AP scan. Correlation between this mode and qualitative computed tomography (QCT) is good (see below). .

Radiation beams of different energies are attenuated differently by each tissue through which the beams pass. The difference in attenuation between bone and soft tissue is greater for the lower energy beam. Because of the more complicated pattern of X-ray absorption, a more sensitive pattern of bone density is obtained.

Usual areas scanned are the lumbar spine, hip, distal radius, calcaneus, as well as the whole body.

Bone mass diminishes both in men and women at and after middle age. Women in particular lose a greater amount of medullary bone, so that less than 50% of the trabecular bone present at skeletal maturity is seen at old age. This loss is greatest at the hip, calcaneus and in the spine, as well as the forearm and wrist.

Bone density assessment at a particular site gives the best prediction for fractures at that site, especially in the case of the spine and the hip, but bone density measurements obtained at the distal radius or calcaneus give good predictions for fractures at any site. The risk of hip fracture doubles with each decade and increases by up to 120% for each standard deviation decrease in bone density.

Qualitative computed tomography (QCT)

The patient is placed on top of a calibration phantom containing liquids of differing densities. The attenuation in the region of interest is compared with standard readings (Figure 1.2). The technique uses a single energy beam and gives excellent artefact-free measurements of cortical or trabecular density anywhere in the skeleton without overlapping artefact (Figure 1.3). Radiation exposure is greater than with DEXA.

Ultrasound assessment of bone density

Measurements can be obtained of (1) the velocity of sound through bone and (2) the increase in attenuation with frequency – the *broadband ultrasonic attenuation* (BUA).

Assessments are usually made of the patella. The machine is portable and the examination quickly

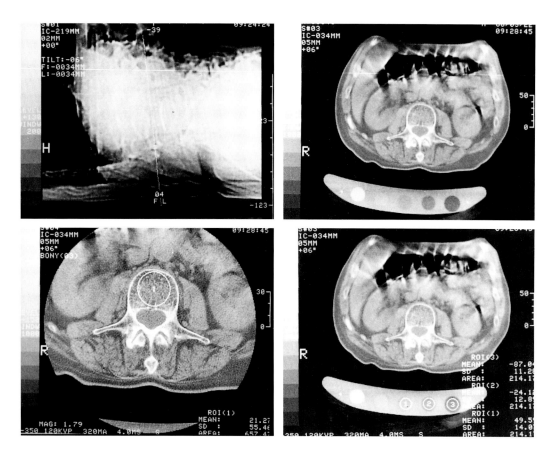

Figure 1.2 *Density readings obtained on the CT scanner are compared with the standard readings obtained on phantoms.*

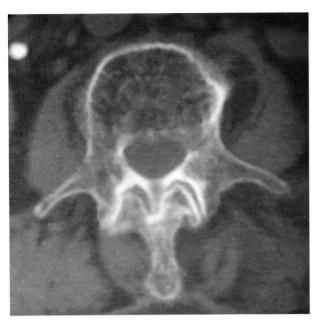

a

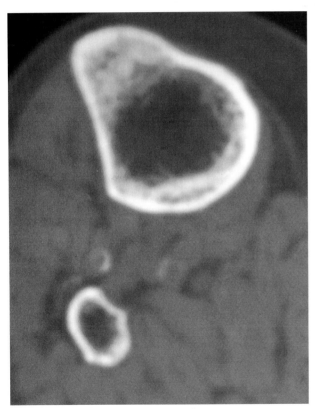

b

Figure 1.3 *CT scans showing osteoporosis (**a**) in a vertebral body, (**b**) in the proximal tibia with cortical thinning and loss of medullary trabeculation.*

performed. It seems that the BUA for the calcaneus accurately reflects decreased bone density in the spine. The test is said to be appropriate in a general medical practice environment.

Magnetic resonance imaging in assessment of bone density

It is thought that the potential exists for MRI to assess bone density, cortical thickness, trabecular distribution and structure using high resolution images.

CORTICAL OSTEOPOROSIS

There are three cortical sites of bone formation and loss – endosteal, periosteal and central cortical. Cortical changes are better visualized using a magnifying glass or macroradiography. Bone resorption within the cortex is seen as an increase in the number of cortical lucent striations (Figure 1.4), which are small cigar-shaped lucencies aligned parallel to the long axis of the cortex. Normally none, or only one or two are seen within the midshaft of the metacarpal cortex. When easily visible, or if three or more are seen across the width of the cortex, excessive bone resorption is taking place. These changes are not usually seen in conditions of decreased bone formation, but occur especially in hyperparathyroidism, thyrotoxicosis, Sudeck's atrophy and following immobilization.

Resorption of cortical bone from its medullary border results in a thin pencil line of cortex around the affected bones (Figure 1.4). The width of the very sharply defined cortex may be less than 1 mm, and indicates that mineralization of the remaining bone is normal, so that cortical margins remain distinct. Areas of endosteal scalloping may be widespread. Local scalloping may be the result of a focal or aggressive process, such as a local tumour.

In the spine the cortices become progressively thinner but remain crisp (Figure 1.5). Eventually the thinned upper and lower end-plates become hairline in thickness. Vertebral margins should be assessed as well as the cortices around pedicles on the anteroposterior view, as these also become thinner and crisper with progressive osteoporosis. There are two major groups of vertebral medullary trabeculae: vertical, along the lines of stress, and horizontal, parallel to the end-plates. These are normally obscured by minor trabeculae and overlying soft tissues. The latter tend to obscure bone detail, especially if the patient

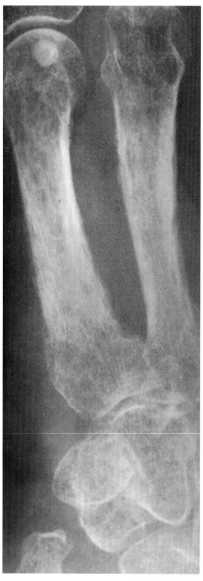

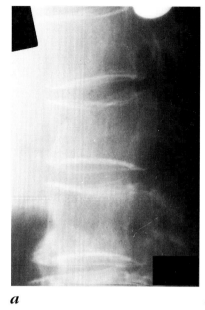

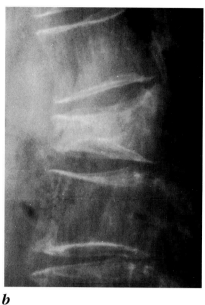

a   *b*

Figure 1.5 *(a) In this osteoporotic patient the initial film was taken immediately after a fall which resulted in back pain. The cortices are thinned but sharply defined against the vertebral centra which contain only sparse vertical weight-bearing trabeculae. There is an anterior cortical fracture of an upper lumbar vertebral body. (b) Six weeks later there is further collapse with sclerosis of the affected vertebral body. The sclerosis may be the result of either trabecular compression or bone necrosis. A vacuum phenomenon may be seen as a lucent cleft in the sclerotic vertebral body after collapse. There is no expansion, and the remaining weight-bearing trabeculae stand out in the adjacent intact vertebral bodies. A kyphosis results.*

Figure 1.4 *Bone resorption in this patient with Sudeck's atrophy appears as loss of definition of the metacarpal cortices with endosteal scalloping and accentuation of the cortical Haversian canals. The subperiosteal bone resorption resembles that seen in hyperparathyroidism. The carpal bones show loss of density centrally, with thin cortices sharply defined against the demineralized centra.*

is obese, or if the film is taken during prolonged breathing (which otherwise blurs out soft tissues). The film then looks grey. Trabecular detail is also lost if the kV used for the exposure is too high.

As osteoporosis increases, the randomly arranged trabeculae are lost, followed by the horizontal trabeculae, leaving only the vertical trabeculae along the lines of stress. Eventually these too may be lost so that the end-stage has only thin, sharp, vertebral margins and sharply pencilled pedicles in contrast to a grey, homogeneous and featureless vertebral centrum (Figure 1.5).

The pathological definition of osteoporosis has been expanded to include the clinical feature of fractures (Figures 1.5, 1.6 and 1.7).

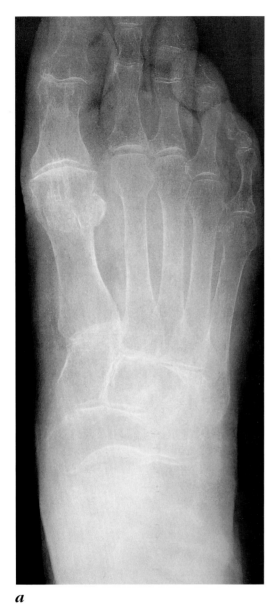

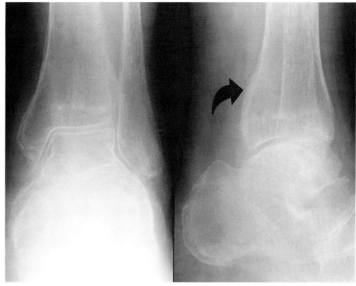

b

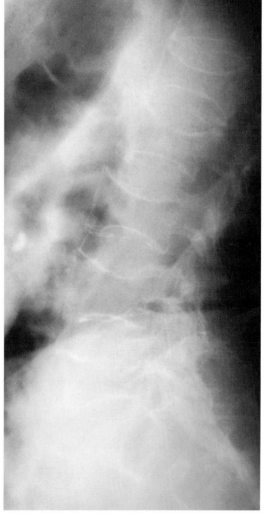

a

Figure 1.6 *Severe osteoporosis. (**a**) In the foot there is marked loss of bone density. Medullary trabeculae are sparse and the cortices are thinned but remain sharp and well defined. (**b**) A stress fracture is demonstrated at the distal tibia on both AP and lateral views. It extends perpendicularly to the cortex and there is an overlying periosteal reaction (arrowed). (**c**) There is marked osteoporosis associated with generalized vertebral deformity of the codfish type. The cortices are again thinned but well defined and little medullary trabeculation is seen.*

c

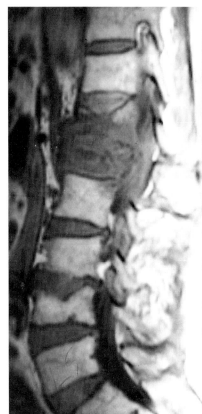
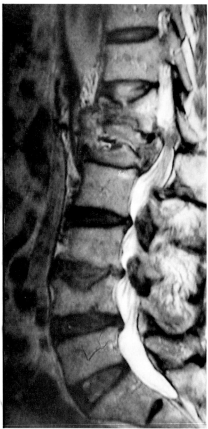

a *b*

Figure 1.7 *Chronic vertebral collapse in osteoporosis. (**a**) This is demonstrated at T12, L1, L3 and L4, where a degree of superior end-plate depression is shown, but at L1 there is more substantial vertebral collapse following trauma with dorsal protrusion of the posterior aspect of the vertebral body into the canal. (**b**) Sagittal T$_1$- and T$_2$-weighted MR images show the chronic deformity of the body of L4; the marrow here consists largely of fat. The bodies of T12 and L1 however show loss of signal due to fibrosis with a minor area of increased signal on the T$_2$-weighted sequences (right) in T12 compatible with oedema.*

CHANGES IN VERTEBRAL BODY SHAPE IN OSTEOPOROSIS

The normal vertebral body has essentially parallel end-plates, although there may be slight end-plate concavity with 1–2 mm of central depression. In the thoracic spine, the anterior height of the vertebral body may be 1–2 mm less than the posterior (Figure 1.8a). This does not imply collapse and may be seen in contiguous vertebral bodies.

Osteoporosis may result in vertebral compression which can be acutely painful or pass unnoticed by the patient. Wedging usually affects the upper end-plate more than the lower, so that the difference in

height between anterior and posterior surfaces of the vertebral bodies is over 2 mm (Figure 1.8b). The radionuclide bone scan shows marked focal increase in uptake (Figure 1.9). Significant collapse results in flattening of the vertebral body which usually does not expand significantly. Expansion in collapse is a feature of Paget's disease (Figure 1.10) and occasionally of primary and secondary bone tumours. In most cases, a collapsed, osteoporotic vertebral body is said to implode. Callus formation is not usually seen in collapsed osteoporotic vertebrae. Collapse in osteoporosis is not generalized throughout the spine and it is unusual to find many vertebral bodies affected by collapse in contiguity.

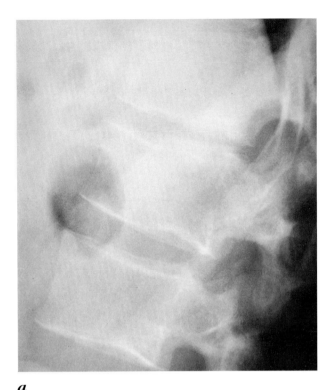

a

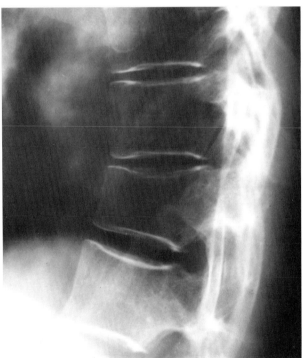

b

Figure 1.8 *(a) Wedging of thoracic vertebral bodies may be a normal feature. (b) Osteoporotic wedging of a lower thoracic vertebral body where the deformity affects the upper end-plate.*

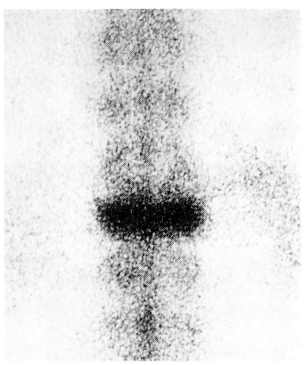

Figure 1.9 *Vertebral collapse in an osteoporotic spine results in focal increase in uptake.*

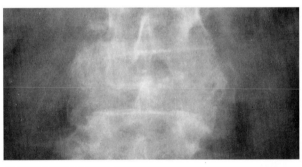

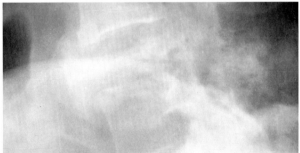

Figure 1.10 *In this example of vertebral collapse in Paget's disease, the body of L4 shows an abnormal sclerotic texture with loss of cortico-medullary differentiation. There is marked flattening of the body, which expands beyond the adjacent vertebrae.*

Table 1.1 Conditions associated with codfish vertebrae.

Normal in young adults
Osteomalacia
Osteoporosis
Idiopathic juvenile osteoporosis
Osteogenesis imperfecta
Sickle-cell disease
Thalassaemia

'Codfish' vertebrae resemble the fish vertebrae in shape, with deep, smooth, biconcave end-plate depressions (Figure 1.6c). This feature is seen in any condition associated with bone softening, including osteomalacia (Table 1.1). In osteoporosis, the depressions may be more marked on the upper end-plates and affected bodies are not always contiguous. In osteomalacia, the change is seen more diffusely throughout the spine.

In young adults, a codfish type vertebral body may be seen, where the upper and lower end-plates show smooth depressions slightly posterior to the coronal midplane. This change lies around the discal nucleus, as can be seen at discography and MRI and usually occurs in the lumbar spine, where the discs are largest (Figure 1.11; see also Chapter 8, page 355).

In children, discal herniation into the gap between the annular ring apophysis and the underlying body results in non or partial union of the ring apophysis in adult life. The defect is contiguous with the nucleus (Figure 1.12).

End-plate irregularities (Schmorl's nodes) occur owing to local discal herniations at sites of previous vascular channels, or cortical defects. The defect is usually well corticated and can be seen on the plain film, tomogram, CT scan, discogram and at MRI scanning (Figure 1.13). The discogram is generally not painful.

Defects at end-plates also occur after trauma, usually vertebro-compressive in nature. Here, a cortical flake is depressed into the adjacent body; the lesions are painful in life and at discography, where contrast medium enters the vertebral body, before healing takes place (Figure 1.14).

Osteoporotic patients form less new bone as part of a degenerative process and are probably more susceptible to vertebral collapse, for example, than those who have normal mineralization or are hyperostotic, as in diffuse idiopathic skeletal hyperostosis (DISH; Forestier's disease; see Chapter 8, page 380).

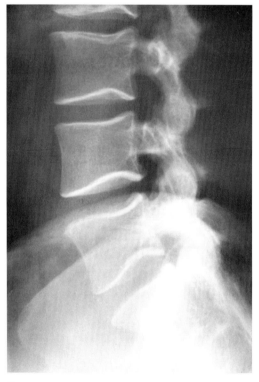

a

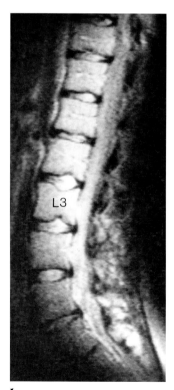

L3

b

Figure 1.11 (*a*) *End-plate depressions are normal in the adult lumbar spine and correspond to the site of the turgid discal nucleus.* (*b*) *In a different patient the T$_2$-weighted MR sequence shows a Schmorl's node on the inferior surface of L3. At the L2/3 disc end-plate changes reflect the shape and position of the nucleus.*

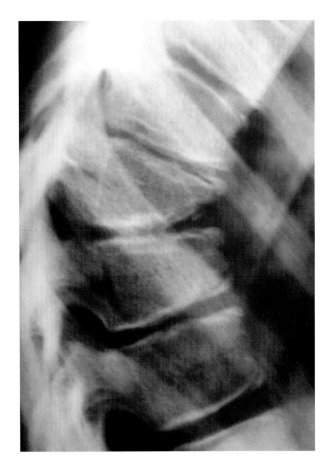

Figure 1.12 *Vertebral deformity has resulted from displacement of the ring apophysis by discal herniation.*

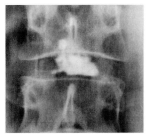 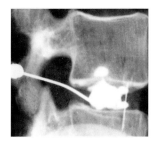

a

Figure 1.13 *Schmorl's node. (**a**) A defect in the cortical margin at the lower end-plate of a lumbar vertebral body is demonstrated to fill with contrast at lumbar discography, indicating a local discal herniation resulting in a Schmorl's node.*

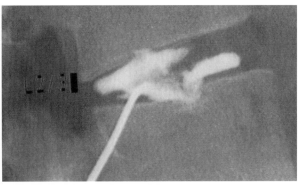

b

*(**b**) Discogram showing contrast medium entering a smooth and well demarcated defect on the upper end-plate of a lumbar vertebral body.*

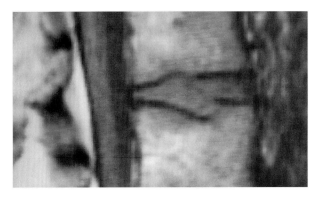

c

*(**c**) The change is well shown at MRI. The defect is corticated.*

CHANGES IN THE APPENDICULAR SKELETON

Two main groups of trabeculae may be identified in the femoral neck: (1) a vertical compressive group ascending from the calcar to the femoral head; and (2) an arcuate tensile group extending from below the greater trochanter to the inferomedial portion of the femoral head (Figure 1.15). As with the spine, these trabeculae initially become more prominent with increasing osteoporosis, due to resorption of the normal, randomly arranged trabeculae. Further resorption progressively absorbs the tensile, and then compressive, group.

In the skull, generalized osteoporosis results in prominence of the sutures and surrounding bone, which appears relatively sclerotic. The squamous temporal bone is naturally thin and shows osteoporosis early (Figure 1.16).

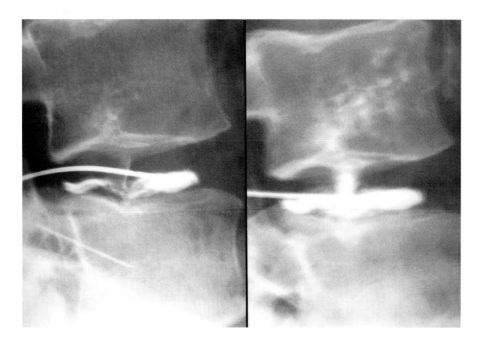

Figure 1.14 *Vertebrodiscal trauma. At discography a superior defect is shown in the annulus. Contrast medium spurts up into the overlying vertebral body through an end-plate defect. The injection caused severe pain in the patient's back, resulting in movement. Vascular filling is also shown.*

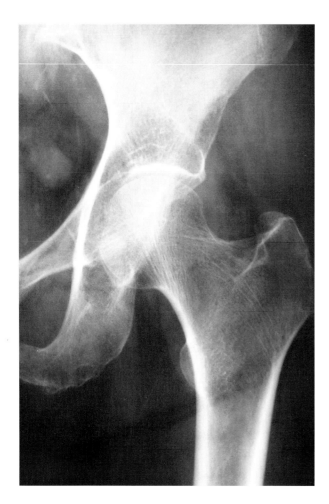

Figure 1.15 *The two main groups of trabeculae are demonstrated in the femoral neck. There is a superior arcuate group and a more medial and vertically directed group of trabeculae extending upwards from the calcar. Ward's triangle lies in the gap between the superior arcuate and the vertical medial primary trabeculae. It enlarges in the osteoporotic femoral neck. Cortical thinning also occurs at the femoral neck in osteoporosis and further predisposes to local fracture.*

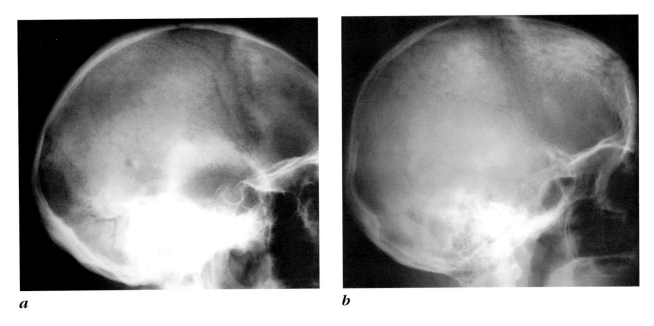

a   *b*

Figure 1.16 *(a) Osteoporosis in the skull results in marked demineralization of the squamous temporal bone and accentuation of the adjacent suture. (b) Another osteoporotic patient in whom the changes are more diffuse. Even hyperostosis frontalis interna is poorly visualized.*

Generalized osteoporosis

This is most commonly seen in the elderly and in the postmenopausal female (Table 1.2). Maximal bone mass is reached between 20 and 40 years of age in both sexes, after which women lose bone more rapidly than men until 80 years of age, when the loss becomes equal.

The changes which occur have been described in the previous section. Cortical thinning and medullary trabecular loss affect the long bones, skull, metacarpals and phalanges, and particularly the

Table 1.2 Causes of generalized osteoporosis in the adult.

Condition	Cause
Osteoporosis of the elderly	?Oestrogen deficiency
Postmenopausal osteoporosis	
Cushing's syndrome	Reduced osteoblastic activity
Steroid administration	
Heparin administration	Possible inhibition of bone formation
Thyrotoxicosis	Increased osteoclastic activity greater than increased osteoblastic activity
Hypogonadism	Related to hypopituitarism
Acromegaly	
Diabetes	Insulin dependent ? Related to protein breakdown
Liver disease and alcoholism	? Related to increased steroid levels
Weightlessness – space travel	Disuse
Osteogenesis imperfecta	Abnormal bone matrix
Hyperparathyroidism	Increased osteoclastic activity
Dietary deficiency	Vitamin C, calcium deficiency

vertebral bodies. Fractures of vertebral bodies produce wedging with loss of height, particularly at the superior end-plates, and end-plate irregularities. Compression fractures are randomly distributed in the lower thoracic and lumbar spine (Figure 1.17). They are not necessarily contiguous and do not heal with callus, which makes them difficult to date. Mild trauma may cause vertebral compression, which produces back pain, but neurological complications are unusual. Height loss may occur with an increased lumbar lordosis and high thoracic smooth kyphosis.

Femoral neck, transcervical and Colles' fractures are also more common in patients with osteoporosis. Upper femoral fractures may be spontaneous through osteoporotic bone, or may follow only minor trauma.

Patients with trochanteric fractures may be more porotic than those with transcervical fractures. Such patients often have little evidence of new bone as part of a degenerative process, even if considerable joint space narrowing is present.

Fractures through the distal radius and ulna, especially Colles' fractures, increase in frequency with age and are related to local loss of bone mass. The older and more osteoporotic the patient, the greater the degree of comminution of fracture parts.

Fractures in osteoporotic bone may be difficult to visualize as there is not enough cortical or medullary bone to show trabecular interruption. Occult fractures, for example, of the hip, knee or calcaneus (Figure 1.18) may be diagnosed at radionuclide bone

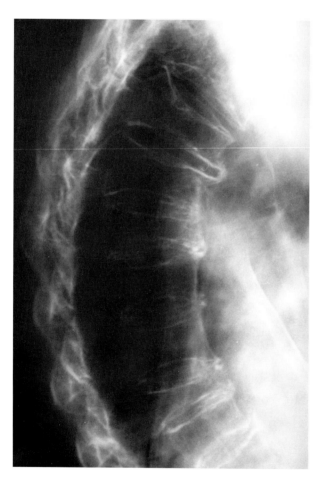

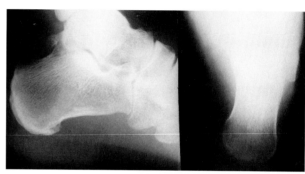

a

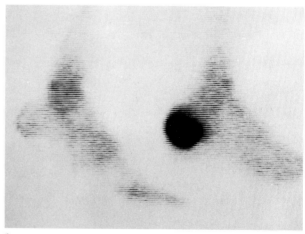

b

Figure 1.17 *Osteoporosis. Marked vertebral compression with end-plate irregularities. The longstanding nature of the change is demonstrated by subsequent bony ankylosis.*

Figure 1.18 *Occult fracture of the calcaneus. (**a**) No major fracture line was demonstrated on the plain film. There is minor irregularity of the cortex at the plantar fascia origin. (**b**) The radioisotope bone scan shows substantial increase in uptake.*

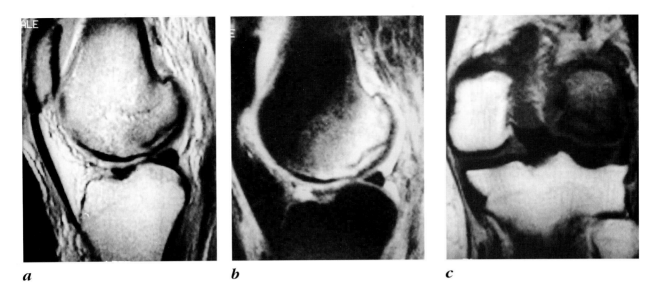

a *b* *c*

Figure 1.19 *Bone bruising with an occult fracture visualized at MRI. (**a**) On the sagittal T₁-weighted image a serpiginous low signal band in the lateral femoral condyle is shown. This is the fracture line and it is surrounded by oedema, seen here as a relatively diffuse area of low signal in the marrow. (**b**) Surrounding bone marrow and soft tissue oedema is demonstrated on the sagittal fat suppression sequence. (**c**) Coronal T₁-weighted sequence shows the fracture line and surrounding marrow oedema.*

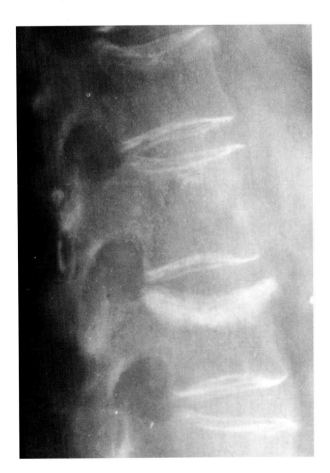

scanning with great sensitivity, but poor specificity. MR imaging, however, shows fractures with great specificity, as well as changes of bone haemorrhage (Figure 1.19).

Cushing's syndrome

This may be due to adrenocortical disease or steroid therapy. Changes may be severe, particularly in the axial skeleton, where vertebral compression leads to end-plate sclerosis with local callus formation, a specific feature of this form of osteoporosis (Figure 1.20). The changes associated with high-dose steroid therapy also include avascular necrosis, particularly of the femoral

Figure 1.20 *In this patient with Cushing's syndrome, osteopenia is associated with wedging of lumbar vertebral bodies and thickening of the upper end-plate of L3 due to hyperplastic callus. This is a feature unique to Cushing's syndrome, as vertebral collapse is not accompanied by callus formation in other conditions.*

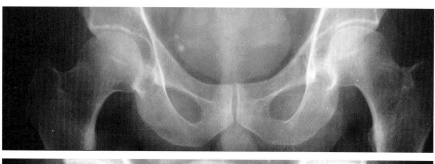

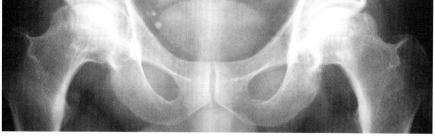

Figure 1.21 *Steroid arthropathy. Avascular necrosis with structural failure has occurred over the course of 8 months.*

head (Figure 1.21) but also of the humeral head (Figure 1.22). Rib 'cough' fractures are also seen, particularly in patients receiving steroids for lung disease. A dose of 10–15 mg/day for 3 years is thought to be required to cause these changes.

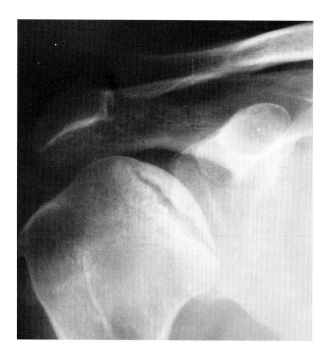

Figure 1.22 *Cushing's syndrome. The humeral head is sclerotic, fissured and deformed, indicating avascular necrosis in a patient receiving steroids.*

Hyperthyroidism

This is a very infrequent cause of radiologically visible osteoporosis; however, the diagnosis will be clear as the clinical disease will be severe.

Heparin osteoporosis

Patients receiving treatment for ischaemic coronary and cerebrovascular disease for up to 15 years, who have received over 15 000 units heparin daily, have been described with osteoporosis and rib and vertebral fractures. However, this is a rare condition. Female patients with a history of thromboembolism in pregnancy may also be on long-term heparin and develop osteoporosis.

Acromegaly

This is often associated with osteoporosis as a manifestation of concurrent hypopituitarism, but the bone and soft tissue changes of acromegaly predominate. Vertebral bodies are elongated in the sagittal plane as part of the general overgrowth of bone, and are osteoporotic (Figure 1.23).

Alcoholism

Alcoholism associated with osteoporosis is not always related to hepatic cirrhosis or malnutrition.

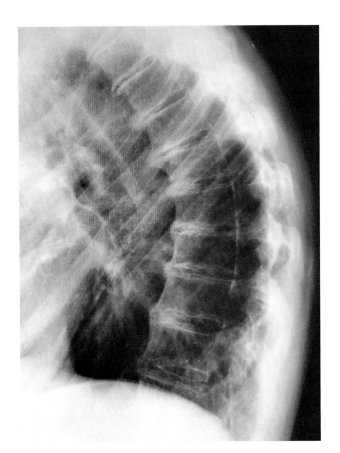

Figure 1.23 *In acromegaly the bones are demineralized with thinning of the end-plate cortices. A smooth thoracic kyphos is associated with new bone anteriorly on the vertebral bodies, in part associated with local buttressing osteophytes.*

Alcohol has been shown to elevate the plasma cortisol levels so that the osteoporosis may be steroid-related.

Osteogenesis imperfecta

This generalized disorder of connective tissue was formerly classified into two main forms – a severe form presenting in utero or early in life, and a late, milder form inherited as a dominant condition (see also Chapter 6, page 330), often not presenting until adult life. This simple, clinical and radiological classification has now been replaced by a more complicated classification (Table 1.3).

Table 1.3 Classification of osteogenesis imperfecta (after Resnick 1995, Sillence 1979).

Type	Osseous deformity	Hearing loss	Dentinogenesis imperfecta	Blue sclerae	Wormian bones
I-A	+	+	–	+	+
I-B	++	+	+	+	+
II-A, B and C	++++ Severe deformity Dwarfism Intrauterine fractures Crumpled long bones Ribs: II-A – broad, continuous beading II-B – broad, discontinuous beading II-C – thin, discontinuous beading	–	–	+	+
III	+++ Progressive dwarfism with platyspondyly Wormian bones Kyphoscoliosis	–	+	+ (becoming normal)	+
IV-A	+ to +++	+	–	–	+
IV-B	+ to +++	+	+	–	+

Type I = autosomal dominant (70%); Type II = dominant new mutation (10%); Type III = dominant new mutation (15%); Type IV = dominant (5%).

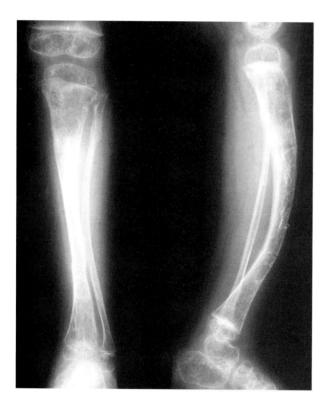

Figure 1.24 *Osteogenesis imperfecta – Type I. There is generalized demineralization of bone, with bowing of the tibia and fibula. The fibula, in particular, is gracile. Transverse pathological fractures are seen in both bones.*

Type I, the mildest form and the most common, is inherited as an autosomal dominant condition. Fractures are increased in number but severe deformity is unusual (Figure 1.24). Patients have blue sclerae; Wormian bones are present. Type IB has associated dentinogenesis imperfecta (Figure 1.25); Type IA does not. Both have hearing loss.

Type II is a lethal dominant new mutation associated with intrauterine fractures, Wormian bones and gross deformity with shortening and telescoped long bones. It is further subdivided into types A – ribs broad with continuous beading (Figure 1.26a), B – lethal at birth, ribs broad but with discontinuous beading (Figure 1.26b) and C – thin ribs with discontinuous beading (Figure 1.26c). The parents are normal and most cases are presumably spontaneous mutations. Blue sclerae are present throughout.

Type III is relatively uncommon and due to a new dominant mutation; it is more severe than Type 1 Most present at birth. It results in severe dwarfism with platyspondyly and multiple fractures. Sclerae are blue at birth but become white in adult life if the patients survive. Wormian bones are present. A kyphoscoliosis may develop. Long bones are gracile (Figure 1.27).

Type IV have white sclerae and hearing loss. Inheritance is dominant. The severity of the disease varies from mild to gross, with fractures and height loss. Type IV-B has dentinogenesis imperfecta. Patients have varying degrees of demineralization; some indeed seem normally mineralized, until it is noted that they have recurring fractures in middle age.

Fractures at long bones tend to be diaphyseal, while in idiopathic juvenile osteoporosis (see page 20) and in non-accidental injury, they tend to be metaphyseal. In non-accidental injury, the children are otherwise normal but both diseases are often the cause of clinical and medicolegal confusion (Table 1.4)

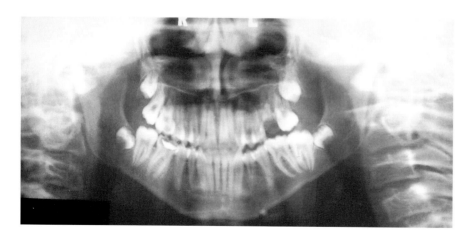

Figure 1.25 *Dentinogenesis imperfecta. Abnormality of the enamel–dentine bond results in local shearing and loss of enamel with subsequent severe caries. The roots are also elongated, curved and the canals thinned.*

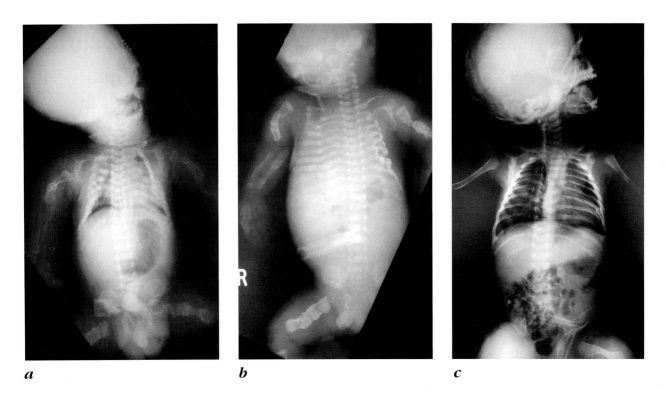

a *b* *c*

Figure 1.26 *Osteogenesis imperfecta —Type II. (**a**) Type II-A. The long bones are broad, crumpled and show multiple fractures that have occurred in utero. There is platyspondyly. The skull is demineralized and shows Wormian bones. The examination was taken shortly after birth. A nasogastric tube is demonstrated in the stomach, but no gas has yet reached the small bowel. A large lower abdominal hernia is present. (**b**) Type II-B. Again, the long bones are broad and show multiple fractures with deformity. The ribs too are broad but the beading is rather more discontinuous. (**c**) Type II-C. The child survives. Multiple Wormian bones are present. The ribs and long bones are generally thin and demineralized. Beading is discontinuous.*

Table 1.4 Differential signs between osteogenesis imperfecta, idiopathic juvenile osteoporosis and non-accidental injury.

Signs	Osteogenesis imperfecta	Idiopathic juvenile osteoporosis	Non-accidental injury
Age	Infants, adults	Around puberty	Infants, children
Long bone fractures	Diaphyseal	Metaphyseal	Metaphyseal (Holland's sign) or diaphyseal
Rib fractures	Beaded, cystic	—	Multiple of different generations
Skull changes	Wormian bones Osteoporosis Dentinogenesis imperfecta	—	Skull fractures
Modelling abnormalities	Can be gross	Severe cases only Vertebral compression fractures Long bone pseudarthrosis	Following fractures

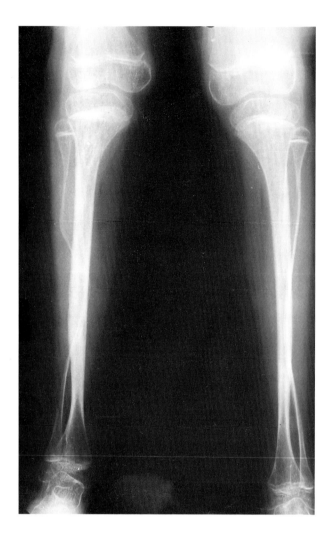

Figure 1.27 *Osteogenesis imperfecta – Type III. There is severe osteoporosis with marked thinning of the bones, especially the fibulae which show severe deformity.*

In mild forms of osteogenesis imperfecta the bones are initially often normal in shape but fracture repeatedly after minor, inappropriate trauma. Osteoporosis may not be marked in adults, but the combination of osteoporosis with bone deformity is strongly suggestive of the disease. The fibula may be bowed (Figure 1.27). This unusual combination also occurs in juvenile chronic arthritis (Figure 1.28a), while in Paget's disease fibular bowing is associated with osteosclerosis and bone expansion (Figure 1.28b). Ribs may be softened, resulting in upward concavity (Figure 1.29). Protrusio acetabuli may be seen (Figure 1.30a), as in rheumatoid arthritis associated with osteoporosis (Figure 1.30b). Osteoarthritis associated with protrusio will often result in normal or increased bone density (Figure 1.30c), similar to the idiopathic or familial forms of protrusio (Figure 1.30d) (Table 1.5).

Scoliosis may be marked (Figure 1.30).

Fractures of the paired long bones (radius and ulna, tibia and fibula) in osteogenesis imperfecta may result in a pseudarthrosis (Figure 1.31), which is also found in neurofibromatosis and idiopathic juvenile osteoporosis. Fractures in osteogenesis imperfecta tend to heal with hypertrophic callus formation (Figure 1.32), occasionally resulting in cross-fusion (Figure 1.33a). The phenomenon of cross-fusion also occurs after Caffey's infantile cortical hyperostosis (Figure 1.33b,c), osteomyelitis (Figure 1.33d), trauma (Figure 1.33e,f) and, partly, in congenital fusions at the proximal radio-ulnar joint.

Many of the fractures are classically diaphyseal, unlike those in idiopathic juvenile osteoporosis (Figure 1.34) which are metaphyseal and not associated with gross callus formation.

Table 1.5 Causes of protrusio acetabuli.

Osteogenesis imperfecta Rheumatoid arthritis	Associated with osteoporosis
Osteoarthritis Idiopathic	Associated with normal bone density
X-linked hypophosphataemic osteomalacia	Associated with increased bone density

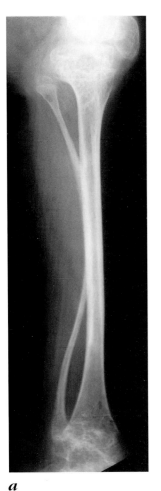 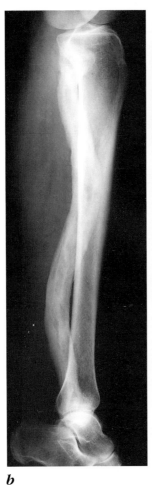 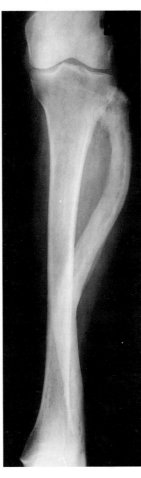

a   *b*

Figure 1.28 *(**a**)Juvenile chronic arthritis also results in fibular bowing, presumably as a result of hyperaemia and overgrowth at the upper and lower growth plates, but with fixation at the proximal and distal joints. (**b**) Paget's disease of the fibula is seen with expansion of the bone. The typical bony texture of Paget's disease extends to both articular surfaces with loss of cortico-medullary differentiation. Non-involvement of the tibia again results in fibular overgrowth and bowing.*

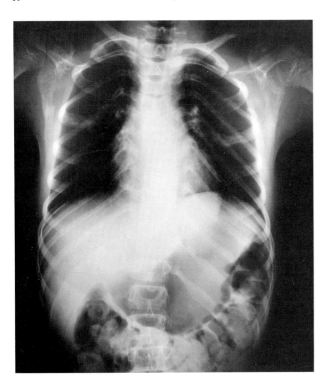

Figure 1.29 *Upward concavity of the ribs in osteogenesis imperfecta may be the result of posterior fractures, or muscle pull on softened bones.*

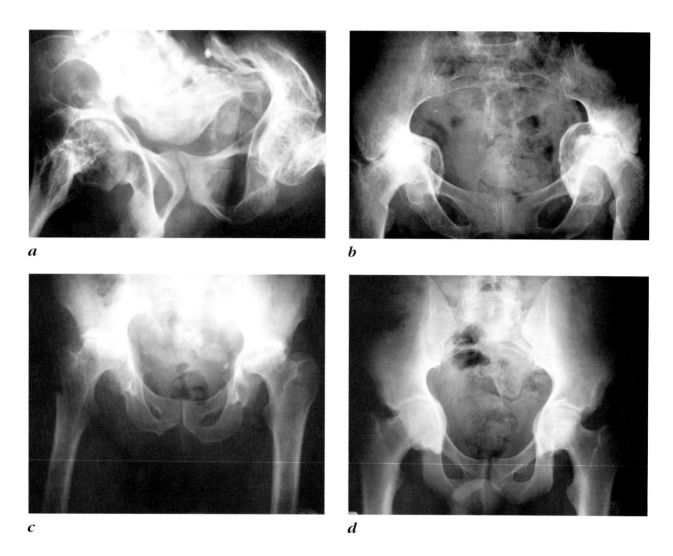

Figure 1.30 (*a*) *In this case of osteogenesis imperfecta, demineralization of bone has produced a scoliosis and protrusio of both hips. The bones around the obturator foramina are also thin, gracile and distorted.* (*b*) *Protrusio in rheumatoid arthritis. The medial walls of the acetabula are grossly displaced internally and vary in thickness. The joint spaces are narrowed superiorly but widened medially; the femoral heads are resorbed, irregular and sclerotic. This patient had severe rheumatoid deformities of the hands.* (*c*) *The appearances in this case of protrusio in osteoarthritis differ from the previous case; the degree of protrusion is less. Both femoral heads have lost bone in the weight-bearing regions, and the joint spaces are narrowed superiorly as well as medially. The acetabular roofs show deepening and reactive sclerosis, but elsewhere bone morphology is normal.* (*d*) *This young patient with congenital protrusio has no underlying arthritis. Bone density is normal.*

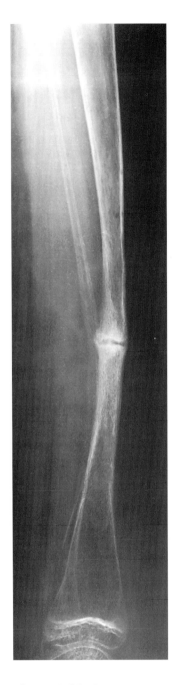

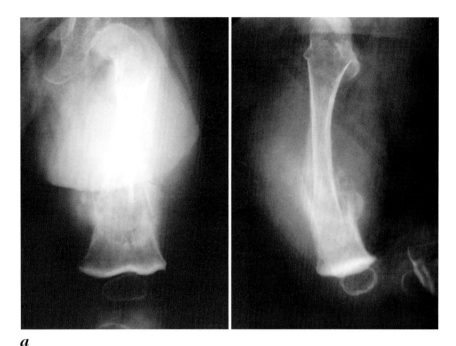

a

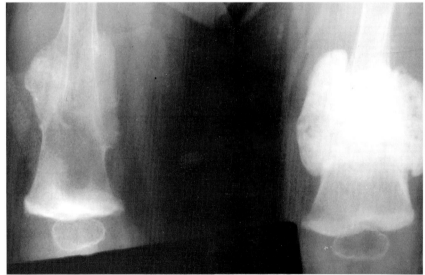

b

Figure 1.31 *Osteogenesis imperfecta – Type III. The bones are decreased in density. The fibula is thin and bowed, and a transverse fracture across the midshaft of the tibia is associated with sclerosis at a pseudarthrosis.*

Figure 1.32 *Osteogenesis imperfecta – hyperplastic callus formation.* (**a**) *Shortly after fracture a large soft tissue mass is demonstrated with evidence of exuberant callus formation in the soft tissues. The bone is demineralized, the fracture is diametaphyseal and shortening results.* (**b**) *A subsequent radiograph, taken less than a month later, shows much ossification around the distal left femoral fracture similar in appearance to an osteogenic sarcoma, but this has occurred much too rapidly and at too young an age for such a diagnosis. There is also evidence of a healed fracture around the distal midshaft of the right femur.*

Figure 1.33 (*a*) *In this case of osteogenesis imperfecta – Type III – there is osteoporosis; the radius and ulna are thin and bowed, and are connected by new bone across the interosseous membrane which is presumably the result of union of callus following fractures. Abnormal modelling of the carpal and metacarpal bones is also shown.* (*b*, *c*) *Caffey's infantile cortical hyperostosis has been severe in this patient. Cross-fusion and growth anomalies are present in the radius and ulna, and left ribs.* (*d*) *Cross-union in osteomyelitis. Following infection, the cloaking layers of periosteal new bone have united across the interosseous membrane.* (*e*, *f*) *Cross-fusion following trauma between the radius and ulna after non-accidental injury.*

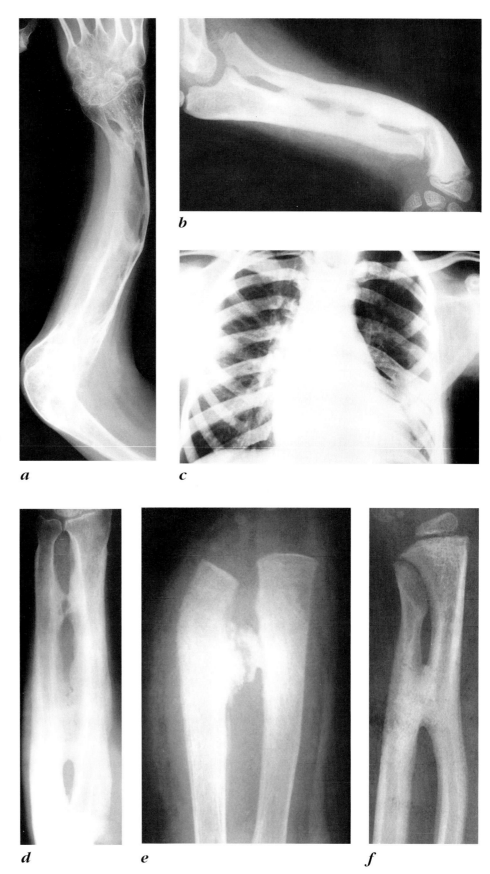

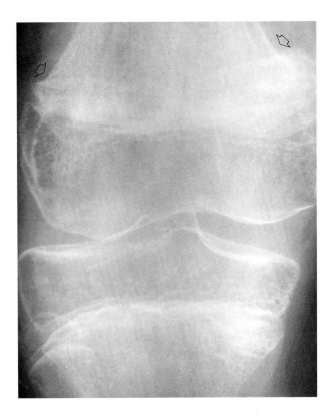

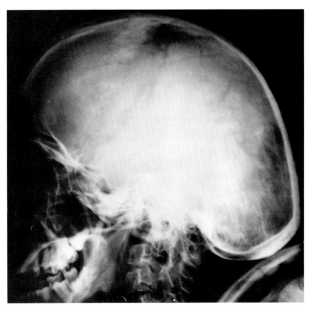

Figure 1.35 *Skull changes in severe osteogenesis imperfecta involve Wormian bone formation and bony softening at the base resulting in a 'tam-o-shanter' deformity.*

Figure 1.34 *This case of idiopathic juvenile osteoporosis shows classical metaphyseal fractures (arrows); the bones are generally demineralized.*

Osteogenesis imperfecta may occur at any age, while idiopathic juvenile osteoporosis only occurs around puberty. The skull changes of osteogenesis imperfecta—osteoporosis and thinned calvarial bones and Wormian bones—are not seen in idiopathic juvenile osteoporosis (Figure 1.35; Table 1.4, page 19).

Non-accidental injury (battered baby syndrome)

Fractures are almost inevitably part of this syndrome; however, these children are seldom generally osteoporotic. Deformity is localized to fracture sites and the fractures, of different generations, are diaphyseal and metaphyseal (Figures 1.36 and 1.37). Fractures are the only visible skull changes on the plain radiograph (Figure 1.38).

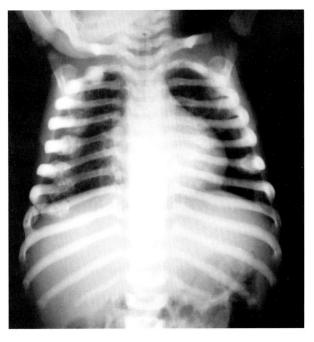

Figure 1.36 *Non-accidental injury. This radiograph of an infant shows multiple rib fractures with hyperplastic callus. The fractures are aligned – a feature of local trauma.*

Figure 1.37 *Non-accidental injury. (**a**) There is lateral subluxation of the left femoral head and massive soft tissue swelling around the shaft; a tiny flake of bone has been detached from the proximal metaphysis of the left femur. (**b**) A subsequent radiograph shows substantial elevation of the periosteum and new bone forming at a considerable distance from the underlying femoral shaft. (**c**) Remodelling of the femur takes place after a short interval. The femoral head appeared normally, ruling out a septic arthritis. There was considerable subsequent shortening.*

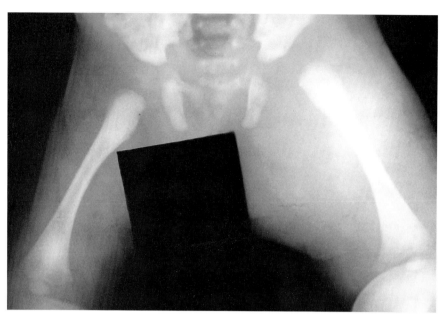

a

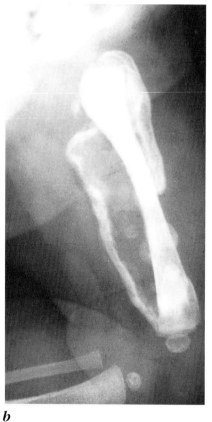

b

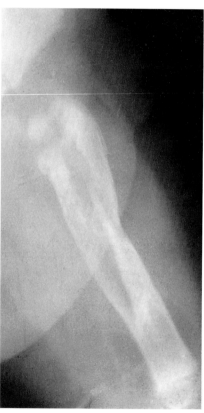

c

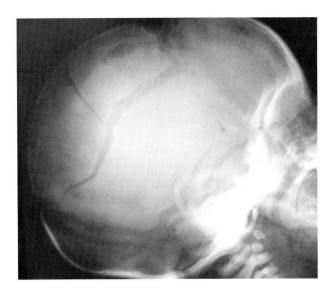

Figure 1.38 *Non-accidental injury. This baby has fractures of the skull.*

Scurvy

This rare disease is currently seen mainly in infants or in elderly, often mentally defective patients. It is caused by a vitamin C deficiency which results in defective collagen synthesis. Patients may present with bleeding due to capillary fragility and, in the elderly, scurvy may also contribute to the overall development of osteoporosis. Bleeding beneath the periosteum results in the formation of a lamellar periostitis which incorporates into the shaft after treatment (Figure 1.39).

In infants with scurvy, osteoporosis produces marked cortical thinning, especially at ring epiphyses, such as those at the knee, where sharp, thin, cortical outlines surround featureless centra (Wimberger's sign). In rickets, epiphyses and metaphyses are poorly defined and without sharply demarcated cortical margins. The well defined, thin band of provisional calcification in scurvy also contrasts with the subjacent metaphyseal bone which shows a local accentuated band of osteoporosis crossing the entire metaphysis (see also Chapter 5, page 291). This zone of osteoporosis may fracture, giving marginal metaphyseal spurring known as Pelkan's spur. A lack of focal destructive osteoporotic lesions elsewhere distinguishes the metaphyseal bands of lucency in scurvy from those seen in leukaemia and neuroblastoma (see page 291).

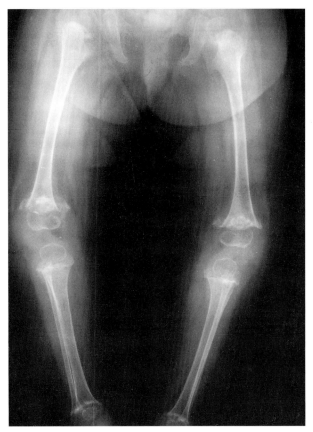

a

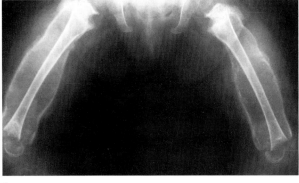

b

Figure 1.39 *Scurvy. (**a**) There is overall loss of bone density with sharply demarcated cortices. This is especially prominent at the epiphyses. Metaphyseal fractures giving marginal metaphyseal spurring are shown. The loss of bone density is uniform. (**b**) Two weeks later, the same patient has formed new bone beneath the elevated periosteum. Metaphyseal fractures are still prominent. Compare with Figure 1.37. In both cases haematoma markedly elevates the loosely applied periosteum beneath which new bone is formed.*

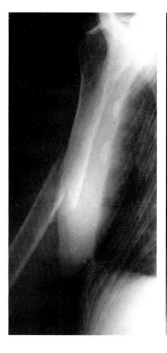
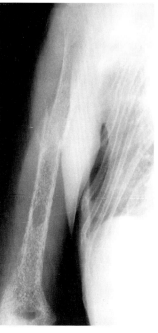
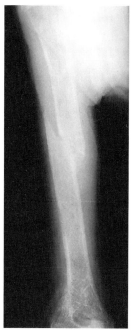

Figure 1.40 *Fracture in hyperparathyroidism. The initial bone density was reduced at the time of the fracture (left). After a short interval and immobilization, intense spotty osteoporosis is seen affecting both the cortex and medulla, and brown tumours are rendered more prominent (centre). The last film shows some recovery of bone density on mobilization, but also shows the resultant soft tissue wasting (right).*

REGIONAL OSTEOPOROSIS (Table 1.6)

Immobilization

This also causes osteoporosis and metaphyseal lucency not usually generalized to all four limbs (see page 291). Osteoporosis after immobilization is most commonly seen following fractures, but may also result from enforced bed rest or paralysis, and has also been described following weightlessness in space travel. Skeletal immobilization is followed by early loss of bone, hypercalcuria and muscle wasting.

Bone loss after a fracture is most marked distal to the fracture, even if the joints above and below are immobilized. The young and old exhibit this change earlier than middle-aged patients. Histologically, there is intense osteoclastic and decreased osteoblastic activity. If the fracture is through bone affected by Paget's disease or hyperparathyroidism, the distal osteoporosis is even more marked (Figure 1.40).

Acute or subacute osteoporosis following a fracture is usually only seen in the limbs, and may be uniform with cortical thinning and medullary trabecular loss. In younger patients other forms may be seen. Cortical striations may become more prominent so that three or four cigar-shaped lucencies may be seen across the cortex (Figure 1.41). Subcortical bone is resorbed in the articular regions, producing pronounced osteoporosis beneath pencilled cortices. Immobilization in children causes bands of lucency extending across

Table 1.6 Regional osteoporosis.

Immobilization
Reflex sympathetic dystrophy syndrome
Transient osteoporosis of the hip
Regional migratory osteoporosis
Inflammatory joint disease

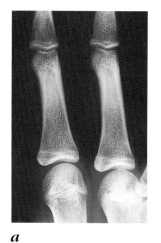
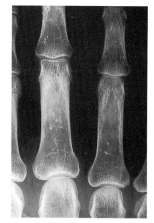

a   *b*

Figure 1.41 *(a) Normal bone with a dense cortex. (b) Osteoporosis with reduction in bone density and prominent cortical striations.*

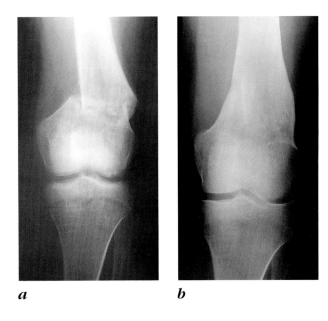

a   *b*

Figure 1.42 *(a) The initial radiograph, taken shortly after a distal femoral fracture, shows quite marked subarticular and metaphyseal radiolucency, even though the growth plate has fused. (b) A radiograph taken 5 years later shows good fracture healing and some restoration of bony density. The submetaphyseal lucency can still be seen in the proximal tibia. Growth arrest lines are also demonstrated.*

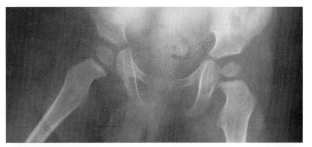

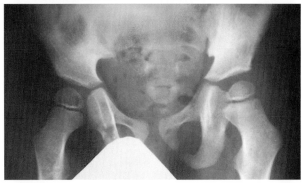

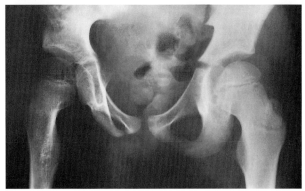

Figure 1.43 *Progressive osteoporosis and bony hypoplasia result from the muscle atrophy of polio.*

the entire metaphysis, and endosteal scalloping may occur (see Chapter 5, page 291). The carpal and tarsal bones are especially affected. Bone loss is not always uniform but may also be patchy or spotty in both the cortex and medulla, the latter change being superimposed upon the overall loss of bone density. This change can be alarming and so pronounced that the fracture line may not be clearly visible. With resumption of function and weight bearing, remineralization occurs but often not to the levels seen in the contralateral normal limb (Figure 1.42).

Polio and other forms of muscular paralysis

When presenting in childhood, these are associated with diffuse chronic osteoporosis and hypoplasia of bone. In addition to cortical thinning and a loss of medullary trabeculation, there is a loss of bone length and width. Foramina, such as those in the pelvis, are smaller on the affected side. Muscle bulk is diminished and subcutaneous and perimuscular fat increased (Figures 1.43 and 1.44) In this disease, and in other diseases of the nervous system, a long, smooth scoliosis may result (see Chapter 8, page 415), concave to the side of active muscle function.

Reflex sympathetic dystrophy syndrome (RSDS)

This is also known as Sudeck's atrophy or osteodystrophy. Changes are usually seen in the extremities

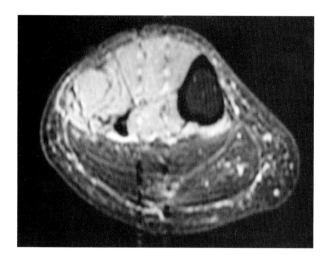
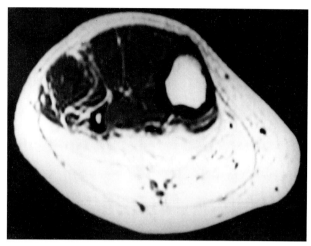

Figure 1.44 *Established polio. At MRI, muscle atrophy and fatty hypertrophy are well demonstrated on fat suppression and T_1-weighted scans.*

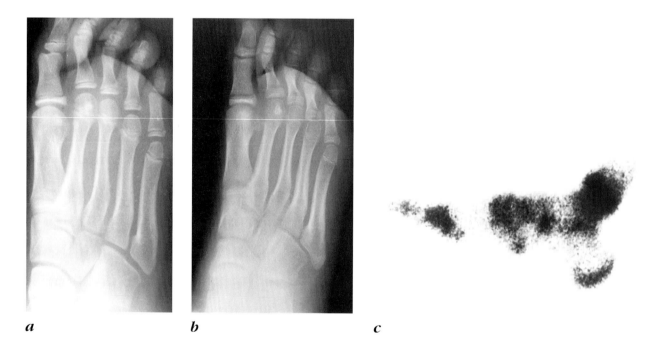

a   *b*   *c*

Figure 1.45 *Reflex sympathetic dystrophy syndrome. (**a**) The initial radiograph shows normal appearances at the time of a proximal injury . (**b**) The subsequent radiograph shows marked demineralization, accentuated around the metatarsophalangeal joints. Bone density in the tarsus is also markedly reduced. A growing bone island is also seen in the second metatarsal head. (**c**) The radioisotope bone scan shows a marked increase in uptake throughout the foot, but especially in the periarticular regions.*

following trauma; however, they may follow compartmental soft tissue infection or limb surgery. Radioisotope bone scans of the affected limb demonstrate increase in both perfusion and bone uptake around all the joints of the affected limb (Figure 1.45), as well as in the contralateral limb in many cases. The diagnosis is based on the history of the injury, the examination of the limb, which may be swollen,

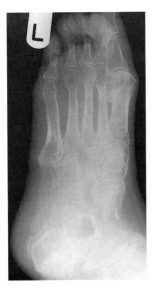
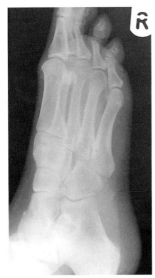

Figure 1.46 *This patient with reflex sympathetic dystrophy syndrome had sustained a fracture of the left leg which was put in plaster and immobilized. The right lower limb retains a normal density throughout, but the gross osteoporosis of the left limb with associated soft tissue swelling is part of this syndrome, which was so painful that the patient had to have her foot amputated.*

painful and tender, and the radiological findings. Osteoporosis is widespread and extreme. The cortices are extremely thin, scalloped, and show excessive Haversian trabeculation, especially in the ring-like bones of the carpus and tarsus. The cortex may even be defective in places and subcortical and metaphyseal bone is hypertransradiant. Medullary bone appears to be patchily resorbed, since it is absent in certain areas and relatively dense elsewhere. Joint spaces are preserved unless another pathology is present, and this preservation can exclude local infective processes. The radiological appearances are those of a severe form of immobilization, with soft tissue swelling and pain, but no joint narrowing (Figure 1.46).

Transient osteoporosis; regional migratory osteoporosis

These entities are characterized by acute pain, usually in the hip, and osteoporosis localized to the painful joint (Figure 1.47a). The radionuclide bone scan is usually strongly positive in the abnormal joint (Figure 1.47b). MR imaging shows changes of bone oedema, especially on T_2-weighted or fat suppression sequences (Figure 1.47c,d).

Transient osteoporosis typically occurs in middle-aged males who have performed unaccustomed exercise—a game of squash or a long walk. Presumably venous occlusion by an effusion in the hip joint is the cause of the change. The effusion may be seen on ultrasound examination. The ESR may be mildly raised. Pain is severe, but the syndrome is self-limiting with partial weight bearing and cessation of athletic activity (Figure 1.47e).

A similar phenomenon occurs in the hip, usually the left, of a woman in the last trimester of pregnancy.

In *regional migratory osteoporosis*, similar changes occur in different joints, often associated with a local periostitis. The changes wax and wane before moving onto another area. Occasionally, only part of a joint may be affected. Again, the radionuclide bone scan is positive and the MR images shows local bone oedema.

RICKETS AND OSTEOMALACIA

This condition is characterized by an increase in the proportion of non-mineralized osteoid in bone. Rickets in children primarily affects the chondro-osseous complex at the epiphysis which is the area of linear growth. After epiphyseal fusion, osteomalacia affects lamellar bone, resulting in different radiological appearances of two diseases with the same aetiology (Table 1.7).

Table 1.7 Causes of rickets and osteomalacia.

Nutritional
Premature infants
Dietary vitamin D deficiency
Inadequate exposure to sunlight
Old age
Malabsorption
Intestinal, pancreatic or biliary disorder
Partial gastrectomy
Metabolic
Drug therapy (anticonvulsants, antituberculous)
Renal disease
Liver disease
Vitamin D dependency

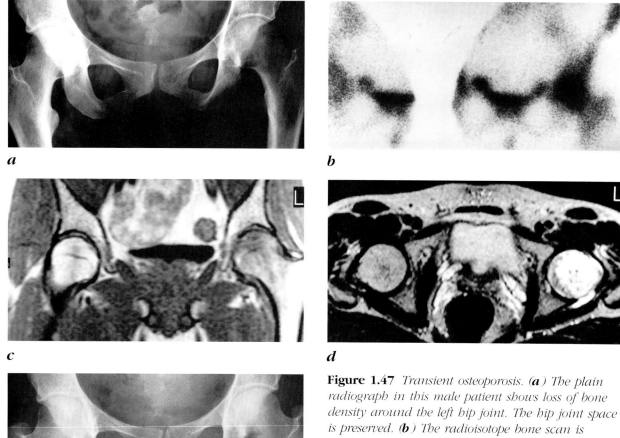

Figure 1.47 *Transient osteoporosis. (a) The plain radiograph in this male patient shows loss of bone density around the left hip joint. The hip joint space is preserved. (b) The radioisotope bone scan is strongly positive in this area. (c) The coronal T₁-weighted MR sequence shows replacement of marrow fat by low signal oedema. (d) An axial T₂-weighted MR image shows increased signal due to bone oedema in the left femoral head, and a hip joint effusion. (e) Nine months later the radiological appearances have reverted to normal and the patient is pain-free.*

Worldwide, the commonest cause of rickets and osteomalacia is vitamin D deficiency. In the UK this is still seen frequently in vegetarian immigrants from Africa and Asia who, in addition, do not receive as much sunlight as in their native lands. Sunlight is needed for the conversion of cholesterol to 1-hydroxycholecalciferol, which is an inactive precursor of vitamin D. If a patient of Indian origin who is a vegetarian presents with local or general bone pain, osteomalacia must be excluded (as incidentally must tuberculous disease, especially in the spine). Among Western populations, the commonest causes of rickets and osteomalacia are congenital or acquired abnormalities of mineral metabolism which are usually resistant to the normal therapeutic doses of vitamin D. These diseases are uncommon in comparison with osteoporosis.

The clinical profile of osteomalacia is one of bone pain and tenderness, with muscular weakness. Back and limb pain may result from fractures and there may be joint pain and deformities. In children, there is bulging of the limbs and ribs at chondro-osseous junctions (rickety rosary).

RADIOLOGY OF RICKETS

Characteristic radiological changes are seen initially and are most prominent at areas of maximum growth and stress. At the wrist, around the knee, and at the

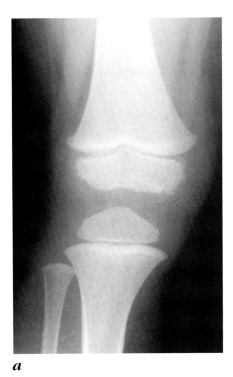

a

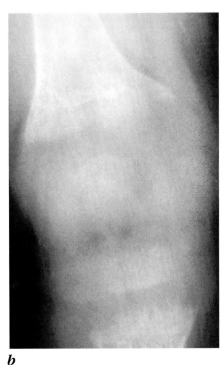

b

Figure 1.48 *Comparison between (**a**) normal and (**b**) rachitic bone. The abnormal joint shows metaphyseal irregularity and splaying, with an increased width of the growth plate. Bone density generally is reduced. Bone definition is generally poor.*

anterior ends of the ribs, the epiphysis loses its sharp outline and becomes fuzzy, as does the adjacent metaphyseal sclerotic line representing the provisional zone of calcification (Figure 1.48). Eventually the metaphysis becomes irregular, radiolucent and widened. This widening is appreciable clinically and is probably a stress reaction at softened bone. The epiphyseal plate appears widened (over 3 mm) due to defective mineralization of the epiphysis and the adjacent metaphysis.

All the epiphyses may be affected and the apophyses also show these changes. Elsewhere lack of mineralization of subchondral bone causes irregularity at the sacroiliac joints and symphysis pubis, so that these joints can become even more difficult than usual to visualize in children.

There is an increase in osteoid in the trabeculae, which consequently are proportionally less mineralized. This leads to radiological blurring of cortical and medullary bone, resulting in a fuzzy or hazy appearance, sometimes with an apparent decrease in radiological density. However, occasionally trabecular coarsening suggests an increase in density.

Softening of the bone may result in bowing in the lower limbs, which may be associated with protrusio acetabuli, and which is especially associated with X-linked hypophosphataemic rickets and osteomalacia (Figure 1.49).

In children, the metaphyseal region is normally the site of increased uptake on the radioisotope bone scan. This change is also seen at the anterior ends of the ribs and at the apophyses. In rickets, this uptake is further increased at these characteristic sites. Pathological fractures may also be seen radiologically and on scintigraphy.

RADIOLOGY OF OSTEOMALACIA

The characteristic, diagnostic radiological feature of osteomalacia is the Looser's zone, although this occurs only in a minority of biochemically diagnosed cases. Looser's zones are short, transverse bands of radiolucency extending inwards from the cortex, particularly at sites of major stress, including the lateral margin of the scapula, ribs, proximal femora medially and around the obturator rings (Figures 1.50 and 1.51). At some sites they may be related to local vascular channels. They consist of osteoid seams and are surrounded by bands of sclerosis, representing healing. The more sclerosis present, the easier the Looser's zone is visualized. They are rarely present in childhood.

With progressive deformity from bone softening, transverse fractures occur in osteomalacia (Figure 1.52). Looser's zones may be curved (Figure 1.53).

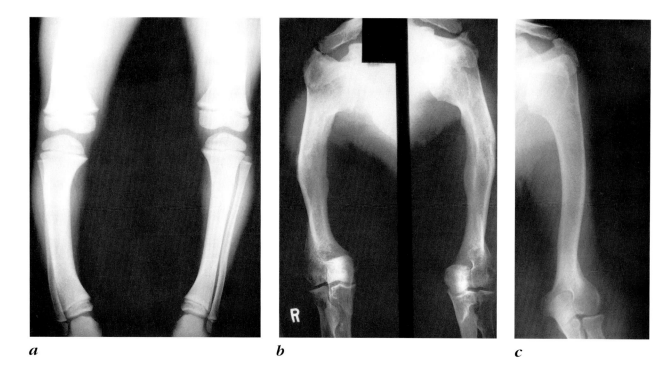

a   *b*   *c*

Figure 1.49 *(**a**) In this patient with X-linked rickets, there is bowing with an increase in bony density. (**b**) X-linked hypophosphataemic osteomalacia. Bowing and sclerosis of the humeri with a generalized increase in density. (**c**) A similar deformity results in cretinism from abnormalities of growth at the proximal humerus. Humerus varus results. The bone is less broad.*

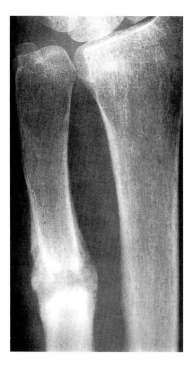

Figure 1.50
Characteristic sites for Looser's zones include the shafts of long bones. The ulna in particular shows diminished bone density. The Looser's zone is healing.

In children the synchondrosis at the ischium remains open until around seven years of age. Looser's zones in osteomalacia arise at the same site, but should not be confused with this synchondrosis (Figure 1.51a). Delay in fusion at the synchondrosis may occur in cretinism and other causes of delay in skeletal maturation. Stress fractures also occur locally (Figure 1.51d).

Looser's zones may also be diagnosed on the isotope bone scan which may be preferable to the radiographic skeletal survey. The distribution of foci of increased uptake ('hot spots') is symmetrical and at the expected sites for Looser's zones, but increase in uptake is seen particularly at the anterior rib ends. Malignant metastatic disease, however, has a totally random distribution in the axial skeleton (Figure 1.54). Changes in osteomalacia reflect:

1   bone softening (Figure 1.55a). Multiple levels of vertebral collapse may be present, often contiguous and codfish in type (Figure 1.55b), as well as limb deformity;

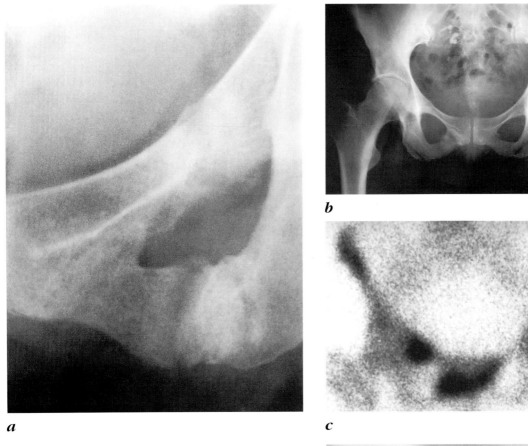

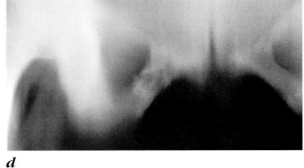

Figure 1.51 (*a*) *Looser's zones are commonly seen around the obturator ring.* (*b*, *c*) *This region is commonly the site of true pelvic fracture. The radionuclide bone scan shows increase in uptake.* (*d*) *Stress fractures occur here too.*

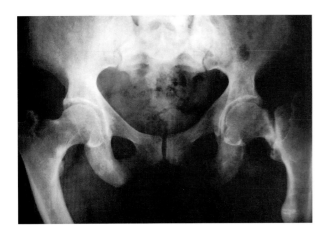

Figure 1.52 *A transverse fracture is seen in the left femoral neck in this patient with osteomalacia. There is varus deformity. Note the healing Looser's zones of the midshaft femora.*

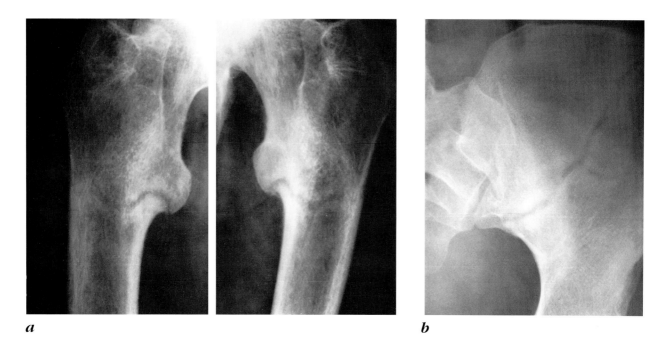

Figure 1.53 *Osteomalacia. Curved Looser's zones are shown in (**a**) the region of the lesser trochanter and (**b**) the left iliac blade.*

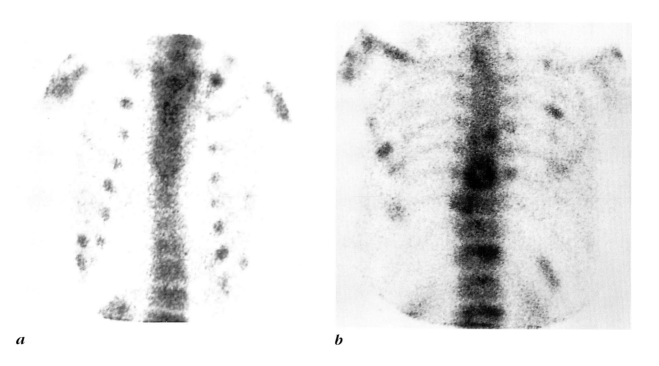

Figure 1.54 *(**a**) Radionuclide scan in osteomalacia. The foci of increased uptake are at costochondral junctions, which are abnormal in rickets (the rickety rosary). The distribution is not random, as in metastatic disease, and is too widespread to suggest trauma. (**b**) Radioisotope bone scan showing metastatic disease, with a random distribution of the foci of increased uptake.*

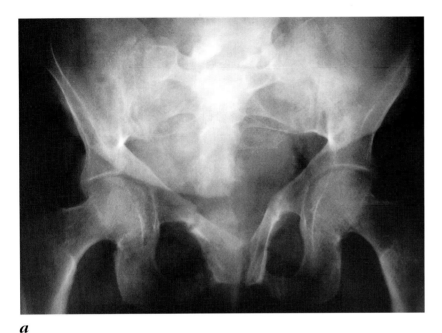

a

b

Figure 1.55 *Osteomalacia. (**a**) A triradiate pelvis is shown — the result of bone softening and Looser's zones. (**b**) Demineralization, poor definition of trabeculae and multiple codfish vertebrae in continuity.*

2   multiple areas of non-mineralized osteoid in cortex and medulla, giving streaky lucency and demineralization;

3   poorly defined trabeculae producing fuzziness due to excessive non-mineralized osteoid on the trabeculae (Figure 1.56);

4   changes of secondary hyperparathyroidism particularly in the hands (see below).

DIFFERENTIAL DIAGNOSIS OF METAPHYSEAL IRREGULARITY

Metaphyseal irregularity with demineralization has a number of causes (Table 1.8) (see also Chapter 5, page 291).

Rickets

The changes are widespread in distribution and extend across the entire metaphysis. The epiphyseal plate is widened and the epiphysis poorly corticated.

Table 1.8 Causes of metaphyseal irregularity.

Rickets
Hypophosphatasia
Enchondromatosis
Metaphyseal dysostosis

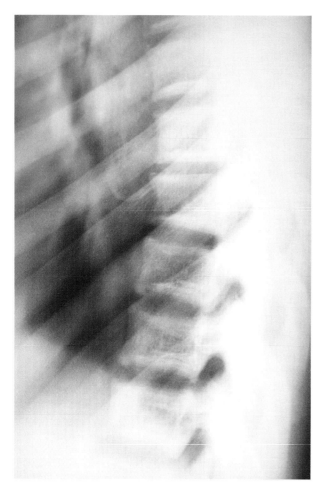

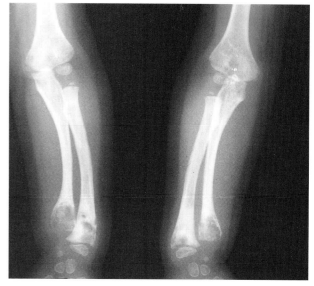

Figure 1.57 *Demineralization is seen in this patient with hypophosphatasia. The ring epiphyses of the wrist are normal. However, there is marked deformity with irregularity of the metaphyses at the wrist (see also Chapter 5, page 301).*

Figure 1.56 *Poorly defined trabeculae in rickets. Note the growth arrest lines.*

Hypophosphatasia

This is a rare condition transmitted as an autosomal recessive disease of varying severity, with bone changes prominent in infants. The metaphyseal changes are similar to those of rickets, but are more severe and associated with gross loss of mineralization. Generalized metaphyseal irregularity is marked and extends far inwards towards the diaphysis, giving a broad, scraggy and poorly mineralized metaphysis in severe cases (Figure 1.57). As well as demineralization, bowing and fractures are found, resulting in shortening and periostitis. Loss of density in the skull is severe and the bones may be scarcely visible. Craniostenosis or Wormian bones may also be seen (Figure 1.58).

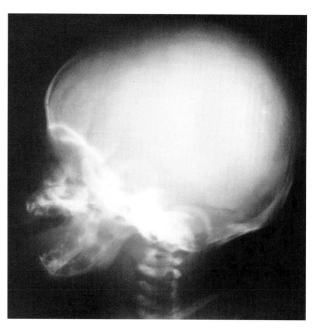

Figure 1.58 *Hypophosphatasia. The sutures are not visualized and the skull vault is poorly mineralized.*

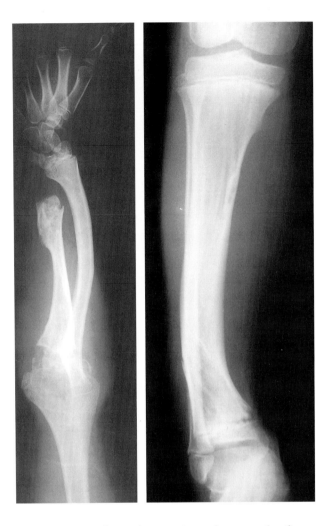

Skull demineralization in osteogenesis imperfecta is accompanied by wide sutures and Wormian bones (Figure 1.35). Craniostenosis does not occur. Fractures are seen in osteogenesis imperfecta and hypophosphatasia but the zone of provisional calcification at the metaphysis is not irregular in osteogenesis imperfecta and the epiphysis is corticated.

Enchondromatosis (Ollier's disease)

This exists in various radiological forms. In one type, long streaky radiolucent islands of irregularly calcified cartilage stream backwards from the zone of provisional calcification; the metaphysis becomes irregular and broadened in appearance (Figure 1.59). Deformities often coexist, especially in the distal radius and ulna (hypoplastic broad ulna, curved broad radius). Similar changes also occur in diaphyseal aclasia (see Chapter 7, page 345). Overall, however, bone density is normal and the epiphysis well defined.

Metaphyseal dysostosis

The most common form of this rare disease is the Type Schmid. Metaphyseal changes are similar to, but less severe than, those seen in rickets. There is mild splaying and irregularity of the metaphyses in childhood (Figure 1.60). Bone density is normal or even increased, Looser's zones do not appear and the skull is normal.

Figure 1.59 *Ollier's disease. Irregular strands of lucency extend backwards into the shaft of the bone from the epiphyseal plate (see also Chapter 7, page 345).*

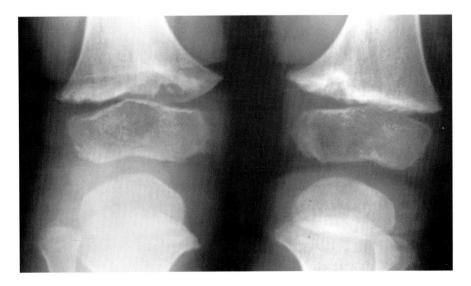

Figure 1.60 *In metaphyseal dysostosis, Type Schmid, bone density is preserved. There is slight irregularity of the distal femoral metaphyses.*

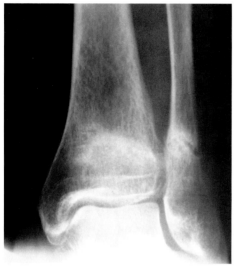
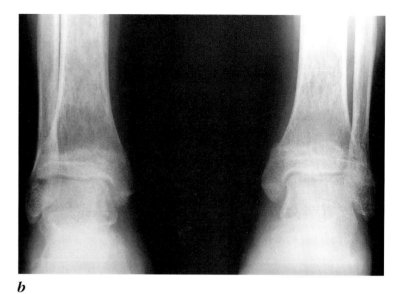

a   *b*

Figure 1.61 *(a) Stress fractures are present at the distal tibia and fibula. (b) Stress fracture in osteomalacia.*

LOOSER'S ZONES AND SIMILAR LESIONS

Looser's zones

These are usually widespread in distribution and often at classical sites (Figures 1.50, 1.51a and 1.54a). Several lesions resemble Looser's zones.

Stress fractures

Stress fractures as shown on a plain radiograph are transverse bands of lucency (the fracture) surrounded by sclerosis (callus) (Figures 1.51d, 1.61, 1.62 and 1.63). Pain is the presenting symptom and the lesion can be seen on an isotope bone scan before it becomes visible on the plain film, as there is an interval between the onset of pain and the formation of callus (Figure 1.64). Characteristic activities give stress fractures at characteristic sites (Figure 1.63b; Table 1.9). The lesions are often symmetrical but not widespread.

Osteoid osteoma, osteoblastoma and Brodie's abscess

These may have a similar appearance and present as painful, focal, often osteolytic lesions with a central

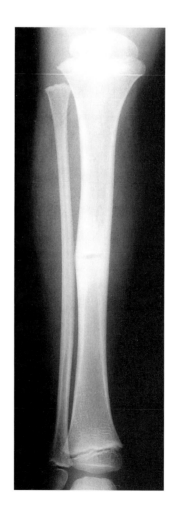

Figure 1.62 *Stress fracture of the midshaft of the tibia. A transverse band of lucency lies at right angles to the thickened cortex.*

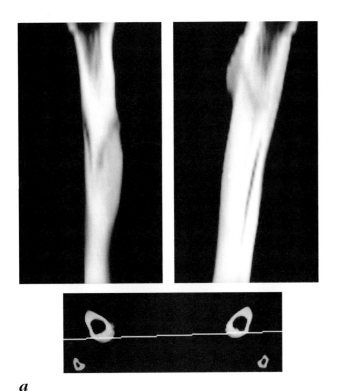

a

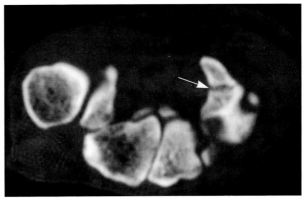

b

Figure 1.63 *(a) CT reformatted image of the tibia in coronal and sagittal planes showing new bone formation around a stress fracture. (b) Stress fracture through the hamate in an obsessive golfer (arrow). The lesion is unilateral. (By courtesy of Mr John Ireland, FRCS.)*

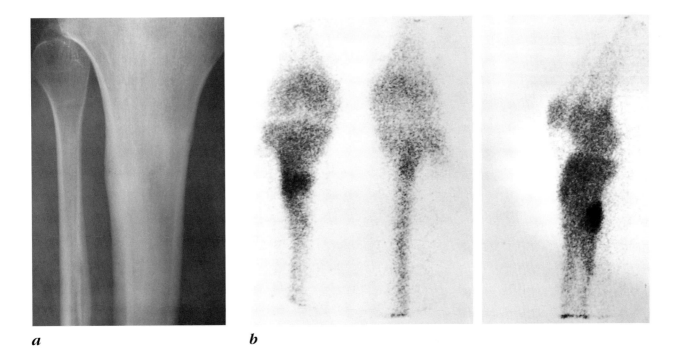

a   *b*

Figure 1.64 *Stress fracture. (a) Localized thickening of the cortex and some increase in density can be seen. (b) A radioisotope bone scan shows a local area of increased uptake corresponding to a stress fracture.*

Table 1.9 Location of stress fracture by activity.

Location	Activity
Sesamoids of metatarsals	Prolonged standing
Metatarsal shaft	Marching; ground stamping
	Prolonged standing
	Ballet
	Postoperative bunionectomy
Navicular	Marching; ground stamping
	Long distance running
Calcaneus	Jumping; parachuting
	Prolonged standing
	Recent immobilization
Tibia—mid and distal shaft	Ballet
	Long distance running
Tibia—proximal shaft (children)	Running
Fibula—distal shaft	Long distance running
Fibula—proximal shaft	Jumping; parachuting
Patella	Hurdling
Femur—shaft	Ballet
	Long distance running
Femur—neck	Ballet
	Marching
	Long distance running
	Gymnastics
Pelvis—obturator ring	Stooping
	Bowling
	Gymnastic
Lumbar vertebra (pars interarticularis)	Ballet
	Heavy lifting
	Scrubbing floors
Lower cervical, upper thoracic spinous process	Clay shovelling
Ribs	Carrying heavy pack
	Golf
	Coughing
Clavicle	Postoperative radical neck dissection
Coracoid of scapula	Trap shooting
Humerus—distal shaft	Throwing a ball
Ulna—coronoid	Pitching a ball
Ulna—shaft	Pitchfork work
	Propelling wheelchair
Hook of hamate*	Holding golf club, tennis racket, baseball bat

* Speculative stress fracture.
Adapted from Daffner RH, Stress fractures, *Skeletal Radiol* (1978) **2**: 221–9, with permission.

lucency in which calcification may or may not be present (Figure 1.65). They are almost inevitably solitary and surrounded by reactive sclerosis which may be so marked that it obscures the underlying lesion (see Chapter 3, page 118).

OTHER FORMS OF OSTEOMALACIA

X-linked hypophosphataemic rickets and osteomalacia

In this condition, which is vitamin D resistant, rachitic changes in infancy and osteomalacic changes in the adult are associated with gross bowing of the long bones, especially in the lower limbs, and an increase in bony density which becomes more pronounced with age (Figure 1.49a,b). The bowed, dense, long bones are increased in width and show gross cortical thickening. In the adult, these features co-exist with changes which suggest a seronegative spondylarthritis, such as ankylosing spondylitis or Reiter's syndrome. There is sacroiliac irregularity and apparent fusion, paravertebral ossification, and ossification at musculo-tendinous insertions (see Chapter 8, page 379). Patients have hypophosphataemia and hyperphosphaturia. Articular erosions are not present and the dense and bowed bones rule out a spondylarthropathy.

Tumoural rickets and osteomalacia

Patients presenting with these conditions are also hypophosphataemic and hyperphosphaturic but do not show bowing or sclerosis of bone. The changes are due to a number of bone and soft tissue tumours which secrete a hormone that inhibits renal tubular phosphate resorption. These tumours include haemangiopericytoma, often of the maxillary antra (Figure 1.66), fibrous dysplasia, neurofibromatosis,

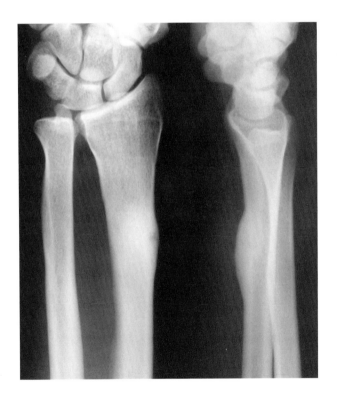

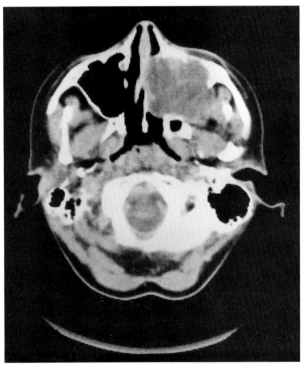

Figure 1.65 *There is 'heaping up' of cortex and periosteal new bone with an associated radiolucency containing ossification. These appearances are typical of a cortical osteoid osteoma.*

Figure 1.66 *Haemangiopericytoma of the antrum (same patient as in Figure 1.50). A large soft tissue mass erodes the left antrum, destroying its wall and extending into the infratemporal fossa as well as the nasal passage.*

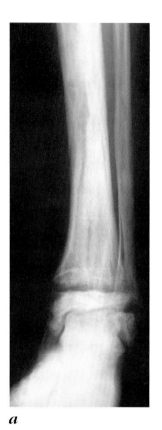 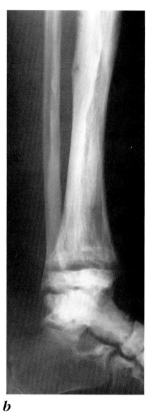

a   *b*

Figure 1.67 *Melorheostosis and tumoural rickets. Widening of the growth plate is associated with areas of sclerosis at the tibia and talus (see Chapter 2, page 87) (by courtesy of Dr S Lee).*

giant-cell tumour, melorheostosis (Figure 1.67), and even osteosarcoma. In patients with characteristic biochemical changes, the bone scan will demonstrate the typical distribution of osteomalacic change, and may also demonstrate the tumour. Otherwise the radiological changes do not differ from those seen in rickets or osteomalacia. The tumour must be totally removed for treatment to be effective.

HYPERPARATHYROIDISM

Most cases of hyperparathyroidism are due to a solitary functioning thyroid adenoma. The disease classically occurs in middle-aged or elderly females whose bones may already be osteopenic.

Parathormone has an anabolic effect which is said to occur if low doses are administered over a long period, while high doses administered over a short period promote a catabolic effect. Catabolism involves the resorption of bone by osteoclasts and osteocytes under parathormone stimulation.

RADIOLOGICAL CHANGES IN HYPERPARATHYROIDISM

Demineralization

Overall, osteopenia is the commonest radiological finding in hyperparathyroidism, but unfortunately it is not specific. Moreover, the disease often occurs with a background of postmenopausal or senile osteoporosis, in which case even after satisfactory treatment the bones never return to normal density.

Subperiosteal bone resorption

This change is almost pathognomonic for hyperparathyroidism and is inevitably present in hyperparathyroid patients with bone disease. It occurs earliest and in its most gross form at the radial aspects of the middle phalanges of the second and third fingers (Figure 1.68). The cortex loses definition and becomes less dense due to enlargement of the cigar-shaped Haversian canals, as in reflex sympathetic dystrophy syndrome (RSDS). Spiculation occurs externally and the distal phalangeal tufts become eroded (Figure 1.69). Subperiosteal bone resorption follows, most commonly at the proximal tibial metaphysis medially (Figure 1.70), along the radial and ulnar shafts, around the acromioclavicular joints (Figure 1.71) and at the musculo-tendinous insertions around the pelvis. The iliac crests, iliac spines and ischia are eroded, as in ankylosing spondylitis (Figure 1.72). Even the sacroiliac joints may be eroded by subarticular osteoclasis. Very occasionally, paraspinal and paradiscal new bone has been described (see Chapter 8, page 360).

There is erosion of the superior aspects of the upper ribs (Figure 1.71), which also occurs in conditions associated with muscle wasting (Table 1.10). These have no cortical irregularity.

Skull changes were very common in patients with bone changes in hyperparathyroidism, with 50% of patients with bone disease having changes in the skull alone. The incidence of skull change in the UK is currently low.

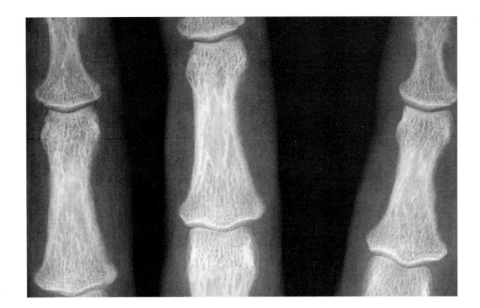

Figure 1.68 *This hyperparathyroid patient has subperiosteal bone resorption, particularly on the radial aspect of the middle phalanges.*

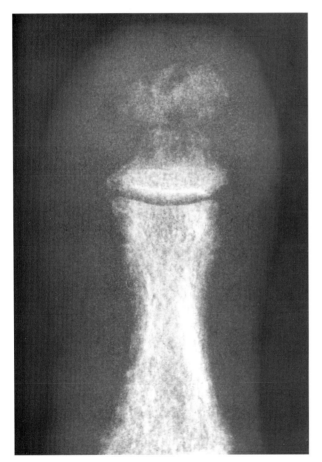

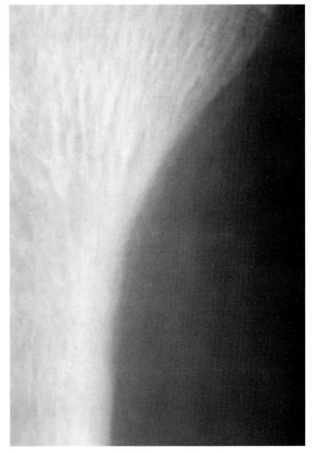

Figure 1.69 *Hyperparathyroidism. This macroradiograph shows resorption of the distal phalanx with associated pseudoclubbing. The cortex has been resorbed by subperiosteal and endosteal bone resorption.*

Figure 1.70 *Resorption of the medial cortex of the proximal tibial metaphysis has occurred in this hyperparathyroid patient.*

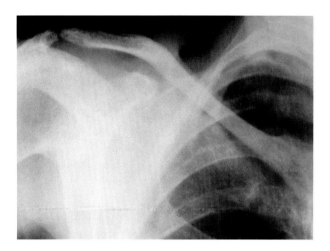

Figure 1.71 *Hyperparathyroidism. Resorption is seen around the acromio-clavicular joint, on the inferior surface of the medial clavicle and on the upper aspects of the ribs.*

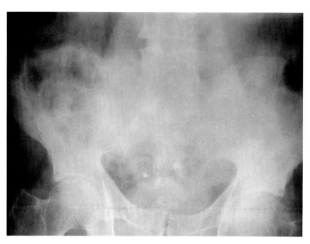

Figure 1.72 *Hyperparathyroidism. Erosions occur at the iliac crests and around the sacroiliac joints.*

Table 1.10 Causes of superior rib erosion.

Hyperparathyroidism (associated with subperiosteal bone resorption)
Rheumatoid arthritis ⎤
Other collagen diseases ⎥ no subperiosteal
Polio ⎥ bone resorption
Muscle wasting in old age ⎦

Changes in the skull include:

1 widespread focal areas of osteolysis, producing a poorly defined 'pepper pot' appearance (Figure 1.73a);
2 loss of definition of tables and meningeal groove markings giving a 'pseudo-Paget' appearance (Figure 1.73b);
3 bone sclerosis in primary hyperparathyroidism, presumably due to calcification in fibrous tissue. Increased density is unusual outside the skull in primary disease (Figure 1.73c).

The purely lytic or mixed sclerotic and lytic pattern must be distinguished from malignant metastatic disease or myeloma, since both sets of conditions may be associated with elevation of the serum calcium level. Patients with skull changes in hyperparathyroidism will inevitably have the hand changes

of subperiosteal bone resorption, whereas those with malignant disease do not. Isotope bone scanning is necessary in either case and further lesions should be examined radiologically.

Subperiosteal bone resorption is also seen in the jaws as loss of the lamina dura, which is the hard cortical line of the socket surrounding the teeth (Figure 1.74). However, this is not as commonly seen as the change in the phalanges. Loss of the lamina dura also occurs with lytic infections, eosinophilic granuloma, dental cysts, metastatic disease and ameloblastoma, and with sclerotic lesions such as Paget's disease and cementoma.

Brown tumours

Brown tumours are related to osteoclastic overactivity, and are generally multiple and often well corticated

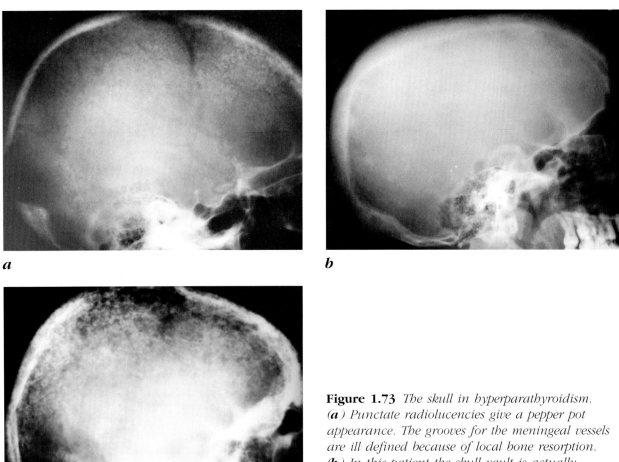

Figure 1.73 *The skull in hyperparathyroidism. (**a**) Punctate radiolucencies give a pepper pot appearance. The grooves for the meningeal vessels are ill defined because of local bone resorption. (**b**) In this patient the skull vault is actually thickened and there is a loss of tabular differentiation, giving a pseudo-Paget appearance. (**c**) In this patient there is a mixture of osteolysis and sclerosis.*

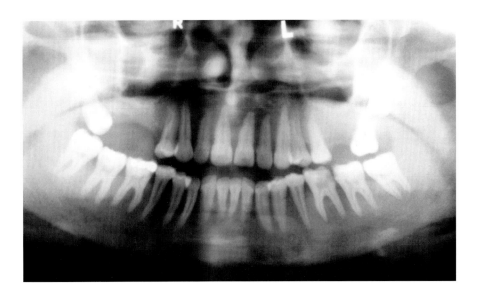

Figure 1.74 *This hyperparathyroid patient demonstrates resorption of the lamina dura around the mandibular dentition. In addition, there is a cyst around the root of the right upper canine tooth.*

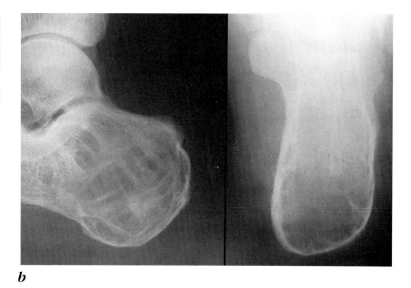

a　　　　　　　　　*b*

Figure 1.75 *(a) Multiple brown tumours in hyperparathyroidism are seen bilaterally in subarticular and metaphyseal locations. Chondrocalcinosis is also present. (b) A large brown tumour is seen in the calcaneus.*

(Figure 1.75). They may be subarticular or in the shaft. Multiple, fairly well demarcated lytic lesions which are not significantly expansile and do not contain calcific flecks always suggest the possibility of hyperparathyroidism. Similar lesions may be seen in fibrous dysplasia (Figure 1.76), but these tend to be unilateral and are not associated with subperiosteal bone resorption. Eosinophilic granuloma also gives multiple lytic lesions in bone but should not be diagnosed over the age of 35 years. Fibrous dysplasia can occur at all ages but lesions tend to calcify with age.

After treatment, lytic lesions in hyperparathyroidism may become dense or remain lytic with increased density only at the margins (Figures 1.77 and 1.78), and the cyst-like lesions may suffer pathological fracture. Tumours do not occur in the absence of subperiosteal bone resorption.

At the present time, primary hyperparathyroidism is not a significant cause of bone disease. The disease is often diagnosed biochemically on routine screening, and patients may not have any bone changes. If they do, they will have subperiosteal bone resorption at the phalanges which is best seen using macroradiography or a magnifying glass. An X-ray of the hands is always indicated in those with suggestive biochemistry.

In hyperparathyroidism an isotope bone scan demonstrates tumoural lesions, while an abdominal X-ray or ultrasound examination shows renal calcification.

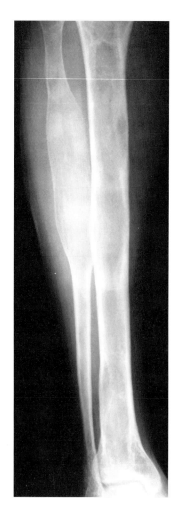

Figure 1.76 *Expansile lesions of the upper tibia and fibula are present in this patient with polyostotic fibrous dysplasia. The cortex is thinned but preserved and sharp. The lesions are widespread throughout both long bones and, in places, show the typical ground-glass appearance of fibrous dysplasia. Bony definition, particularly at the cortices in areas not affected by the lesions, is much more normal than in hyperparathyroidism where there is usually a degree of demineralization and cortical erosion. The disease tends towards a unilateral distribution.*

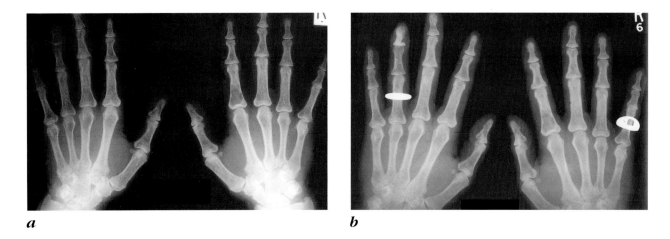

Figure 1.77 *Hyperparathyroidism. (**a**) The initial radiograph shows a brown tumour in the distal phalanx of the left ring finger and another in the proximal phalanx of the right index finger. (**b**) Following parathyroidectomy, the lesion in the left hand heals with sclerosis while the right-sided lesion becomes dense at its margin.*

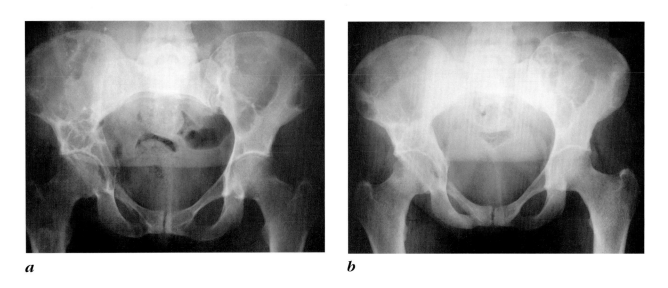

Figure 1.78 *Hyperparathyroidism. (**a**) In this patient of the late Professor Dent, the initial radiograph shows multiple brown tumours involving the left iliac blade, the pubic bones bilaterally and the right lower iliac bone and ischium. (**b**) After surgery the lesions on the right have healed mainly by sclerosis, while those on the left have become smaller and better defined.*

Chondrocalcinosis

Calcification, especially at the menisci in the knees and wrist, but also at articular cartilages elsewhere, occurs in the elderly as part of the aging process. Hyperparathyroidism should be excluded in patients of 55 years of age and below who exhibit multiple joint involvement with chondrocalcinosis (Figure 1.79) (see also Chapter 9, page 437). Calcium pyrophosphate dihydrate (CPPD) crystal deposition disease and gout also cause calcification and may be painful (see Chapter 9, Table 9.2, page 437). Gout is associated with large erosions and soft tissue swelling, but overall bone density is usually preserved.

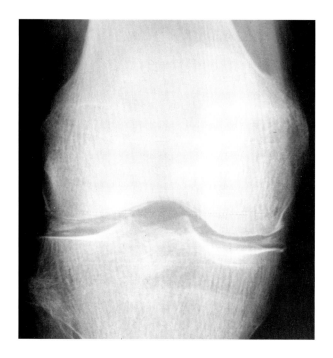

Figure 1.79 *Chondrocalcinosis in hyperparathyroidism. Both the articular and meniscal cartilages are affected.*

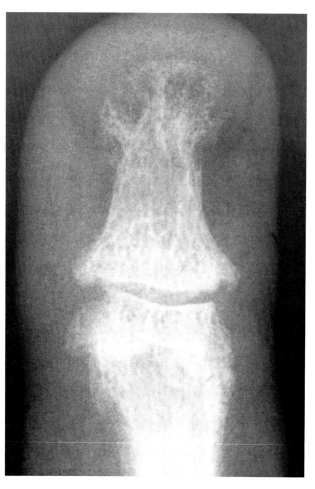

Figure 1.80 *Hyperparathyroidism. There is resorption of the distal tuft with para-articular erosions. Subperiosteal bone resorption is also seen along the shaft of the middle phalanx.*

Joint erosions

These occur in hyperparathyroidism due to subcortical osteoclastic resorption of bone in subarticular regions. In patients with an overall loss of bone density, the lesions are poorly defined and occur at the sacroiliac and acromioclavicular joints and symphysis pubis. The carpus, metacarpo- and metatarsophalangeal joints are affected specifically and the appearances may resemble those seen in rheumatoid arthritis, but always occur in the presence of subperiosteal bone resorption (Figure 1.80).

SECONDARY HYPERPARATHYROIDISM

Hyperparathyroidism may also be seen in patients with pre-existing osteomalacia. Parathyroid hyperplasia compensates for high serum phosphate and low serum calcium levels.

RENAL OSTEODYSTROPHY

The term describes the bone changes in patients with chronic renal failure. The changes of osteomalacia or rickets arise as the diseased kidneys are unable to hydroxylate 25-hydroxycholecalciferol. Secondary hyperparathyroidism then occurs, with some differences possibly due to the anabolic effects of parathormone (see Chapter 2, page 99).

Periostitis on long bone shafts is generally absent in primary hyperparathyroidism but occurs in renal osteodystrophy (Figure 1.81). Brown tumours, osteoclast aggregates and chondrocalcinosis are less common in renal osteodystrophy. Visceral, periarticular and vascular soft tissue calcification occur more commonly in renal osteodystrophy than in primary hyperparathyroidism (see also Chapter 9, page 445).

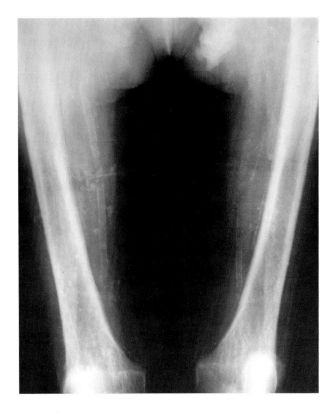

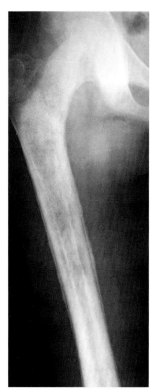

Figure 1.82 *Sickle-cell disease with thalassaemia. The overall effect is one of bone infarction without significant expansion of bone. Periostitis is demonstrated. There is old cortical infarction, as shown by a very extensive internal split cortex, and the dead old cortex is very dense. There is also evidence of a septic arthritis at the right hip. The joint space is narrowed and there is bone destruction.*

Figure 1.81 *Periostitis is uncommon in primary hyperparathyroidism but does occur in renal osteodystrophy. There is also gross vascular and soft tissue calcification in this osteodystrophic patient.*

WIDESPREAD OSTEOPOROSIS DUE TO MARROW INFILTRATION

SICKLE-CELL DISEASE AND THALASSAEMIA

These are haemolytic anaemias, to which the body responds by marrow hyperplasia. The degree of hyperplasia depends on the severity of the disease. Sickle-cell disease occurs in patients of African descent and thalassaemia in those of Mediterranean descent; as a result of interbreeding, some patients have both sickle-cell disease and thalassaemia, but it seems that the radiological features of sickle-cell disease predominate (Figure 1.82). Changes in thalassaemia predominate in the areas of the body containing red marrow. In severe thalassaemia the entire skeleton may be affected and extramedullary haemopoiesis may occur (Figure 1.83), with thoracic and abdominal soft tissue masses, as well as splenomegaly. Thalassaemia, which causes more severe anaemia, may have the most pronounced bone change. In sickle-cell disease, thalassaemia and Gaucher's disease, marrow hypertrophy causes loss of medullary trabeculation and cortical thinning. Gaucher's disease is said to be more common in Jews of European origin. The number of weight-bearing trabeculae are reduced but they are rendered prominent. In thalassaemia particularly, marrow hypertrophy leads to bone expansion. In the skull, changes include thickening of the vault bones which spares the basi-occiput and squamous temporal bone. Obliteration of the facial sinuses by blood-producing marrow, sparing the ethmoids, is said to be due to a local lack of marrow. A 'hair-on-end' appearance is associated with frontal bossing in thalassaemia (Figure 1.84). Vertebrae and ribs are expanded by marrow hypertrophy (Figures 1.85 and 1.86). Generalized malignant infiltration does not expand bone. In thalassaemia, expansion of vertebral bodies

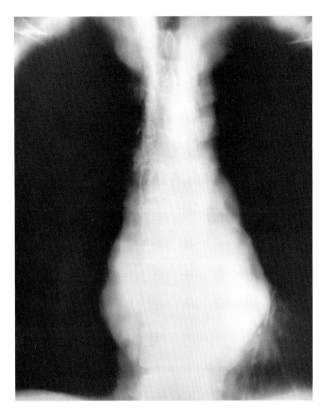

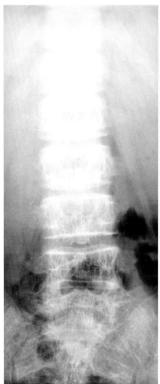

Figure 1.85
Thalassaemia. Lumbar spine in a patient of Greek Cypriot origin. There is quite marked loss of bone density and cortical thinning. The vertebral bodies are expanded in the coronal plane but show early vertebral compressive changes, for instance, at L4. The remaining trabeculae are very prominent and the appearances not unlike those seen in haemangiomatosis.

Figure 1.83 *In thalassaemia, extramedullary haemopoiesis results in a paraspinal soft tissue mass. The vertebral bodies are expanded and demineralized, and the cortices are thinned. There is also a loss of medullary trabeculation.*

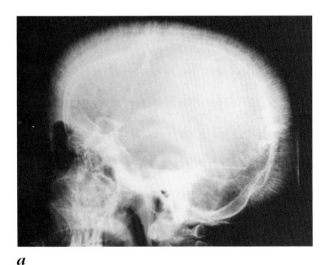

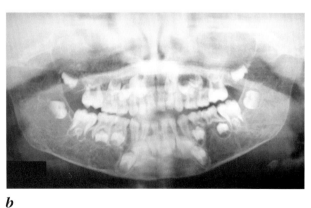

a　　　　　　　　　　　　　　　　　　*b*

Figure 1.84 *Thalassaemia. (a) The skull shows a marked hair-on-end appearance affecting the entire vault, but sparing the basi-occiput. The maxillary antra are obliterated by trabecular bone, and similar changes occur in the sphenoid. The squamous temporal bone, however, shows a simple loss of bone density. (b) The mandible is similarly affected.*

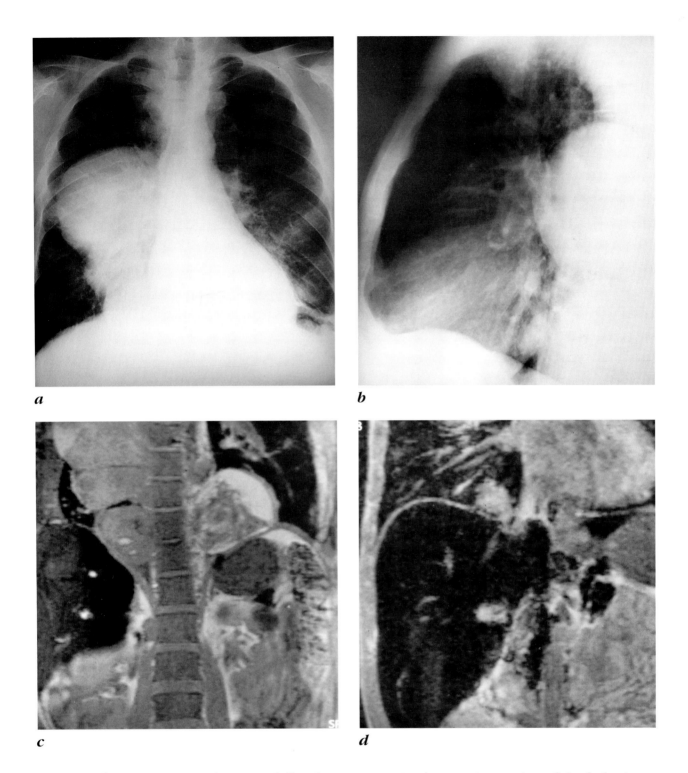

a

b

c

d

Figure 1.86 *Thalassaemia with extramedullary haemopoiesis. Another case in a patient of Greek Cypriot ethnic origin. (**a**) The chest X-ray shows large paraspinal paramediastinal masses. The bones are abnormally expanded, the cortices thinned and medullary trabeculation diminished. These changes are all in keeping with a diagnosis of thalassaemia. (**b**) The lateral view confirms that the soft tissue masses are posteriorly situated, well defined but lobulated. (**c**) Coronal T$_1$-weighted MR sequences show the multi-lobulated glandular hyperplasia on the right. (**d**) The paraspinal masses in the thorax are continuous with, and surround, the thoracic vertebral bodies. Deposition of iron in the liver is shown by low signal.*

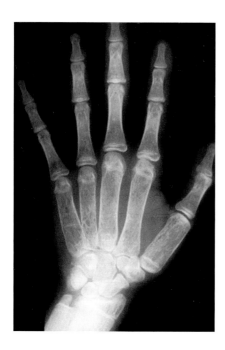

Figure 1.87 *In this thalassaemic patient there is undertubulation with gross diaphyseal expansion in the metacarpals. The cortices are thinned and medullary trabeculation diminished. The nutrient foramina are increased in size, particularly in the middle phalanges.*

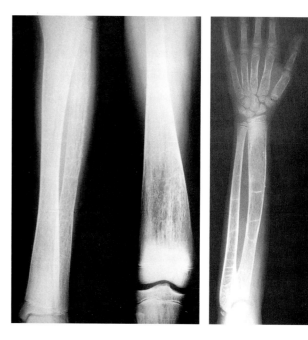

Figure 1.88 *Thalassaemia. Expansion of the tubular long bones, particularly at the metaphyses, results in an Erlenmeyer flask appearance. The cortices are thinned and the medullary trabeculation is deficient. The fibula is expanded and the cortex on its lateral aspect has been broken through, presumably by marrow hyperplasia, and a hair-on-end appearance has resulted.*

may be associated with multiple levels of collapse, often of the codfish type. Expansion of long bones leads to a rectangular appearance of the osteoporotic metacarpals, metatarsals and phalanges (Figure 1.87) and an 'Erlenmeyer flask' appearance at the ends of the major long bones (Figure 1.88) (see Chapter 5, Table 5.4, page 299 and Chapter 7, page 348). Expansion of ribs with cortical thinning is associated with notching of the undersurface due to locally increased circulation (Figure 1.89; Table 1.11).

Heart failure and cardiac enlargement are also seen in thalassaemia and the enlarged liver may show an increased density, particularly on the CT scan, due to increased iron deposition following haemolysis. Areas of functioning marrow hyperplasia may be shown using bone-marrow-seeking isotopes.

Marrow hypertrophy is the predominant radiological pattern in thalassaemia. However, sickle-cell disease has infarction as the predominant feature. Marrow hypertrophy is not as pronounced, so that bone expansion is not a prominent feature and may even be absent. Any osteoporosis due to marrow

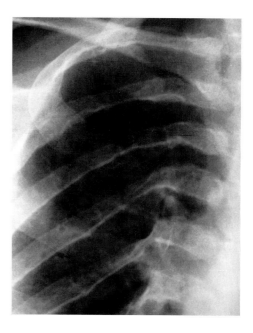

Figure 1.89 *This thalassaemic patient has rib notching due to a local increase in vascularity.*

Table 1.11 Causes of notching on the undersurfaces of ribs.

Arterial	**Venous**
Aortic obstruction:	Superior vena caval obstruction
Coarctation	Inferior vena caval obstruction
Subclavian obstruction:	
Taussig–Blalock operation	**Arteriovenous**
Obstructive arteritis	Arteriovenous fistulae (pulmonary and/or parietal)
Pulmonary oligaemia:	
Pulmonary artery atresia	**Neurogenic**
Pulmonary stenosis	Neurofibromatosis
Fallot and Ebstein's anomalies	
Thalassaemia	**Idiopathic**
	Unknown cause

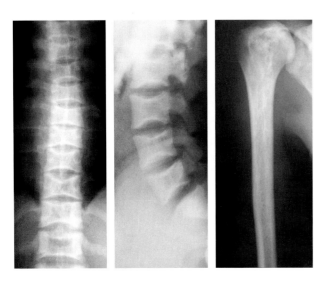
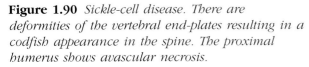

Figure 1.90 *Sickle-cell disease. There are deformities of the vertebral end-plates resulting in a codfish appearance in the spine. The proximal humerus shows avascular necrosis.*

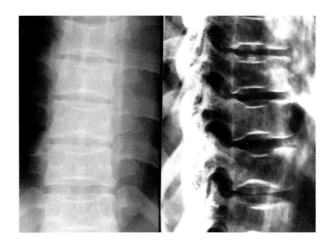

Figure 1.91 *Sickle-cell disease. Cortical infarcts at the vertebral end-plates have resulted in failure of growth in the affected areas, while growth proceeds normally in the remainder of the vertebral body.*

expansion may be obscured by the widespread infarction which results in osteosclerosis.

In sickle-cell disease, there is trabecular loss, cortical thinning and collapse in the vertebral column (Figure 1.90) and sharply right-angled step defects in the end-plates, probably due to local infarcts (Figure 1.91). Similar changes occur in Gaucher's disease.

Avascular necrosis of articular surfaces is seen (Figure 1.92) and cortical infarcts cause a 'split cortex' (Figure 1.82). This 'bone-within-a-bone' appearance is due to the 'tombstone' of the old cortex lying within the new (Table 1.12).

Table 1.12   Causes of cortical splitting.

Osteomyelitis
Sickle-cell disease
Gaucher's disease

Changes in sickle-cell disease can occur early in life. Sickle-cell dactylitis occurs in babies, when focal expansile lesions of phalanges are associated with soft tissue swelling, periostitis and pathological

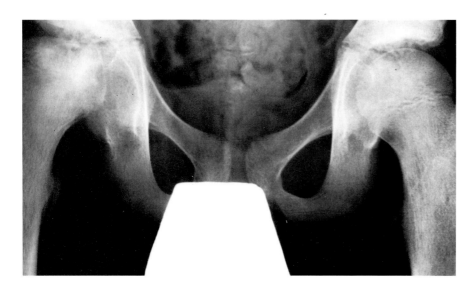

Figure 1.92 *Avascular necrosis in sickle-cell disease. The right femoral head shows reactive sclerosis around an area of structural failure of the articular cortex following infarction. The left femoral head is quite markedly demineralized but not yet collapsed.*

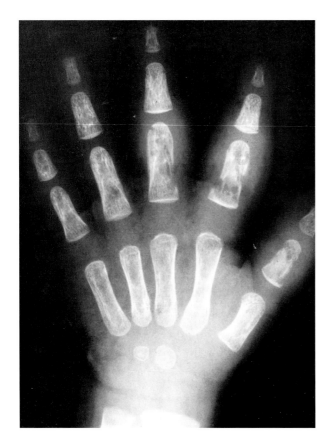

Figure 1.93 *Sickle-cell dactylitis involves soft tissue swelling over areas of bone destruction in many of the phalanges. The phalanges are expanded, bullet-shaped and demineralized. Split cortices can also be seen in many of the metacarpals. Pathological fractures occur throughout the areas of osteomyelitis.*

fractures in the affected bone (Figure 1.93), which may be compounded by blood-borne infection by *Salmonella* or *Escherichia coli.*

Involvement of affected epiphyses may lead to premature fusion and local growth arrest. In the chest, heart failure may follow anaemia, and pulmonary infarcts may lead to pulmonary arterial hypertension.

The radioisotope bone scan shows the acute infarction before plain radiographic changes and can also be used to assess healing. In sickle-cell disease, the spleen is usually small due to repeated infarction.

SARCOIDOSIS

Changes in bone occur in up to 15% of patients with sarcoid; most have evidence of lung changes and skin disease.

The hand is the most commonly involved part of the skeleton (Figure 1.94), the loss of bone density may be generalized or localized, including:

1   Punched-out, well defined lucent areas in the phalanges, due to deposition of sarcoid tissue. Nutrient foramina may be prominent. This change is also seen in leprosy and thalassaemia.
2   A diffuse, lace-like pattern of resorption.
3   Distal tuft and cortical resorption associated with soft tissue masses.
4   A local periostitis.
5   Periarticular calcification in patients with hyper-calcaemia.

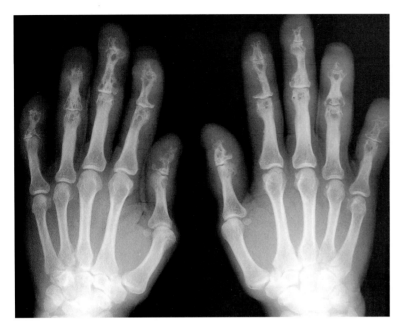

Figure 1.94 *Hands in sarcoid. Many of the changes found in sarcoid are present in the hands of this patient. There is some tissue thickening and pseudo-clubbing. Resorption of much of the distal phalanges has taken place. This is all well defined. Punched-out areas of focal bone destruction are demonstrated, together with a more diffuse pattern of infiltrative bone destruction, for instance, in the middle phalanx of the right little finger. Articular erosions are also demonstrated at the bases of phalanges (see the base of the middle phalanx of the left little finger and of the right ring finger). There are also large cortical defects. Note the patient has sesamoids at all the metacarpal heads of the right hand; this is a rare finding (Bizarro, 1921).*

6 Sarcoid arthritis in up to 37% of patients occurring in an acute form with a synovitis and local osteoporosis, and in a more chronic form when articular collapse results from underlying granulomatous change.

7 Bone sclerosis (see Chapter 2, page 106).

GAUCHER'S DISEASE

There is an accumulation of abnormal lipid in the reticulo-endothelial cells (Gaucher cells), giving hepatosplenomegaly, marrow infiltration and hypertrophy. The infiltration of the marrow may be diffuse, producing cortical thinning, often with endosteal scalloping, and loss of medullary trabeculation, or focal, giving a more 'bubbly' change which may resemble myeloma (Figure 1.95). Infiltration gives bone expansion, producing an Erlenmeyer flask appearance (see Chapters 2, 5 and 7) but the Gaucher cell infiltrate also causes occlusion of blood vessels in bone by extrinsic compression, resulting in some of the infarctive changes seen in sickle-cell disease (Figure 1.96).

Patients with Gaucher's disease may show avascular necrosis of articular surfaces (Figure 1.97), cortical infarcts giving split cortices and end-plate infarcts of vertebral bodies with general or focal lytic lesions, but sclerosis of infarcted bone is also seen (Figure 1.98a)

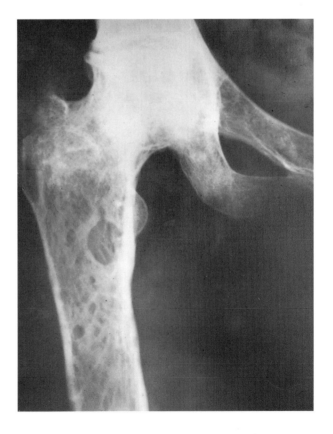

Figure 1.95 *Gaucher's disease. Widespread well defined medullary infiltration with collapse of the femoral head. Osteoarthritis is present.*

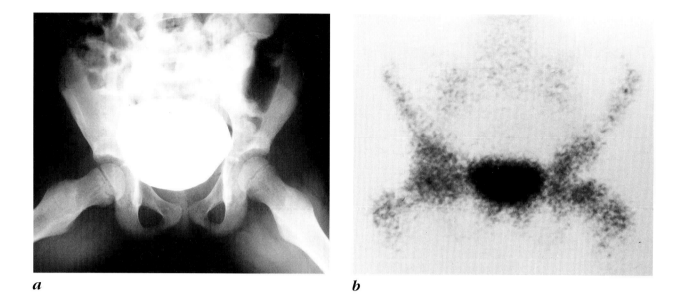

a   *b*

Figure 1.96 *Gaucher's disease. (**a**) There is early flattening of the left femoral head. The tip of the greatly enlarged spleen is seen in the left flank. (**b**) The radioisotope bone scan in the same patient shows a defect in the left femoral head region.*

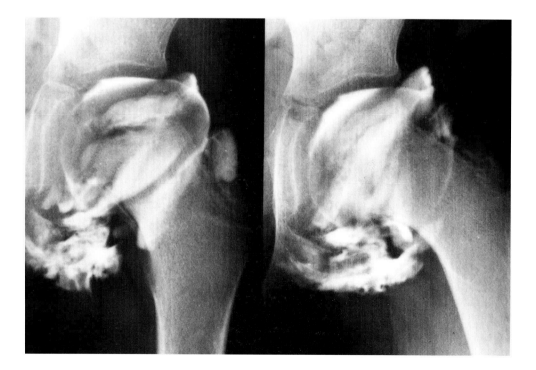

Figure 1.97 *Gaucher's disease. Avascular necrosis of the femoral head is demonstrated at arthrography. There is flattening of the ossific nucleus and, as a result of this, also of the cartilage.*

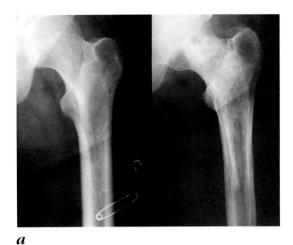
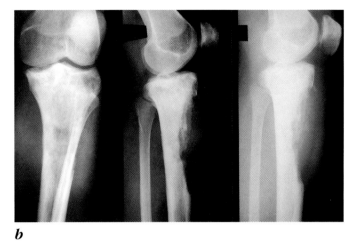

a   *b*

Figure 1.98 *Gaucher's disease. (**a**) Avascular necrosis and infarction. There is progressive change in the upper left femur with a split cortex and evidence of proximal femoral infarction. (**b**) Fibrosarcoma superimposed upon the changes of medullary infarction; a large, destructive and irregular osteolytic lesion is seen with a soft tissue extension.*

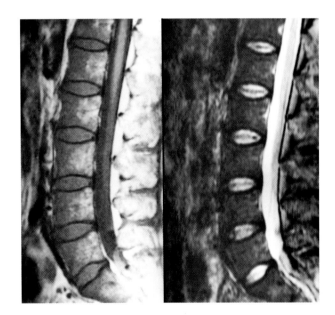

Figure 1.99 *Gaucher's disease in the lumbar spine showing loss of signal on sagittal T$_1$- and T$_2$-weighted images due to infiltration with Gaucher cells.*

(see also Chapter 2, page 104). There may be bone infections and pathological fractures. Fibrosarcoma is a rare complication of infarction in both sickle-cell and Gaucher's diseases (Figure 1.98b). Marrow infiltration is shown at MR imaging (Figure 1.99)

DIFFUSE MALIGNANT DISEASE

In theory, widespread malignant disease causes extensive demineralization. In infants, leukaemia and neuroblastoma and, in the elderly, myeloma and metastatic cancer of the breast are the most common causes of this change. However, in practice, a purely generalized osteoporotic pattern is unusual. In infantile leukaemia and neuroblastoma, widespread bone destruction does occur, but there is usually metaphyseal accentuation of the destructive process (see Chapter 5, page 291). A 'raindrop' pattern of bone destruction emphasizes the malignant nature of the process which will not be present with other causes of childhood osteoporosis (Table 1.13).

Sutural diastasis due to hydrocephalus and tumour deposition in the sutures may also be found and should not be confused with Wormian bones. In addition, neuroblastoma may be associated with spinal erosion and abdominal calcification.

In adults, breast malignancy and myeloma are probably the cause of most cases of widespread malignant infiltration resulting in osteopenia. These patients are usually elderly and will therefore already have a reduced bone density. Myeloma is thought not to cause destruction of vertebral pedicles, although metastases do. It is usual for widespread myelomatosis and carcinomatosis to produce focal destruction of bone in addition to generalized demineralization

Table 1.13 Causes of generalized demineralization in children.

Leukaemia
Neuroblastoma
Scurvy
Rickets
Idiopathic juvenile osteoporosis
Osteogenesis imperfecta
Thalassaemia
Homocystinuria
Hypopituitarism
Mucopolysaccharidosis
Histiocytosis

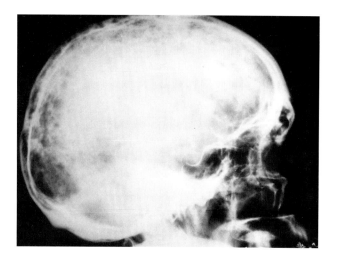

Figure 1.101 *Myeloma. Focal destructive lesions in the skull vault.*

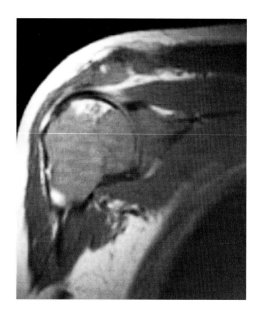

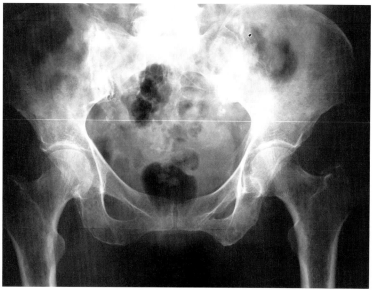

Figure 1.100 *Myeloma. Coronal T₁-weighted MR sequence demonstrating extensive loss of signal in the humeral head, in the adjacent glenoid and around the acromioclavicular joint in this patient with disseminated myeloma. The normal marrow remains bright.*

Figure 1.102 *In myelomatosis there is an overall loss of bone density with a slight accentuation in the upper femora and ischia. A raindrop pattern of radiolucency can be seen. These appearances may be the sole manifestation of myelomatosis.*

(Figure 1.100). Pedicular or cortical destruction may be difficult to visualize in an already demineralized axial skeleton, but must be investigated. The radioisotope bone scan is invaluable in the detection of metastases. Only rarely is malignant disease so widespread and uniform that uptake on the scan is uniformly increased, and therefore mistaken for normal. Occasionally this change is seen with widespread sclerotic metastases in both breast and prostatic malignant disease.

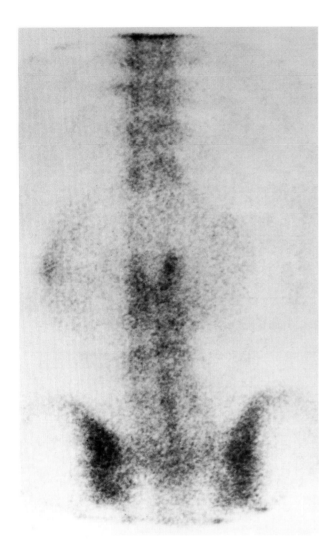

Figure 1.103 *This radioisotope bone scan shows a total absence of uptake in a vertebral body of the lumbar spine affected by myelomatosis.*

Myeloma may produce diffuse osteoporosis, but again focal lesions or a raindrop pattern of destruction should be looked for (Figures 1.101 and 1.102). Cortices around the vertebral bodies, sacral foramina and cortical lines on the pelvis or acetabula should be assessed for integrity (Figure 1.102). The isotope scan is not always positive in myeloma as deposits may present with focal 'cold' areas of uptake as defects on the scan (Figure 1.103).

BIBLIOGRAPHY

Bizarro AH (1921) On the sesamoid and supernumerary bones of the limbs. *J Anat (Cambridge)* **55**: 256.

Bloem JL (1988) Transient osteoporosis of the hip. MR imaging. *Radiology* **167**: 753–5.

Grampp S, Jergas M, Glüer CC et al (1993) Radiologic diagnosis of osteoporosis. Current methods and perspectives. *Radiol Clin North Am* **31**: 1133–45.

Langton CM (1994) The role of ultrasound in the assessment of osteoporosis. *Clin Rheumatol* **13** (Suppl 1): 13–17.

McGowan JA (1993) Osteoporosis. Assessment of bone loss and remodelling. *Aging: Clinical and Experimental Research* **5**: 81–93.

Majumdar S, Genant HK (1995) A review of the recent advances in MRI in the assessment of osteoporosis. *Osteoporos Int* **5**: 79–92.

Sartoris DJ, Resnick D (1990) Current and innovative methods for noninvasive bone densitometry. *Radiol Clin North Am* **28**: 257–78.

Sillence D (1981) Osteogenesis imperfecta: an expanding panorama of variants. *Clin Orthop* **159**: 11–25.

Sillence DO, Senn A, Danks DM (1979) Genetic heterogeneity in osteogenesis imperfecta. *J Med Genet* **16**: 101–16.

Wahner H, Fogelman I (1994) *The Evaluation of Osteoporosis.* London: Martin Dunitz.

Yao L, Lee JK (1988) Occult intraosseous fracture. Detection with MR imaging. *Radiology* **167**: 749–51.

Chapter 2 **Osteosclerosis**

An increase in bone density may be generalized and diffuse, widespread but focal, or due to a solitary lesion. The diagnosis of osteosclerosis is perhaps more easily made than that of osteopenia, particularly if the changes are focal. Most of the radiographic image of a bone, and its density, is due to the cortex. Cortical thickening and periosteal new bone therefore will cause an increase in radiological bony density. These changes may result from stress and hypertrophy, which occur, for example, in athletes.

Focal medullary osteosclerosis is perhaps more easily recognized, because a focal lesion, such as a solitary bone island, is clearly seen against surrounding medullary bone. If the increased density is widespread, cortico-medullary differentiation may be lost. However, widespread sclerosis may be difficult to assess. Thick or bulky soft tissues, or an underexposed film, may cause bones to look diffusely dense. Even an isotope bone scan may show an increase in uptake which is so diffuse that differentiation from normal may be difficult (see page 60).

Increase in bone density (Tables 2.1 and 2.2) may be assessed by the same techniques used in the measurement of osteoporosis (see page 1).

OSTEOSCLEROSIS WITH EXPANSION

OSTEITIS DEFORMANS (PAGET'S DISEASE)

This is a common disease in the elderly which is usually found incidentally, and is slightly more common in men (Figure 2.1). In both men and women, incidence at autopsy rises from 3% at 40 to around 10% at 85 years of age. It is more common in the UK and USA than in Scandinavia and is less

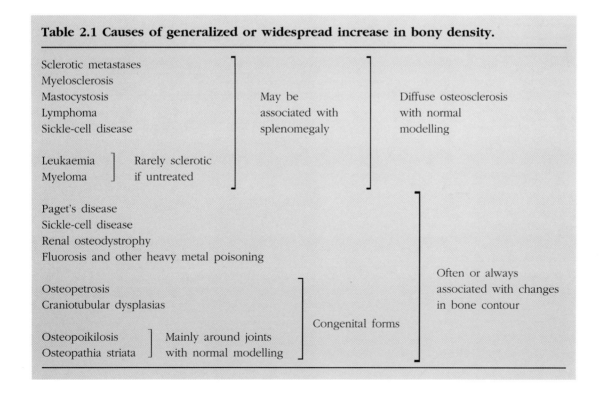

Table 2.1 Causes of generalized or widespread increase in bony density.

Sclerotic metastases
Myelosclerosis
Mastocystosis   May be   Diffuse osteosclerosis
Lymphoma   associated with with normal
Sickle-cell disease   splenomegaly   modelling

Leukaemia] Rarely sclerotic
Myeloma   ] if untreated

Paget's disease
Sickle-cell disease
Renal osteodystrophy
Fluorosis and other heavy metal poisoning

Osteopetrosis   Often or always
Craniotubular dysplasias   associated with changes
                                                       in bone contour
                               Congenital forms
Osteopoikilosis   ] Mainly around joints
Osteopathia striata] with normal modelling

Table 2.2 Causes of focal multiple or solitary sclerotic lesions.

Paget's disease*
Infarcts*
Osteomyelitis*
Fibrous dysplasia*
Metastases*
Lymphoma*
Mastocytosis
Leukaemia
Myeloma*
Healing benign or malignant bone lesions*
Osteomas*
Bone islands*
Osteopathia striata
Osteopoikylosis
Melorheostosis
Tuberous sclerosis
Diffuse idiopathic skeletal hyperostosis
Mixed sclerosing bone dystrophy

*May be solitary.

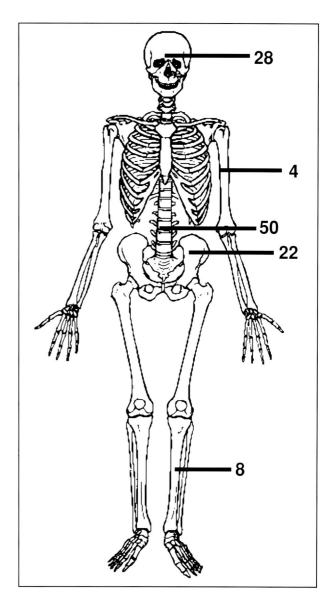

Figure 2.1 *Paget's disease: percentage distribution at major sites only. (After Hamdy, 1981)*

common in Africa and Asia. This may be because populations in these continents are younger, and investigated less often. There are also regional variations within the UK and, in Australia, the incidence declines in those generations longer in the country.

The initial stage of the disease is one of active resorption of bone which is not usually seen radiologically in the weight-bearing skeleton. However, it is seen in the skull vault as an advancing front of osteolysis, known as osteoporosis circumscripta (Figures 2.2 and 2.3), and may also be seen in the anterior tibia (Figure 2.4a). In long bones the lytic process starts at an articular surface, extending in continuity to the other end of the bone behind a flame-shaped front of osteolysis (Figure 2.4a). This is associated with cortical resorption and loss of cortico-medullary differentiation so that only a few cortical trabeculae remain. The radionuclide bone scan is strongly positive (Figure 2.5).

The resorptive phase is followed by the laying down of new bone with an abnormal pattern so that lucency is progressively replaced by a dense, woolly sclerosis with loss of normal cortico-medullary differentiation (Figures 2.4b, 2.6 and 2.7). In the spine, bone condenses beneath vertebral end-plates, giving

a 'picture-frame' appearance. The newly laid down bone may show a mixed sclerotic and lytic pattern but, with time, the disease progresses towards total sclerosis and total involvement of a bone, particularly if small (Figure 2.8). Initially the bone scan shows increased uptake even if radiological changes are minimal (Figure 2.9); however, the end-stage of total sclerosis may be quiescent on the scan, although bone expansion is present.

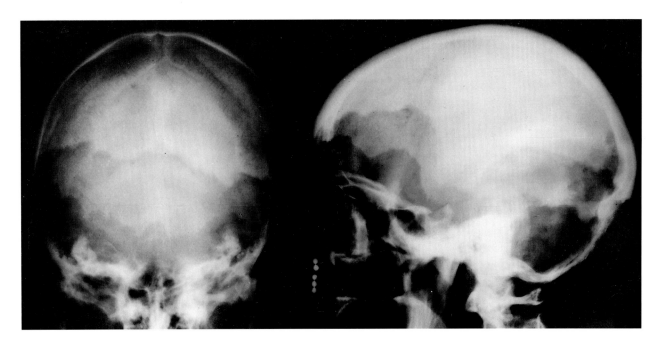

Figure 2.2 *Osteoporosis circumscripta. An unusual feature of Paget's disease of the skull is gross loss of bone density with a geographical margin.*

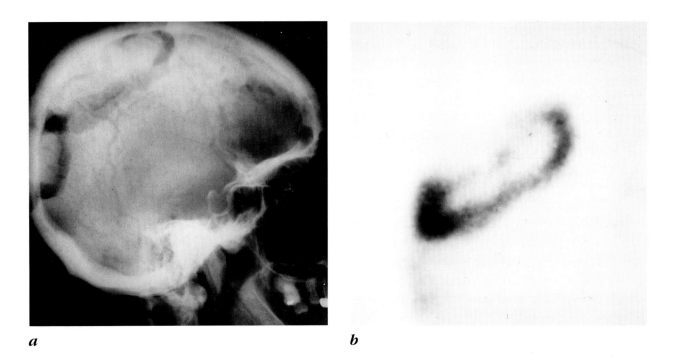

a   *b*

Figure 2.3 *Osteoporosis circumscripta. Two circular focal areas of active osteolysis in Paget's disease (**a**) are reflected as areas of increased uptake on the radioisotope bone scan (**b**).*

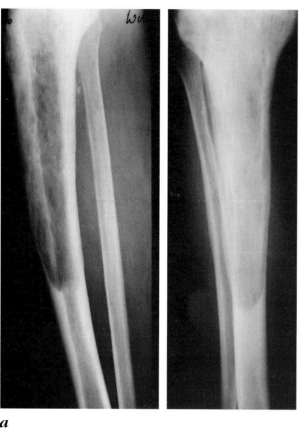

a

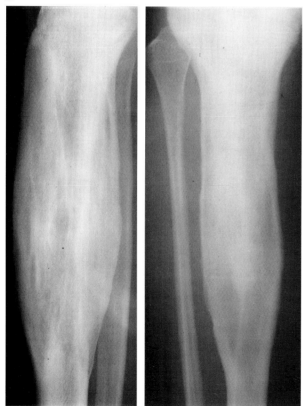

b

Figure 2.4 *Paget's disease of the tibia. (**a**) Quite marked radiolucency is seen in the anterior tibia extending to the proximal articular surface and ending inferiorly in a flame shape. This precedes the osteosclerotic phase and, in this patient, is associated with expansion of the bone and cortical thickening. (**b**) The later film shows further expansion of bone and subsequent sclerosis with an amorphous texture. The pathological process still ends inferiorly in a flame shape.*

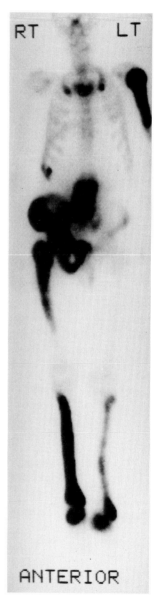

Figure 2.5 *Paget's disease is demonstrated by a radioisotope bone scan. Areas of active disease are shown as foci of increase in uptake and bone expansion.*

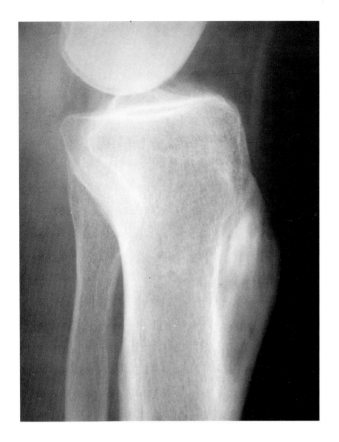

Figure 2.6 *There is an area of Paget's disease related to the previous tibial tuberosity apophysis with local expansion, alteration of bone texture and a flame-shaped inferior margin.*

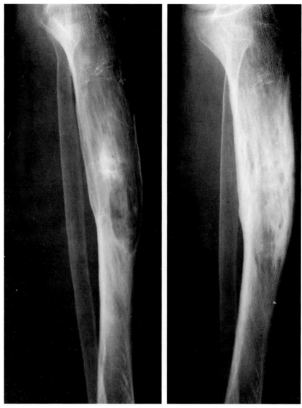

Figure 2.7 *The progression of Paget's disease is shown in two films taken 1 year apart.*

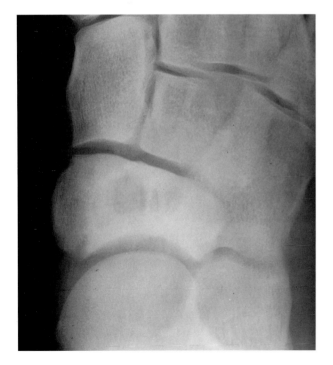

Figure 2.8 *Paget's disease of the tarsal navicular. A characteristic end-stage of Paget's disease is shown by expansion of the bone with total sclerosis, cortical thickening and an almost uniform bone texture. The whole bone is affected.*

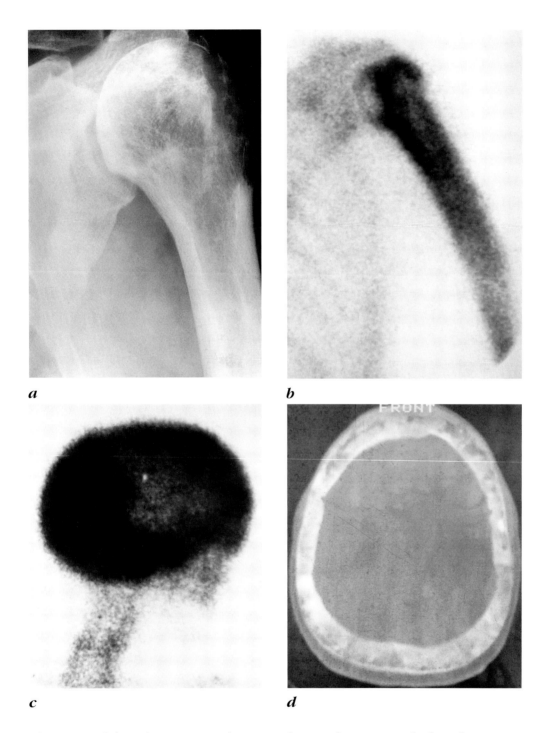

a *b*

c *d*

Figure 2.9 *(a) In this patient with Paget's disease, the cortex is thickened, cortico-medullary differentiation is poor, and there is an increase in density in the medulla. There is a typically coarse trabecular pattern which extends to the proximal articular surface. (b) In the same patient, a radionuclide bone scan shows the gross increase of uptake in the affected area, extending to the articular surface. (c) A bone scan shows a diffuse increase in uptake in the skull with vault thickening. (d) The CT scan demonstrates the thick vault and loss of cortico-medullary differentiation.*

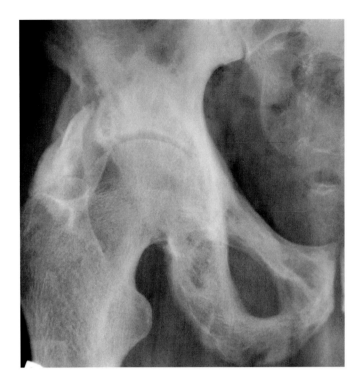

Figure 2.10 *Paget's disease. The right innominate bone shows expansion, cortical thickening, loss of cortico-medullary differentiation and a coarsened medullary trabecular pattern. A large exostosis is shown in the region of the anterior inferior iliac spine, which has the same abnormal bone texture of Paget's disease and which may be compared with the normal proximal femur. This lesion follows tendinous avulsion of softened bone.*

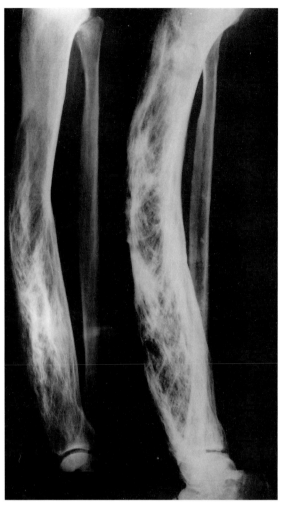

Figure 2.11 *This patient with Paget's disease has gross expansion of the tibia with a typically coarsened trabecular pattern and loss of cortico-medullary differentiation, initially extending upwards to the proximal midshaft with a flame shape, but eventually reaching the upper tibial articular surface. There is bowing as a result of softening. The fibula is rarely the site of Paget's disease and is unaffected in this patient.*

In the reparative stages of the disease, new bone is laid down beneath the periosteum on the cortex, producing an increase in the external diameter of the bone, and also endosteally, encroaching upon the medullary cavity. Cortico-medullary differentiation remains poor, the external contours of the bone remain smooth or slightly undulant, and occasionally a tendon pulls off an exostosis at its insertion (Figure 2.10).

Paget's bone is soft, so that bowing (Figure 2.11), deformity and pathological transverse (Figure 2.12) or insufficiency fractures occur (Figure 2.13, Table 2.3). In the spine, vertebral expansion in the sagittal and coronal planes is associated with vertebral collapse which may cause spinal cord compression, often in association with a picture-frame appearance (Figures 2.14 and 2.15). Paget's disease affecting adjacent vertebral bodies causes expansion (Figure 2.15) and

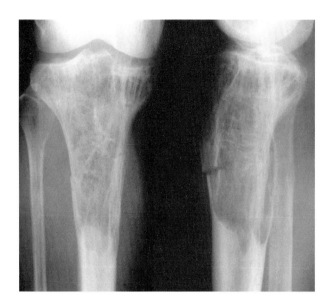

Figure 2.12 *A transverse pathological fracture is seen in an area of active lysis in Paget's disease. The bone is expanded and has a flame-shaped advancing front of demineralization.*

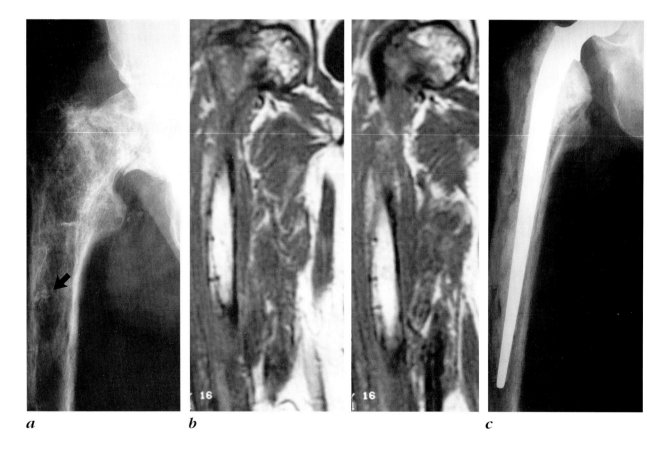

a   *b*   *c*

Figure 2.13 *Pathological and insufficiency fractures in Paget's disease. (**a**) The proximal femur shows all the changes of Paget's disease and a transcervical fracture has occurred. A transverse insufficiency fracture (arrow) is shown in the lateral femoral cortex. (**b**) Coronal T_1-weighted scans of the right femur demonstrate changes related to the fracture at the femoral neck—there is varus deformity and quite marked alteration of fatty marrow signal due to haemorrhage. In addition, multiple insufficiency fractures are demonstrated in the lateral femoral cortex. (**c**) The insufficiency fractures are very well seen in the post-operative films.*

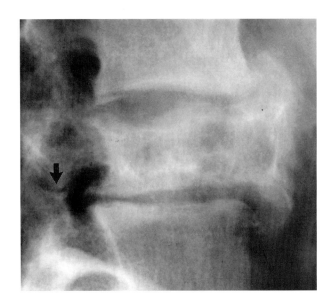

Figure 2.14 *Paget's disease. On the lateral view there is collapse of a lumbar vertebral body, which is associated with expansion of the bone anteriorly, and a picture-frame appearance due to condensation of bone beneath the end-plates. A pathological fracture of the lamina is seen (arrow).*

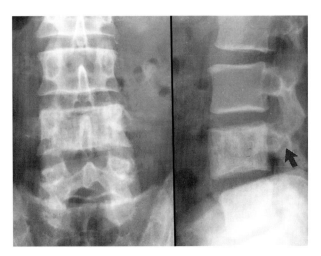

a

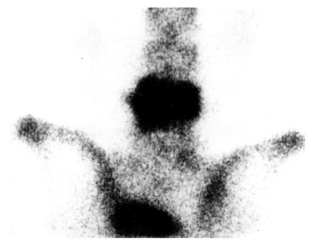

b

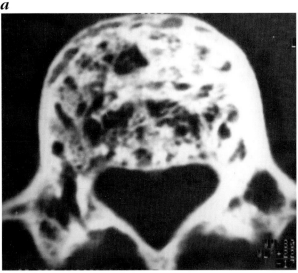

c

Figure 2.15 *Paget's disease. (**a**) There is expansion of the body of L4. The anterior concavity of the vertebral body is lost. The end-plates are rendered prominent. There is a pathological stress fracture in the lamina (arrow). (**b**) The radioisotope bone scan confirms the presence of active bone disease together with expansion of the vertebral body. (**c**) CT scan shows an expanded vertebral body with a mixture of sclerotic and lytic changes in the medulla of the body extending into the appendages.*

Table 2.3 Causes of bone softening and deformity.

Fibrous dysplasia
X-linked and other forms of osteomalacia
Osteogenesis imperfecta
Osteopetrosis
Still's disease (juvenile chronic arthritis) in the paired long bones
Neurofibromatosis in the paired long bones
Protrusio acetabuli is seen in rheumatoid arthritis and osteoarthritis
    and as a congenital lesion

NB These are unusual changes in disorders other than Paget's disease.

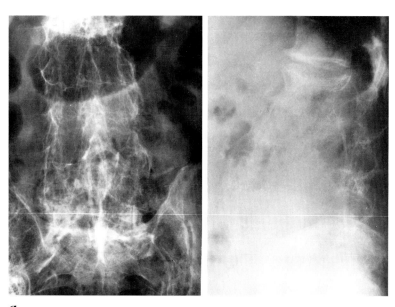

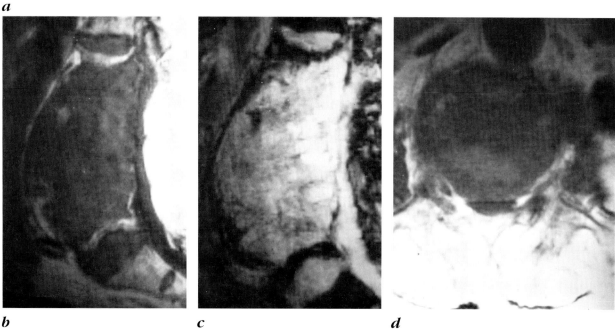

Figure 2.16 *Paget's disease with ankylosis and spinal stenosis. (**a**) The plain radiograph shows fusion of the lowest three lumbar vertebral bodies. There is expansion and substantial loss of bony density. (**b**) The sagittal T$_1$-weighted MR image demonstrates the presence of fusion and block vertebral bodies with canal stenosis. There is now no fatty marrow but a diffuse inhomogeneous decrease in signal. On the fat suppression image (**c**) diffuse increase in signal is shown, indicating hypervascularity. There is almost total canal stenosis. (**d**) The axial T$_1$-weighted MR sequence shows marked vertebral expansion and canal stenosis.*

a

b   *c*   *d*

fusion across discs (Figures 2.16 and 2.17). Similar changes occur with other vascular lesions, e.g. aneurysmal bone cyst (Figure 2.18) and myeloma. Paget's disease occurs in the mandible much less commonly than in the skull (Figure 2.19). Occasionally the process may commence at the site of a former apophysis (Figure 2.6).

After a fracture and immobilization, the bone distal to the fracture line becomes extremely demineralized.

A similar phenomenon is seen in hyperparathyroidism. Callus shows all the features of Paget's disease.

Pain in Paget's disease should alert the radiologist to the presence of a fracture or tumour. Associated tumours include osteogenic sarcoma (Figures 2.20 and 2.21), chondrosarcoma and fibrosarcoma, as well as giant-cell tumour.

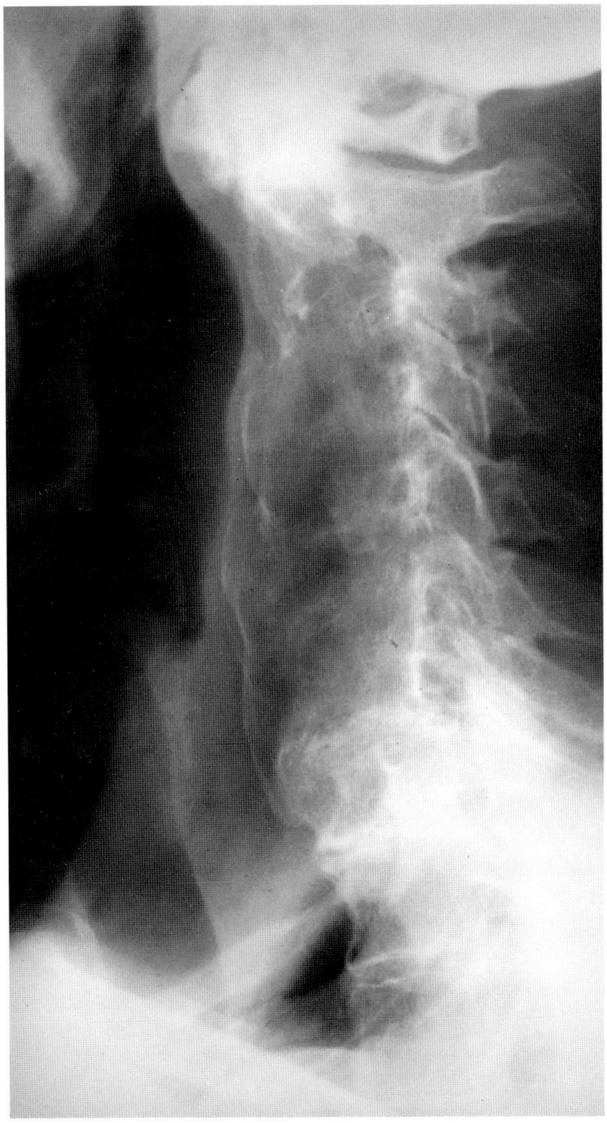

OSTEOSCLEROSIS WITHOUT EXPANSION

SCLEROTIC METASTATIC DEPOSITS IN BONE

As Paget's disease occurs primarily in the elderly, it is most likely to be radiologically confused with widespread sclerosing osseous metastases. The most common malignant tumours of bone are metastases, only 10% of which are solitary. However, a solitary metastasis is more common than a solitary malignant primary bone tumour. Metastases usually occur after 45 years of age, whereas most primary bone tumours (benign and malignant) are seen in younger patients.

In an autopsy study (Galasko 1986), 57% of patients with breast malignancy and 55% of those with prostatic malignancy developed bone metastases, while lung cancer metastasized to bone slightly less often (44%).

Metastases are most commonly present in the vertebral column, ribs, skull and proximal long bones (Figure 2.22), but are unusual distal to the knee or elbow. They occur, therefore, in areas of red marrow formation which have a high local blood flow.

Metastatic spread from the pelvis (prostate, bladder, uterus) to the ribs, vertebral column and pelvic bones is facilitated by the valveless system of paravertebral veins of Batson. Occasional metastases to the hand or foot often have their origin in the lung and are usually lytic.

The distribution of metastases within the axial skeleton is random, and is better seen using skeletal scintigraphy (Figure 2.22) than plain films. MRI is most sensitive in the diagnosis of skeletal metastases (Figure 2.23).

As the sclerosing process spreads, the medulla becomes obliterated and the bone may become uniformly sclerotic, with loss of cortico-medullary differentiation and visible trabeculation (Figure 2.24).

Figure 2.17 *Paget's disease. A similar appearance occurs in the cervical spine.*

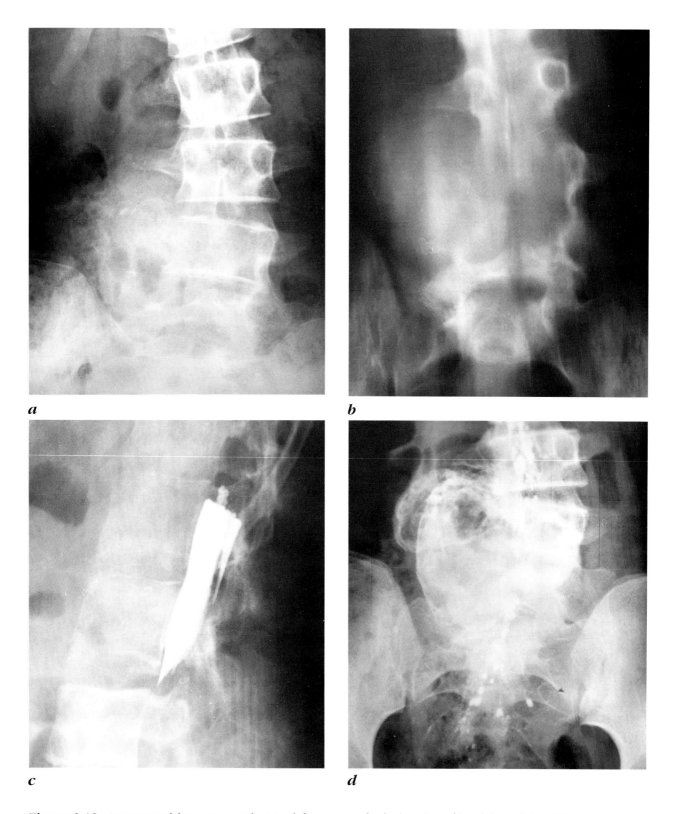

a

b

c

d

Figure 2.18 *Aneurysmal bone cyst with spinal fusion. On both the plain film (**a**) and the AP tomogram (**b**) as well as the lateral myelogram (**c**) there is fusion at the posterior elements of L4 and L5 associated with bone destruction and expansion. The margins of the lesion can barely be seen. There is occlusion of the canal. (**d**) After treatment the margins of the lesion mineralize and their true extent can be perceived.*

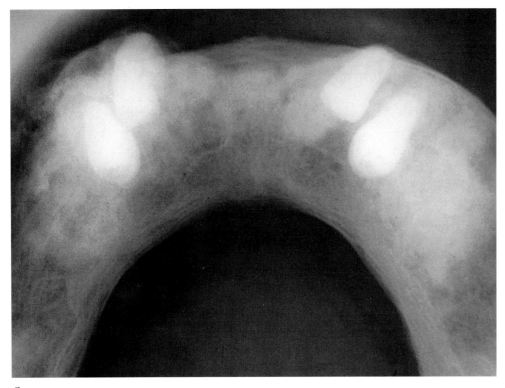

a

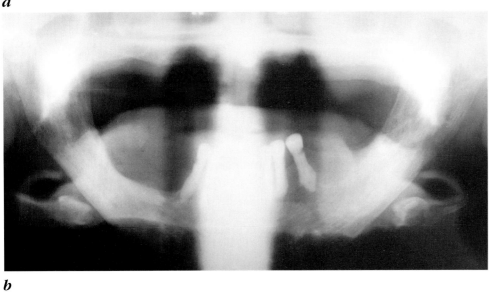

b

Figure 2.19 *(a, b) Paget's disease. Expansion, sclerosis and loss of cortico-medullary differentiation are seen.*

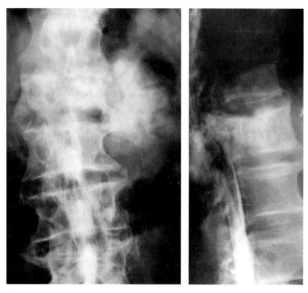

a

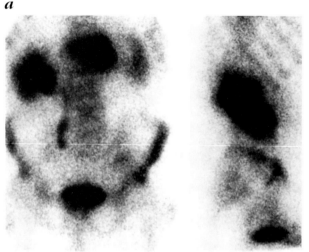

b

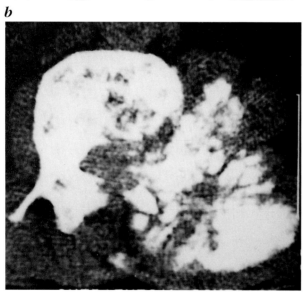

c

Figure 2.20 *Paget's sarcoma. (**a**) The body of L2 shows an increase in density and anterior expansion, as do the posterior elements. There is a large osseous mass arising from the vertebral body and spreading into the local soft tissues. There is obstruction to the flow of contrast at radiculography. The appearances are those of malignant degeneration in Paget's disease. (**b**) The radioisotope bone scan shows increase in uptake in the affected, expanded vertebral body, and also uptake in the soft tissue tumour mass to the left of the spine. There is also an obstructive uropathy on the right side due to metastatic adenopathy. (**c**) The CT scan shows the abnormal bone texture of the vertebral body and the sarcomatous mass on its left side.*

Sclerotic metastases arise mainly from primary malignancy in the breast, prostate and gastrointestinal tract. These primary sites may also result in lytic or mixed sclerotic and lytic metastases, but most lesions in bone due to prostatic metastases are sclerotic.

New bone formation in metastases develops:

1 in the fibrous stroma associated with certain metastases, particularly prostatic, where the stroma ossifies in the presence of osteoprogenitor cells;
2 as a reactive phenomenon secondary to bone destruction. Destruction by a tumour on one side of a trabeculum may be associated with woven bone deposition on the other side.

This phenomenon occurs in almost all metastases, with the exception of myeloma, lymphoma, leukaemia and highly anaplastic and aggressive lytic metastases, where destruction occurs more rapidly than any sclerosing reaction.

In normal adult vertebral bodies, less than 1% of bone is woven; however, in most metastases, with the exceptions mentioned above, there is often up to 40%, which implies active repair.

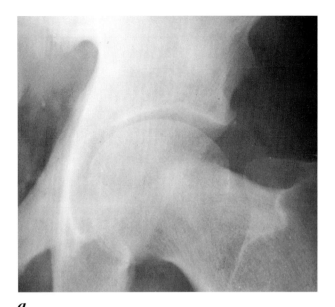

a

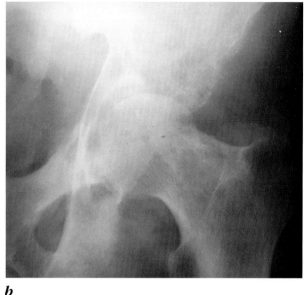

b

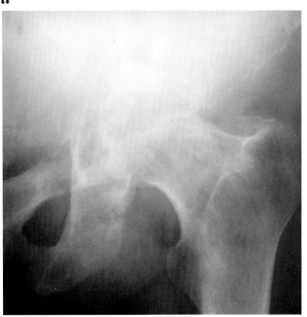

c

Figure 2.21 *Paget's disease of the left innominate bone developing sarcomatous change. (**a**) The appearances are really quite unremarkable apart from showing sclerosis and slight expansion of the acetabulum. (**b**) Four years later there is now an area of osteolysis with cortical destruction and a large pelvic soft tissue mass. (**c**) The subsequent radiograph shows progressive destruction of the acetabulum and enlargement of the soft tissue mass. The appearances are those of malignant degeneration in Paget's disease.*

In malignant sclerotic metastatic disease from breast, and particularly prostate carcinoma, the initial site of change in the axial skeleton is medullary. In the vertebral body, the pedicles are involved. Progression of the lesions leads to developing obliteration of the medullary cavity with loss of cortico-medullary differentiation and trabecular architecture (Figure 2.24), while lytic areas of bone destruction cause cortical scalloping. Medullary lucency may infrequently be present in prostatic metastases but is more common with breast metastases (Figure 2.25). Areas of preserved bone density remain, so that changes are not uniform.

Periostitis and expansion of bone is unusual in metastatic disease. The degree of expansion which occurs in Paget's disease is generally not seen. Occasionally a periosteal reaction may produce an

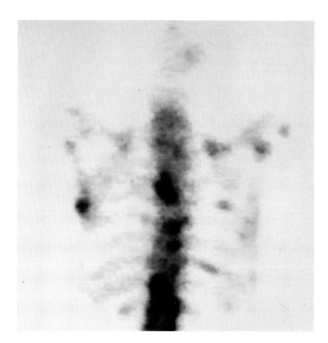

Figure 2.22 *A radioisotope bone scan shows the widespread and random distribution of skeletal metastases.*

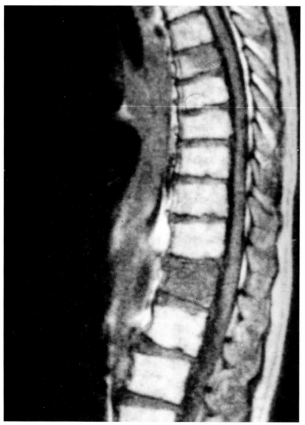

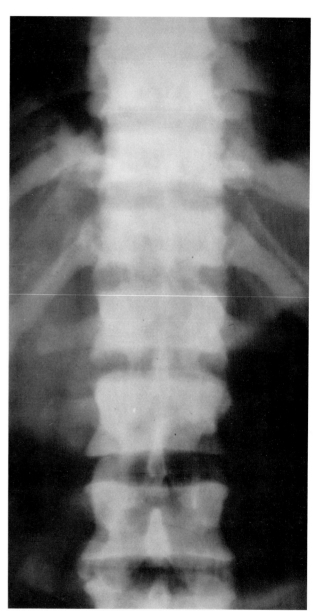

Figure 2.23 *Skeletal metastases. At MRI, tumour replaces fat on the* T_1*-weighted sequence. (Reproduced from* Exercises in Diagnostic Imaging *by S. Burnett and A. Saifuddin, Harwood Academic Publishers, Amsterdam, 1997, by kind permission of the authors and publishers.)*

Figure 2.24 *Secondary deposits from carcinoma of the prostate. No expansion of the vertebral bodies is seen. The pedicles and spinous processes are also affected. Cortico-medullary differentiation is diminished or lost.*

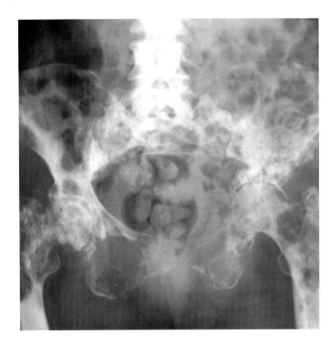

Figure 2.25 *This patient has metastatic disease from carcinoma of the breast, with widespread areas of osteolysis throughout the pelvis and in the proximal femora. There is also some reactive sclerosis. The patient therefore has a mixed pattern of disease which is predominantly lytic.*

undulant outer margin. Malignant sunray spiculation, which occasionally occurs with malignant deposits (Figure 2.26), only occurs in Paget's disease if it undergoes malignant degeneration.

In the axial skeleton, the ribs are less generally involved in Paget's disease than in prostatic disease, so that widespread rib sclerosis is more likely to be due to prostatic metastases (Figure 2.27). Softening and bowing do not occur with malignancy but pathological fractures do.

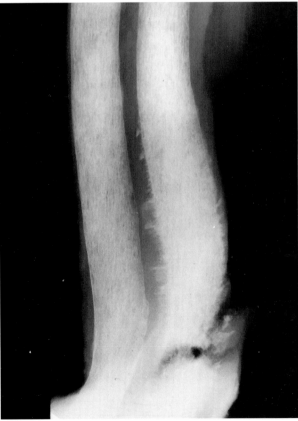

Figure 2.26 *Metastatic disease. Sunray spiculation with bone expansion in sclerotic metastatic deposits from carcinoma of the bladder.*

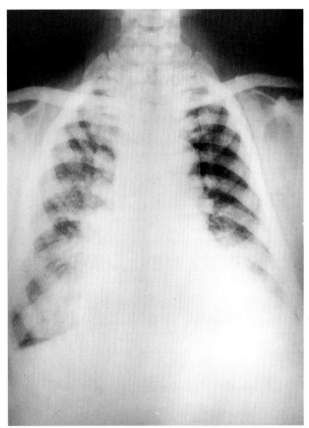

Figure 2.27 *This patient with metastatic disease from carcinoma of the prostate has widespread sclerosis of the ribs which makes Paget's disease less likely. In addition, the bones are not expanded.*

Table 2.4 Causes of diffuse sclerosis in malignant disease.

Sclerotic metastases—prostate, lung, bladder, breast, carcinoid, uterus

Following therapy for malignant disease

Myelosclerosis
Mastocytosis ⎤
Lymphoma ⎥ Osteosclerosis with splenomegaly
Leukaemia ⎦

The skull is not expanded by prostatic metastases and the disease tends to be less uniform than the changes in Paget's disease, although tabular differentiation may be lost.

Other organs are affected in malignant disease. Pulmonary metastases and lymph node enlargement may be present, as well as splenomegaly (Table 2.4).

OSTEOSCLEROSIS WITH SPLENOMEGALY

MYELOSCLEROSIS

This is a disease of unknown aetiology in which the marrow is initially replaced by a fibrous ground substance (myelofibrosis), which becomes progressively ossified. Dense bone may finally occupy up to 70% of the marrow as calcium is deposited in the fibrous matrix.

In the myelofibrotic stage, the skeleton is of normal density but, with progressive ossification, the thoraco-lumbar spine, ribs and pelvis show an increase in medullary density which is often uniform, though foci of extra sclerosis may be present (Figure 2.28). Cortico-medullary differentiation and trabecular detail are lost. The peripheral skeleton and skull are less frequently involved and may even show signs of marrow hyperplasia. The long bones of the axial skeleton are not abnormally modelled as periostitis is absent. MRI shows

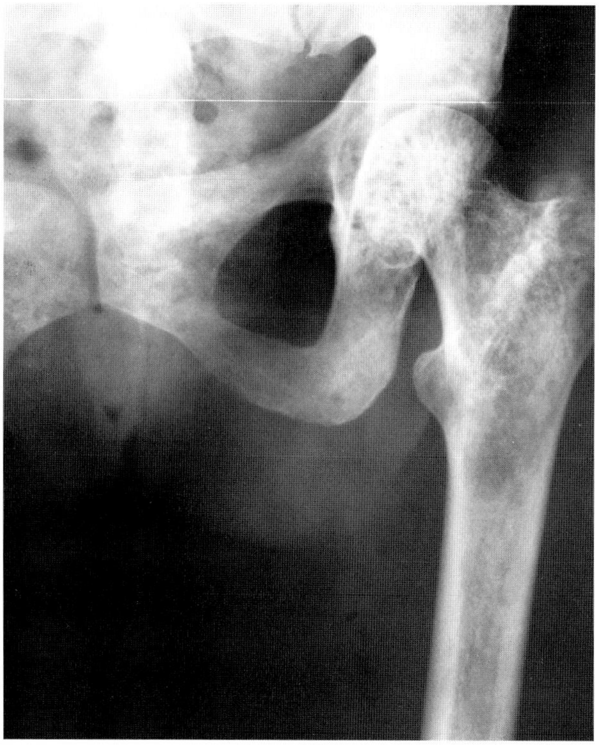

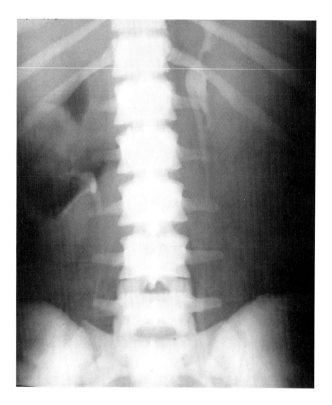

Figure 2.28 *Myelosclerosis. A diffuse increase in density is seen in the medullary cavity of the femur and pelvic bones. In places, there is resorption of the cortex with endosteal scalloping.*

Figure 2.29 *In this patient with myelosclerosis there is widespread diffuse uniform osteosclerosis without bone expansion. Massive splenomegaly displaces the left kidney and ureter towards the midline.*

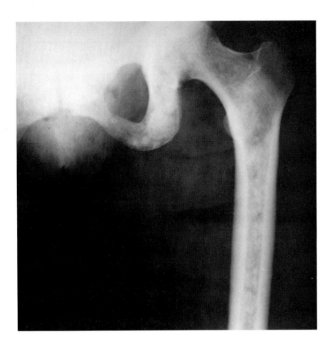

Figure 2.30 *Mastocytosis showing a widespread diffuse increase in medullary density.*

replacement of marrow by a diffuse change of low signal intensity as fibrous tissue and subsequent mineralization replace fat or haemopoietic tissue in the marrow.

Massive splenomegaly and, to a lesser extent, hepatomegaly are inevitable (Figure 2.29). Soft tissue masses elsewhere are due to extramedullary haemopoiesis, and there may be varices and ascites. Secondary gout is a prominent feature, and pneumonia is a major cause of death.

URTICARIA PIGMENTOSA (MASTOCYTOSIS)

Large numbers of mast cells are present in the skin and may produce skin nodules. In both infants and adults, wheals are produced by histamine release when the skin is traumatized.

In the bones, mast cell aggregates can cause focal osteolysis, but usually new bone formation results in thickened trabeculae with medullary sclerosis (Figures 2.30 and 2.31). Hepatosplenomegaly and

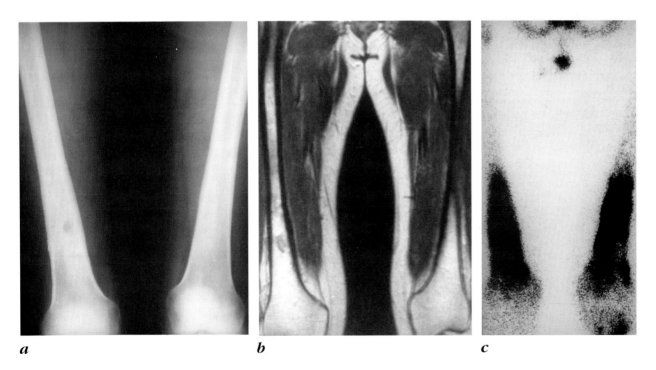

a   *b*   *c*

Figure 2.31 *Mastocytosis. (a) Focal lytic lesions are associated with reactive bone sclerosis and cortical thickening. (b) The changes are also shown at MR imaging. Fatty marrow is replaced by lower signal material, presumably mineralized, on this T_1-weighted sequence. The cortex is seen to be thickened medially. (c) The radionuclide bone scan shows generalized, diffuse increase in uptake.*

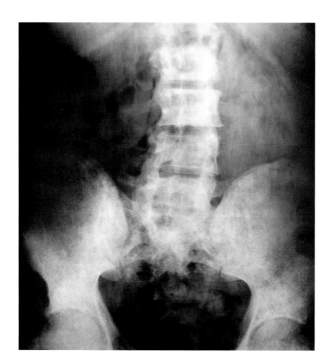

Figure 2.32 *Sclerosing myeloma with a widespread increase in trabecular density in the lumbar spine, sacrum and innominate bones. This is a rare manifestation in untreated myeloma. Lytic lesions in myeloma may sclerose following chemotherapy or radiotherapy.*

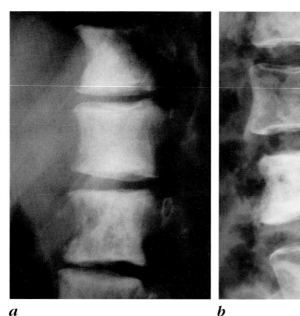

a   *b*

Figure 2.33 *Anterior vertebral scalloping. (**a**) Hodgkin's disease. The vertebral bodies show general reactive sclerosis. There is displacement of gut gas shadows away from these vertebral bodies, presumably because of overlying lymph node masses, with erosion of the anterior surfaces of these vertebral bodies. (**b**) A similar appearance is demonstrated in a patient with tuberculosis. A mid lumbar vertebral body shows anterior erosion and reactive sclerotic change because of anterior subligamentous infective disease.*

lymphadenopathy follow. In children, bone changes in the long bones are said to predominate but, in adults, mainly the central skeleton is affected, as active marrow is centrally confined.

In mastocytosis, splenomegaly is rarely as marked as in myelosclerosis, where the spleen often tips in the iliac fossa. Marrow and peripheral blood examination also distinguish the two diseases. Lack of bone modelling deformities distinguish them both from haemolytic anaemias, Gaucher's disease and particularly osteopetrosis. Generalized osteosclerosis is rare in myeloma and the lymphomas (Figure 2.32).

LEUKAEMIA

Osteosclerosis is rare in leukaemic children, nearly all of whom have changes of bone destruction, which are also seen in adults.

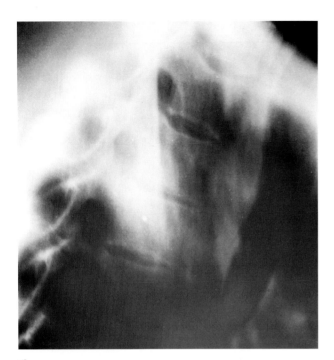

a

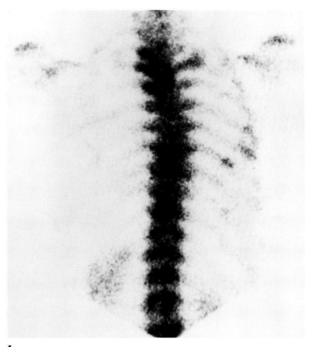

b

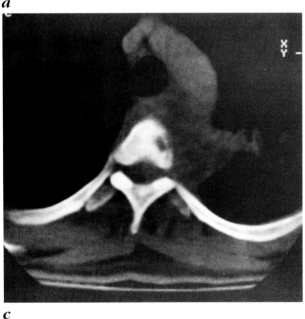

c

Figure 2.34 *Tuberculosis.* **(a)** *The lateral tomogram shows a soft tissue mass displacing the tracheal translucency anteriorly and eroding the anterior aspects of adjacent vertebral bodies. There is early discal narrowing.* **(b)** *In the radioisotope bone scan there is increased uptake in the upper thoracic spine and adjacent ribs in the region corresponding to the plain film change.* **(c)** *The CT scan shows a local erosion on the vertebral body with irregularity of the cortex and an overlying soft tissue mass.*

LYMPHOMAS

Bone involvement is either direct, from adjacent nodes, or by haematogenous spread resulting from splenic involvement. Contiguous erosion of bone from diseased lymph nodes primarily affects the region of the sacroiliac and para-aortic nodes, therefore the spine and pelvis are most commonly involved in this form of the disease. Haematogenous metastases can occur anywhere in the axial skeleton. Two-thirds of the bony lesions are multiple and may be lytic, sclerotic or both. The incidence of sclerotic lesions varies greatly (between 20 and 45%) because lytic lesions sclerose on therapy and sclerotic lesions may become lytic with progressive destruction. Widespread sclerosis is rare and generally only the pelvis and spine are affected. Anterior spinal erosions and fluffy periosteal reactions are seen (Figure 2.33). Erosions on the anterior aspects of contiguous vertebral bodies are seen in Hodgkin's disease due to pressure or invasion by anteriorly situated abnormal lymph nodes.

A similar phenomenon may occur as a result of pressure from an aortic aneurysm or invasion from tuberculous lymph nodes (Figure 2.34). In the latter condition the adjacent disc spaces are more usually involved and narrowed than in lymphoma.

Destruction of vertebral bone in malignant disease is occasionally followed by radiological evidence of

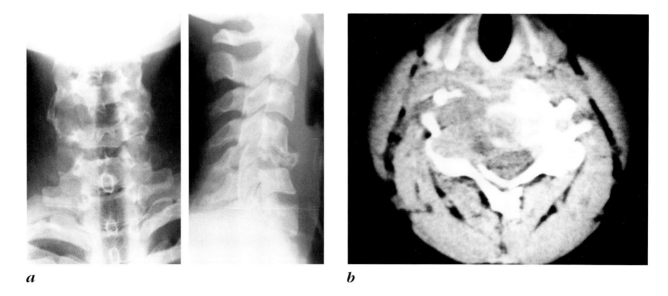

a   *b*

Figure 2.35 *In this patient with osteogenic sarcoma, (**a**) the vertebral body of C5 is collapsed, and there is some anterior displacement of bony fragments. The adjacent discs vary in height and, anteriorly, they are narrowed due to herniation into the affected vertebral body. There is a local soft tissue mass. (**b**) The CT scan shows destruction of the vertebral body, encroachment upon the neural canal and some local expansion.*

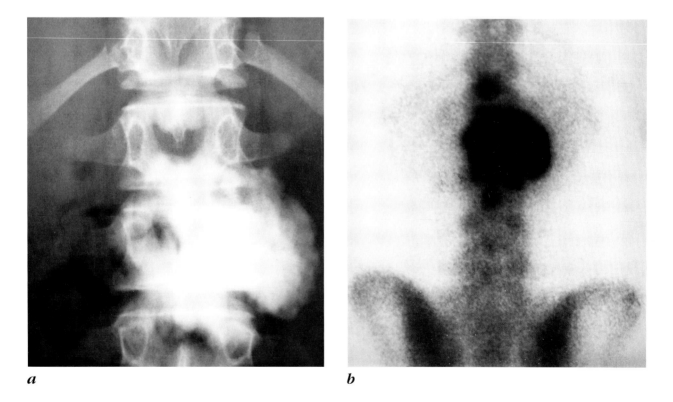

a   *b*

Figure 2.36 *Osteosarcoma. (**a**) A large well defined sclerosing mass arises from the left of L2. (**b**) The radioisotope bone scan shows diffuse increase in uptake in this expanded body. There is a metastatic lesion in the arch of T12, seen both on the plain film and on the radioisotope bone scan.*

discal narrowing as disc material herniates into softened vertebral bone (Figure 2.35). Osteogenic sarcoma in the spine is usually sclerotic and expansile (Figure 2.36). Assessment of the paraspinal pathology causing spinal erosion is made by MRI, CT, ultrasound and biopsy.

FOCAL AREAS OF BONE SCLEROSIS (TABLE 2.5)

OSTEOPOIKILOSIS

This is discovered as an incidental finding and is of no clinical significance. Genetically, the disease is caused by an autosomal dominant gene, and lesions may be present at birth and during infancy. The histology was first described by Schmorl. Small (2–5 mm), well circumscribed, round or ovoid areas of uniform sclerosis are distributed in the bone around the major joints

Table 2.5 Focal areas of bone sclerosis.

Bone islands Osteopathia striata Osteopoikilosis	Innocent conditions with no adverse features and normal bone modelling
Melorheostosis Tuberous sclerosis Multiple osteomas	Widespread osteosclerosis in symptomatic disorders with abnormal bone contours

(Figure 2.37). The skull is not usually involved and bone remote from the articular regions is usually spared. The lesions are multiple at each site and only rarely change under observation during adult life and so are distinguishable from sclerotic metastases. Increased density is the result of bone trabeculae which are slightly thicker than normal and regularly spaced in a parallel arrangement.

OSTEOPATHIA STRIATA

This condition resembles osteopoikilosis and a mixture of the two types of lesion is found in some patients. Parallel, longitudinal rays of increased bony density stream backwards along the shafts of the long bones from the metaphyses in the immature skeleton, but appear to approach articular surfaces after fusion (Figure 2.38). Small bones are affected in their entirety. These asymptomatic lesions do not alter with time.

Streaks of abnormal bony density passing proximally from the growth plates are also seen in Ollier's disease. These are lucent rather than sclerotic and are usually associated with modelling abnormalities (Figure 2.39).

Vertical striations at the metaphysis are also seen in rubella (Figure 2.40) and in osteopetrosis (Figure 2.41). In this latter disease, the bones are expanded and sclerotic (see page 95).

BONE ISLANDS

These may be solitary or multiple, are commonly situated in the femoral neck or acetabulum, and may be regarded as a forme fruste of osteopoikilosis, although the lesions are rather larger. They may occur anywhere and may increase in size under

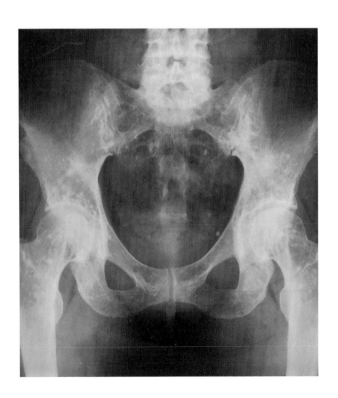

Figure 2.37 *Osteopoikilosis. Discrete islands of increased bone density are seen with a periarticular distribution around the sacroiliac and hip joints, and the symphysis pubis.*

Figure 2.38
*Osteopathia striata.
Vertical parallel
strands of increased
bony density extend
backwards from the
articular surfaces in
a mature skeleton.*

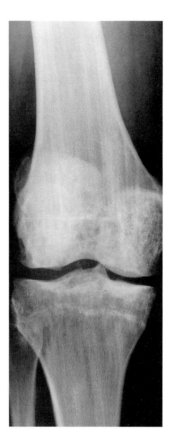

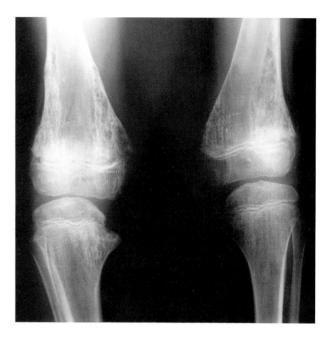

Figure 2.39 *In Ollier's disease, abnormal bone
texture is seen in the metaphyseal regions, consisting
of strands of radiolucent cartilage streaming
backwards from the epiphyseal plates. The changes
are associated with abnormal modelling.*

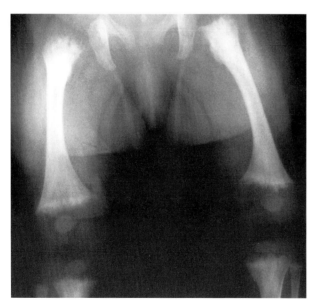

Figure 2.40 *Rubella syndrome. There is
metaphyseal flaring and irregularity with vertical
lucencies.*

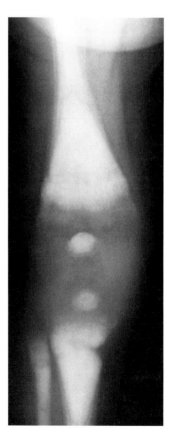

Figure 2.41
*Osteopetrosis.
Expansion and
sclerosis and a bone-
within-a-bone
appearance are the
features of this
disease. The
abnormally
mineralized
metaphysis shows
poorly defined
vertical channels,
which are vascular
in origin, extending
backwards from the
metaphyses.*

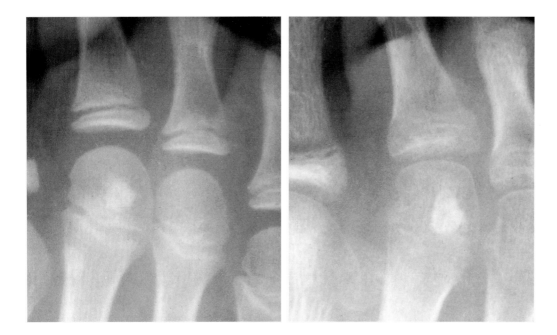

Figure 2.42 *Growing bone island in the second metatarsal head.*

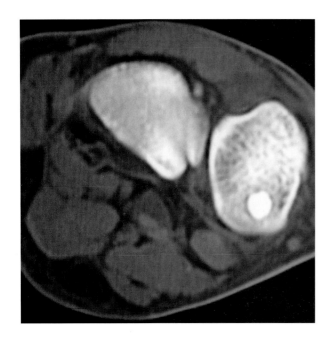

Figure 2.43 *Sclerotic bone island seen at CT scanning; it is a well demarcated lesion.*

observation (Figure 2.42). They show some uptake on a bone scan and may cause slight confusion with focal metastases. Both lesions blend in with surrounding bone and may show peripheral infiltration into the adjacent medulla.

Focal areas of bone sclerosis are well displayed on CT scanning (Figure 2.43) and at MRI are seen as focal areas of low signal.

WIDESPREAD OSTEOSCLEROSIS IN SYMPTOMATIC DISORDERS WITH ABNORMAL BONE CONTOUR

MELORHEOSTOSIS

Clinically this condition is associated with pain in the limbs and skin contractures. Sclerotic bone is deposited on the internal and external aspects of the cortex of tubular bones, usually in the distribution of the sclerotomes, which are the sensory nerve supply to skeletal structures.

The external surfaces of the affected bones have a lobulated, undulant appearance similar to flowing

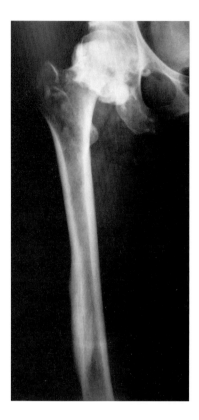

Figure 2.44
Melorheostosis. Marked new bone formation is seen on the lateral aspect of the midshaft femoral cortex, and around the femoral neck. The proximal lesion resembles an osteoma.

candle wax. The lesions cross joints (Figures 2.44 and 2.45), and ossification is seen in local soft tissues (Figure 2.46). Bones are both thickened and lengthened. (For other causes of bone lengthening, see Table 7.2, page 348.)

Often, only one half of a tubular bone is involved. It elongates along its long axis and a bowing deformity results. Large sclerotic lesions resemble osteomas and may cause gross expansion of bone. The ribs and vertebral bodies are rarely affected (Figure 2.47) but the skull is apparently not affected.

MIXED SCLEROSING BONE DYSTROPHY

Sclerosing changes in bone, melorheostosis, osteopoikilosis and osteopathia striata may co-exist in a mixed form with overlapping features of each disease. Thus, the sclerosis at a bone end may be both linear and nodular (Figure 2.48). Vascular lesions, arteriovenous malformations and haemangiomas co-exist in the adjacent soft tissues.

TUBEROUS SCLEROSIS

This is one of the neurocutaneous syndromes or phakomatoses and has widespread manifestations, including facial adenoma sebaceum, mental defect and epilepsy. A fine honeycomb lung results in chronic pneumothorax and pulmonary arterial hypertension. Renal angiomyolipoma and lung, liver and adrenal hamartomas may also be present.

In the skull, the intracranial hamartomas or tubers may calcify and the vault itself undergoes a patchy increase in density (Figure 2.49). The long tubular bones show undulant cortical thickening, both endosteally and periosteally, and the metacarpals, metatarsals and phalanges show similar features with narrowing of the medulla (Figure 2.50). Corticomedullary differentiation is preserved. In the pelvis, large flame-shaped areas of density occupy both iliac blades (Figure 2.51) and the vertebral bodies may show sclerosis affecting both bodies and appendages.

Hand changes are often associated with small lytic defects, often at the distal phalanges, due to local hamartomas or fibromas (Figure 2.52). Skull sclerosis and hand lesions are found in 60–65% of cases and together are characteristic of the disease.

FLUOROSIS

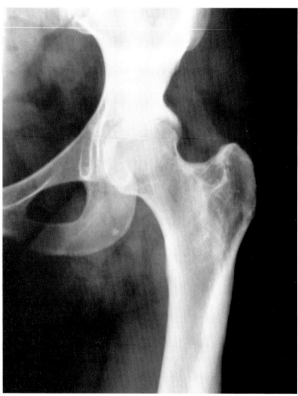

Figure 2.45 *Another patient with melorheostosis showing acetabular and femoral sclerosis.*

Ingestion of water containing 8 parts per million fluorine, or exposure to industrial waste, leads to

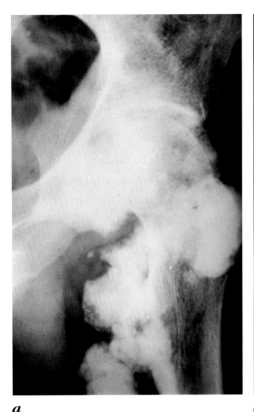

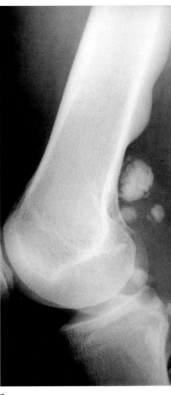

a

b

Figure 2.46 *(a, b)*
*Melorheostosis. Soft tissue lesions
may occur around joints and
these are painful. The appearances are not specific, but will be
associated with changes of
melorheostosis elsewhere in the
adjacent skeleton (see also Figure
7.39). (c) In another case of
melorheostosis, the plain film
shows eccentric and irregular
sclerosis along the medial aspect
of the distal femur, crossing the
joint into the adjacent tibia.
There is new bone on the outer
aspect of the cortex and also in
the soft tissues. (d) On the radioisotope bone scan increase in
uptake is demonstrated in the
areas of bone sclerosis. (e) The
coronal* T_1*-weighted MR sequence
shows sclerotic bone, as expected,
as areas of low signal lying
within the marrow, on the
periosteum and in the soft tissues.*

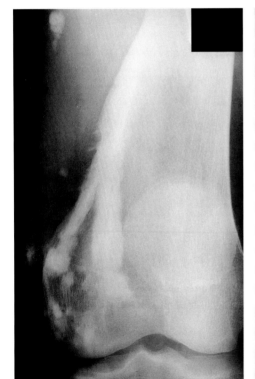

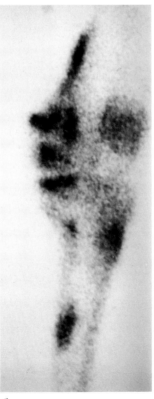

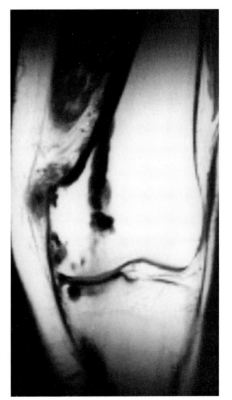

c

d

e

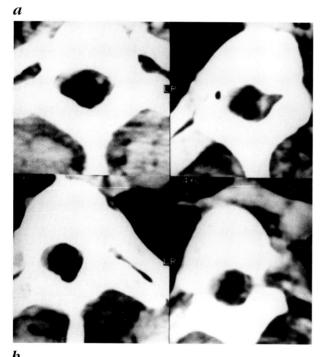

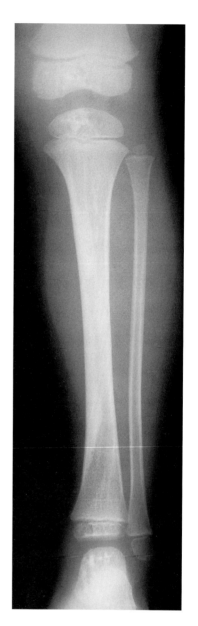

Figure 2.47 *Melorheostosis.* (*a*) *A rare example of change in vertebral bodies and adjacent ribs. The appearances are strikingly similar to those seen with metastatic disease. The distribution follows the sclerotomes.* (*b*) *The CT scan shows generalized bone thickening and sclerosis, sparing a right rib.*

Figure 2.48 *Mixed sclerosing bone dystrophy. Stippling of the epiphyses is shown together with linear sclerosis of the metaphyses.*

fluorosis. Although low fluorine concentrations appear to protect teeth from caries, concentrations greater than 2 parts per million lead to dental enamel mottling and pitting.

Bone sections in fluorosis show cortical thickening and prominent medullary trabeculation. Radio-

logically, there is a pronounced, diffuse increase in bone density in the axial skeleton, with relative sparing of the cranium and peripheral bones. Cortico-medullary differentiation is lost and the bones become uniformly dense (Figure 2.53). There is marked 'fringing' or ossification of musculo-

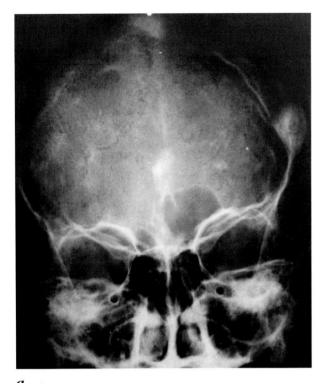

a

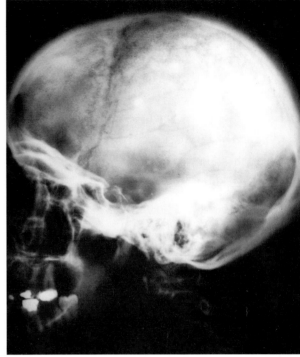

b

c

Figure 2.49 *Plain radiographs (**a**, **b**) and CT (**c**) show periventricular tubers and areas of increased density in the skull vault of this patient with tuberous sclerosis.*

tendinous insertions into bone, resulting in lesions resembling the neostosis of ankylosing spondylitis and of diffuse idiopathic skeletal hyperostosis (DISH; ankylosing hyperostosis) (Figure 2.54; see Chapter 8, page 380). Ligaments ossify, even in the spinal canal, and periostitis in the hands is always a feature of gross and widespread disease.

The combination of sclerosis and fringing also occurs in X-linked hypophosphataemic osteomalacia (Figure 2.55). Bowing, Looser's zones and often sacroiliac joint fusion are seen in X-linked hypophosphataemic osteomalacia but not in fluorosis. The sclerosis in fluorosis does not seem to lead to bone weakening, softening or fracture, therefore fluorine therapy has been used in the treatment of osteoporosis.

HEAVY METAL POISONING

Apart from fluorine, other chemical elements cause changes in bone density and modelling. However

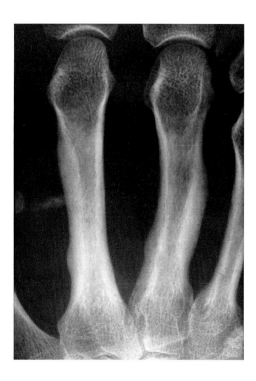

Figure 2.50 *Tuberous sclerosis. Cortical thickening almost obliterates the medullary cavity. There is a smooth and undulant periosteal reaction.*

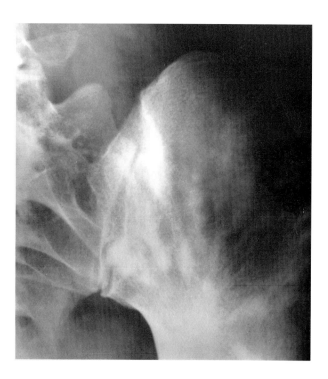

Figure 2.51 *Large flame-shaped areas of osteosclerosis are seen in the iliac blade in this case of tuberous sclerosis.*

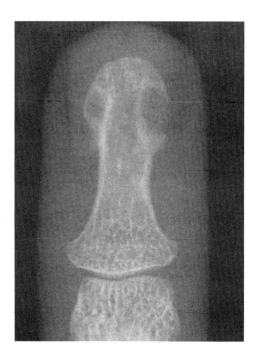

Figure 2.52 *Tuberous sclerosis. Small, well corticated defects occur in the distal phalanges, related to subungual fibromas or hamartomas within the bone.*

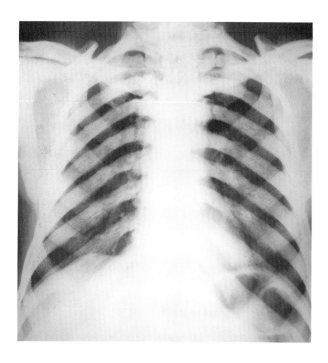

Figure 2.53 *In this patient with fluorosis, there is an overall increase in bony density and the margins of the ribs are undulant due to ossification of muscle insertions.*

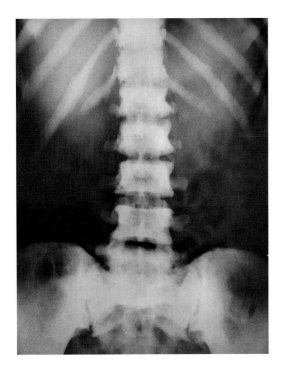

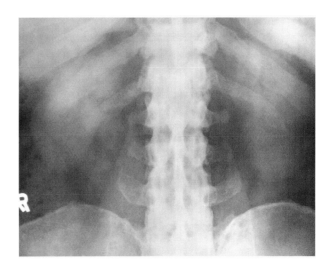

Figure 2.55 *X-linked hypophosphataemic osteomalacia. Increase in bony density is associated with thickening and fringing of the ribs.*

Figure 2.54 *A widespread diffuse increase in bone density with obliteration of cortico-medullary differentiation can be seen in this fluorotic patient. The ribs show osteosclerosis and are expanded with ossification of musculotendinous insertions.*

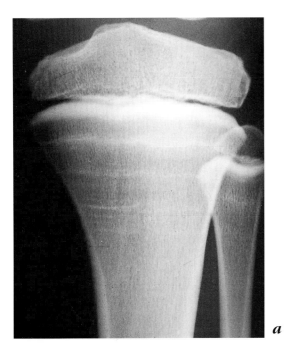

a

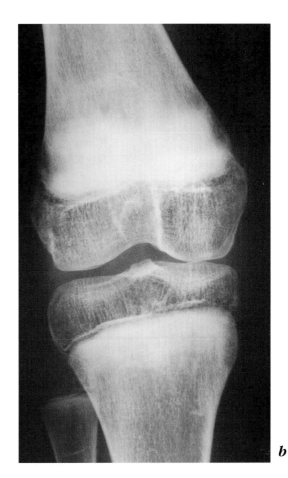

b

Figure 2.56 *(a) Metaphyseal bands of density are associated with local undertubulation in this patient with lead poisoning. (b) Bismuth poisoning followed treatment for syphilis.*

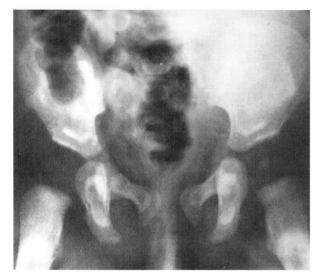

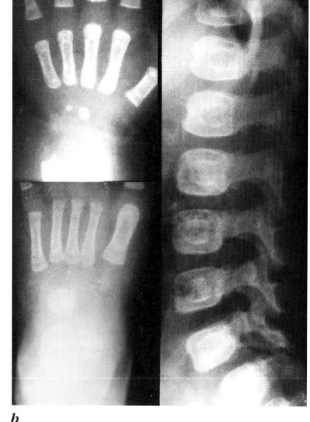

a

Figure 2.57 *Phosphorus poisoning. (**a**) Maternal ingestion results in the bone-within-a-bone appearance in the pelvis of this newborn infant. (**b**) The spine, hands and feet also show a bone-within-a-bone appearance.*

b

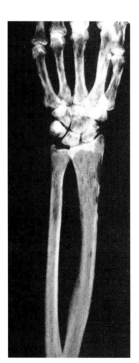

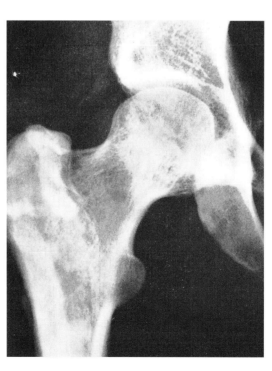

Figure 2.58 *Ingestion of radium by a watch-dial painter led to areas of osteonecrosis, with resultant sclerosis and bone destruction.*

these changes are generally epiphyseal and metaphyseal, and reflect ingestion during growth, so that isolated episodes limited in time cause local band-like metaphyseal and epiphyseal densities, more similar to osteopetrosis than fluorosis. An increase in metaphyseal density with undertubulation is seen in children with lead poisoning and in bismuth intoxication (Figure 2.56; see Chapter 5, pages 296 and 301; Chapter 7, page 348). Maternal ingestion of heavy elements, for example, in matches, during pregnancy may give a similar change in the fetus due to phosphorus transmission across the placenta (Figure 2.57).

With radium poisoning, widespread areas of infarction and necrosis may produce areas of sclerosis and bone destruction (Figure 2.58).

OSTEOSCLEROSIS, ABNORMAL MODELLING, HEPATOSPLENOMEGALY AND PATHOLOGICAL FRACTURES

OSTEOPETROSIS

Bone changes occur due to failure of resorption of the primary spongiosa, which is normally resorbed by vascular mesenchyme. Absence of this process leads to preservation of fetal bone with a high concentration of calcium and therefore increased bone density and metaphyseal undertubulation. The increased density may be uniform and all bones may be affected. In many patients, however, the process is intermittent so that normal bone is laid down between zones of abnormal bone. The bands parallel the surfaces laying them down, so that arcuate dense curves are seen beneath the iliac crests, and cuboid densities are seen in vertebral bodies and tarsal and carpal bone—the bone-within-a-bone phenomenon (Figure 2.59; Table 2.6).

Four different types are described:

1 A severe *congenita* form inherited as an autosomal recessive (Figure 2.60). Blindness, deafness and hydrocephaly are found due to encroachment upon nerve foramina by expanded bone. Obliteration of marrow results in anaemia and retardation of growth. Chronic infection results in an early death. In this form, anaemia results in hepatosplenomegaly, retardation of growth and widening of bone, particularly in the diametaphyseal regions, give an appearance resembling an Erlenmeyer flask (see Table 5.4, page 299).

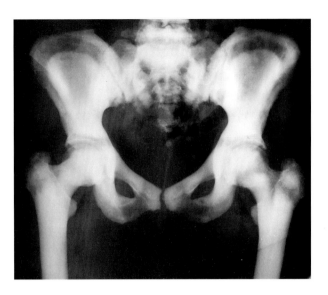

Figure 2.59 *Osteopetrosis. A bone-within-a-bone appearance is shown, reflecting the intermittent nature of the pathological process. This is associated with undertubulation, which is particularly apparent in the upper femora.*

Table 2.6 Causes of a bone-within-a-bone appearance.

Osteopetrosis
Paget's disease
Sickle-cell disease
Heavy metal poisoning
Stress lines

Multiple fractures occur even in utero and contribute further to small stature and deformity. Metaphyseal changes include longitudinal striations due to local blood vessels, as well as undertubulation (Figure 2.41). Identical changes are seen in the mandible; the dentition is disordered (Figure 2.61). Dental infection and severe mandibular osteomyelitis are found.

2 A delayed or *tarda* type, with an autosomal dominant inheritance, as described by Albers-Schönberg. This form is generally less severe. A bone-within-a-bone appearance is seen (Figure

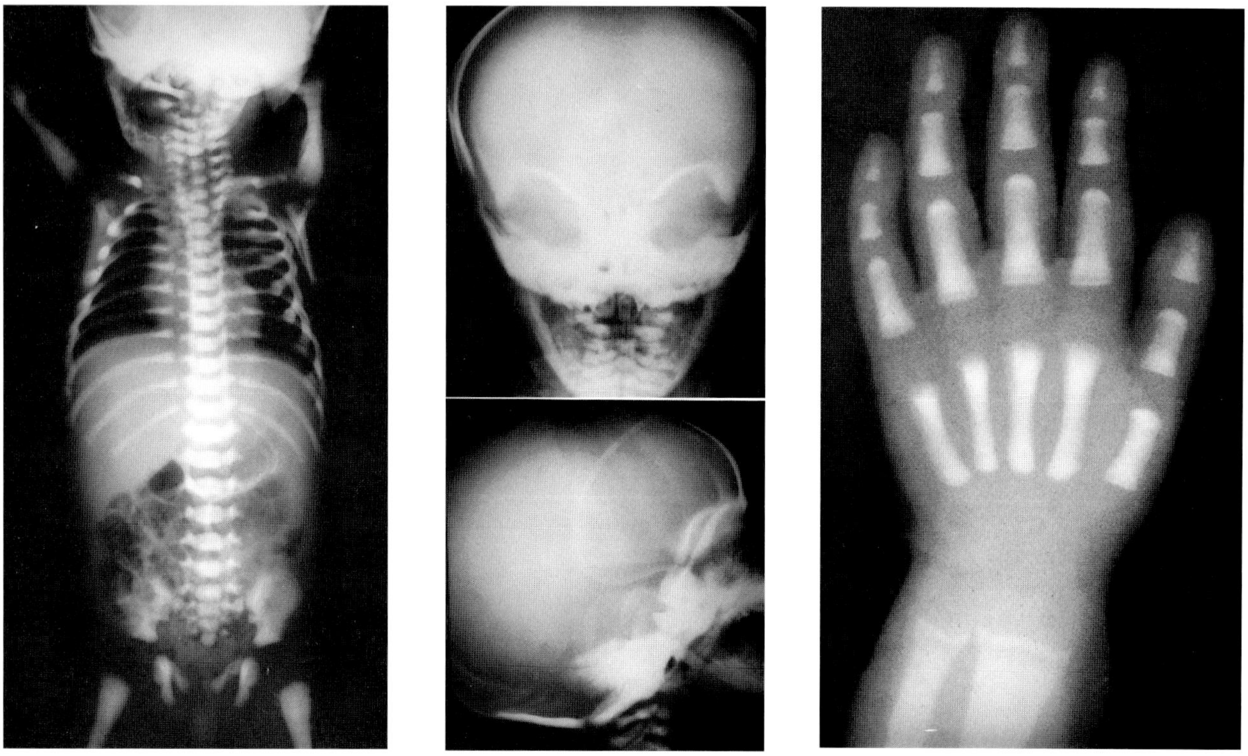

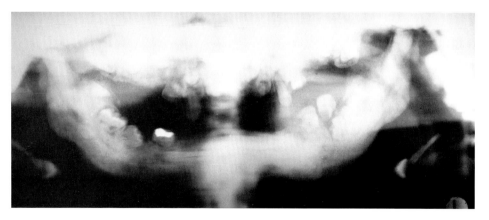

a   *b*   *c*

Figure 2.60 *Osteopetrosis—severe congenital form. (**a**) There is widespread sclerosis of bone which is almost uniform, although a bone-within-a-bone appearance is seen at the iliac crests and in the humeri. There is undertubulation of the long bones, especially affecting metaphyseal regions. (**b**) The skull shows quite marked sclerosis of the facial skeleton and of the base of the skull. There is intense sclerosis of the supra-orbital ridges. Abnormal skull development leads to abnormally shaped orbits. (**c**) The bones of the hands are expanded, sclerotic and a bone-within-a-bone appearance is seen at birth.*

Figure 2.61

Osteopetrosis of the mandible in a child. There is expansion and a bone-within-a-bone appearance is seen in the mandibular condyles. Dentition is disordered. Most teeth will not form because the germinal centres have been destroyed by the process. The abnormal bone in the mandible is prone to severe infection.

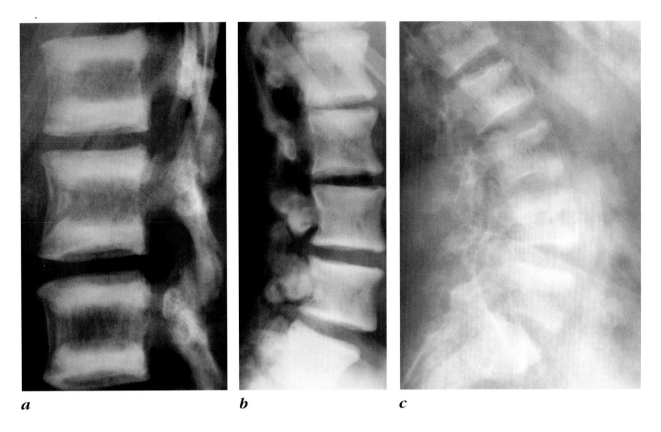

a   *b*   *c*

Figure 2.62 *(a) Osteopetrosis—a bone-within-a-bone appearance. The appearances are those of a rugger-jersey spine. The bone trabeculae are better defined than in renal osteodystrophy. (b) Pyknodysostosis. An increase in bony density is seen in the vertebral bodies of the lumbar spine. Anterior and posterior defects are also present, giving an appearance similar to a cotton reel. Pathological stress fractures have occurred in the pars interarticularis. (c) Renal osteodystrophy. There is generalized loss of bone density but subendplate condensation of bone results in a rugger-jersey spine. The trabeculae are poorly defined.*

2.62a), as well as an Erlenmeyer flask appearance (see page 298).

3 A less severe *recessive* type.

4 Osteopetrosis with *renal tubular acidosis*. This has an autosomal recessive inheritance. Cerebral calcifications are also seen and some patients are mentally retarded.

The tarda form is generally less severe and may not be noticed until two or three fractures are sustained in middle age due to inappropriate or minor trauma (Figure 2.63). Bone deformity due to softening occurs, and may be seen in the ribs, which can lose their normal upward convexity and slope downwards. Similar deformity exists with osteogenesis imperfecta and osteomalacia.

PYKNODYSOSTOSIS

This rare form of increased bony density was distinguished from osteopetrosis by Maroteaux and Lamy in 1962. The patients are severely dwarfed, and the bones are intensely osteosclerotic, lack cortico-medullary differentiation and are susceptible to fracture.

The modelling abnormalities resemble those of cleidocranial dysplasia. Wormian bones, acro-osteolysis and hypoplastic clavicles are seen, on a background of increased bony density (Figure 2.64). In addition, the angle of the mandible is lost (Figure 2.65), the paranasal air sinuses do not develop and hepatosplenomegaly is prominent. The bones are abnormally modelled, not expanded, but rather

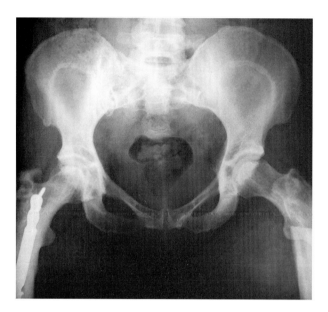

Figure 2.63 *Osteopetrosis with pathological fractures. The sclerosing bone dysplasia here is obviously of a less severe type, but nonetheless transverse fractures have occurred in the femora.*

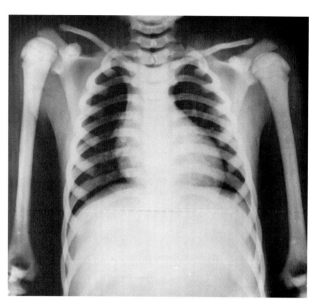

Figure 2.64 *Pyknodysostosis with uniform increase in bony density.*

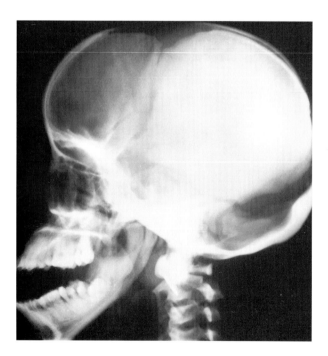

Figure 2.65 *In pyknodysostosis, dwarfism is associated with an increase in bony density which is apparent in the parietal and occipital bones. The mandible does not have a normal angle.*

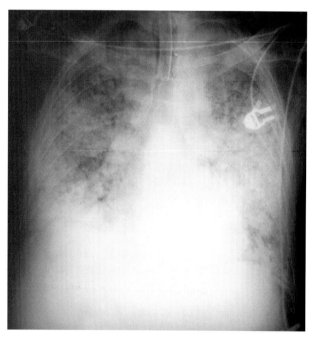

Figure 2.66 *Lungs in renal osteodystrophy. Widespread calcification is seen throughout both lungfields.*

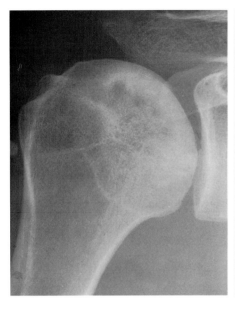 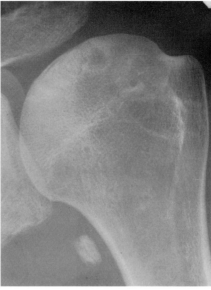

Figure 2.67 *Avascular necrosis. Crescentic lucencies may be seen beneath the cortex of the humeral heads associated with subarticular density in this patient receiving steroids. A loose body is also present.*

gracile. In particular, the vertebral bodies have large anterior and posterior defects, and resemble cotton reels (Figure 2.62b).

RENAL OSTEODYSTROPHY

In this condition, changes of secondary hyperparathyroidism are superimposed on those of osteomalacia.

An anabolic effect of parathormone on bone tends to occur if levels are mildly elevated over a long period of time, in contrast to the bone destruction seen with higher levels of hormone in primary hyperparathyroidism (see Chapter 1, page 44). The anabolic effects include:

1 excessive maturation of osteoblasts leading to new bone formation;
2 increased laying down of osteoid, particularly in areas which have a relatively high blood supply. This osteoid calcifies under the influence of the secondarily elevated serum calcium levels.

Increased bone density in the axial skeleton and beneath the vertebral end-plates gives a 'rugger jersey' or 'sandwich spine' appearance (Figure 2.62c). Trabeculae remain hazy and are not as well defined or as dense as those seen in osteopetrosis, for

instance (Table 2.7). Diffuse sclerosis, with poor definition of affected trabeculae, is seen. Subperiosteal bone resorption also occurs at the usual sites, and cortico-medullary differentiation is poor. The major long bones may have cortical thickening, and Looser's zones may be visible. Soft tissue calcification may be seen in blood vessels, in and around joints, and occasionally in the lungs (Figure 2.66) and other viscera.

Avascular necrosis in renal osteodystrophy occurs at major articular surfaces and also at the condyles of the temporomandibular joints. This may be related to drug therapy rather than the disease and is particularly prominent at the humeral head (Figure 2.67), which is otherwise only rarely affected by avascular necrosis.

Table 2.7 Causes of the rugger-jersey appearance (sandwich spine or subend-plate condensation).

Osteopetrosis
Renal osteodystrophy
Heavy metal ingestion
Paget's disease
Growth arrest line

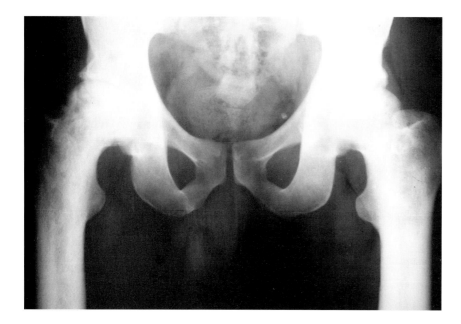

Figure 2.68 *Sickle-cell disease. An increase in bone density is associated with cortical thickening and obliteration of the medullary cavity. This particularly affects the proximal femora.*

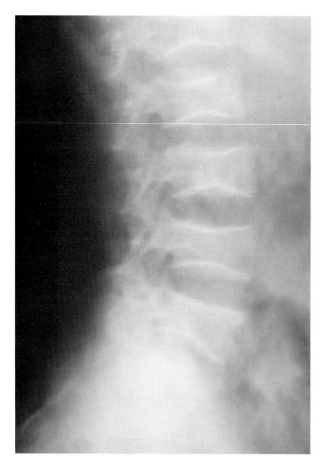

Figure 2.69 *Sickle-cell disease with bone softening results in vertebral collapse and deformity of the codfish type.*

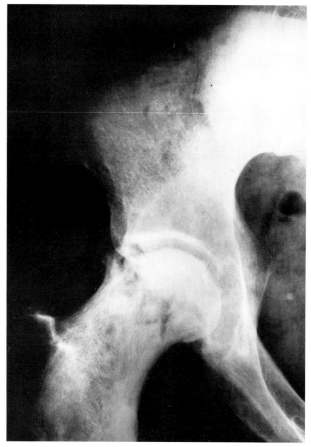

Figure 2.70 *In this patient with Gaucher's disease there is widespread reactive sclerosis in the proximal femur and avascular necrosis of the femoral head.*

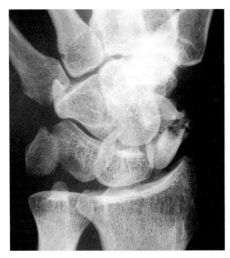 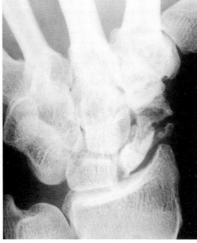

Figure 2.74 *Avascular necrosis of the scaphoid follows a waist of scaphoid fracture. The proximal pole shows an increase in density. The radiographs are taken 4 years apart.*

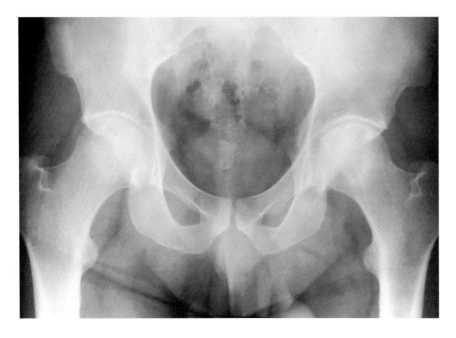

Figure 2.75 *Avascular necrosis of the femoral head. Relative radiolucency in both femoral heads is surrounded by a serpiginous zone of density, the zone of creeping substitution.*

AVASCULAR NECROSIS AND INFARCTION OF BONE (see also Chapter 4)

Cell death in the epiphysis following local cessation of blood flow is known as avascular necrosis. Infarction is the term used when the bone shafts are affected by medullary or cortical periosteal changes.

Cellular elements within bone die 36–48 hours after loss of blood supply, but initially the basic trabecular framework remains unaltered. Radiological change is not to be expected in the acute stage of ischaemia although later, reactive hyperaemia in surrounding vital bone causes the vital bone to become osteoporotic. This process does not involve avascular bone which, therefore, appears relatively sclerotic (Figure 2.74). Its density is initially unaltered. Subsequent healing takes place from the periphery of the infarcted area, with neo-vascularity, fibroblast proliferation and laying down of new bone on the framework of the old. The infarcted area of the medulla becomes surrounded by a serpiginous or ring-like zone of reactive sclerosis, termed the 'zone of creeping substitution', which represents the advancing front of neo-ossification (Figure 2.75).

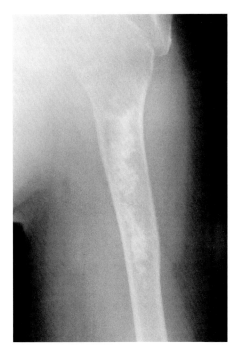

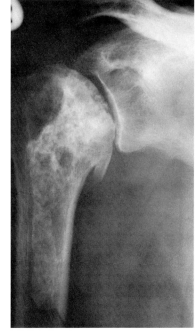

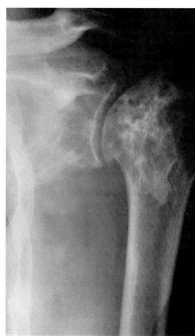

Figure 2.76 *This large medullary infarct could be confused with an enchondroma or chondrosarcoma. However, the overlying cortex is preserved and the surrounding bone shows no radiolucency to suggest the presence of non-mineralized cartilage.*

Figure 2.77 *In this patient with caisson disease, avascular necrosis of the humeral heads has resulted in collapse with secondary degeneration. Well demarcated medullary infarcts are visible and split cortices are also shown.*

These changes are classically seen in the diametaphyseal regions of long bones.

Causes of diametaphyseal infarction

Prominent infarctive changes are seen in sickle-cell disease, dysbaric osteonecrosis and Gaucher's disease, when large serpiginous densities are prominent, associated with cortical and epiphyseal infarctive changes (Figures 2.76 and 2.77).

Diametaphyseal sclerosis is commonly seen in the humeral and femoral necks of elderly patients. Fine, localized, medullary stippling is usually seen at multiple sites, and the surrounding medulla is normal in density with the cortex intact and the bone normally modelled (Figure 2.78). This stippling, which was thought to be due to local infarction, has been said to be related to reinforced remaining trabeculae in osteoporotic bone.

Enchondromas and chondrosarcomas may occasionally be seen in the areas typical for infarc-

tion, particularly the femoral and humeral necks. The basic chondral matrix is radiolucent and lies around areas of speckled mineralization; that is, areas of trabecular resorption and mineralization co-exist. However, chondrosarcomas are unlikely to be distributed at the multiple and symmetrical diametaphyseal sites of infarction. More importantly, the bone is likely to be expanded locally, the cortex scalloped endosteally and possibly thickened periosteally (Figure 2.79). Expansion does not occur with medullary infarcts, which will also tend not to change on serial films. If no change occurs over 6–12 months, the lesion is almost certainly benign, and the ultimate diagnosis of little clinical importance. In the absence of change, biopsy can be avoided. The local cortex may well be preserved, thick and hard, and penetration difficult (Figure 2.80). Chondrosarcomas may be expected to show features of malignant change. Sarcomatous change does occur in infarcts but it is rare. Cortical infarcts result in a bone-within-a-bone appearance or split cortex.

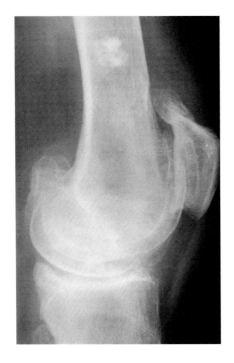

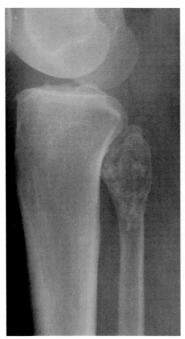

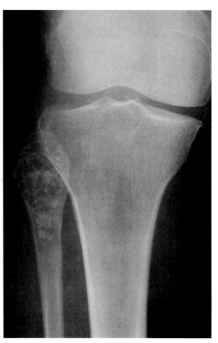

Figure 2.78 *In this example of a distal femoral infarct, there is spotty calcification of the distal femur; however, the surrounding bone shows normal density and the cortex is preserved. Note the defect on the distal femur caused by the patellar osteophyte.*

Figure 2.79 *This example of enchondroma shows expansion of the proximal fibula with thinning of the cortex which is not breached. The abnormal matrix shows the speckled calcification which is characteristic of benign cartilaginous tumours.*

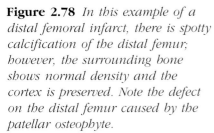

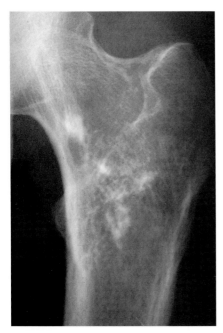

b

a

Figure 2.80 *Infarct (biopsy proven).* (**a**) *The speckled mineralization lies in an area typical for infarction, cartilage tumours (see Figure 2.79) and osteoporotic stippling. There is however no significant area of non-mineralization to suggest a chondral aetiology.* (**b**) *The CT scan confirms the presence of speckled mineralization in the proximal femur, especially medially, in the region of the lesser trochanter. The cortex is preserved and the bone is not enlarged.*

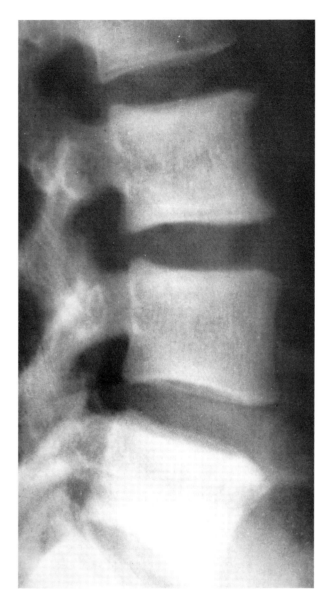

Figure 2.81 *Sclerosing sarcoid. The lateral view of the lumbar spine shows a diffuse sclerosis affecting the vertebral bodies without expansion.*

Causes of cortical splitting

The dead cortex remains within the medulla due to apposition of bone beneath the elevated periosteum, and is separate from the new vital cortex (Figure 1.82). It appears dense and cannot be resorbed or become osteoporotic because of local avascularity. This density represents the tombstone of the old cortex. A split cortex may be the result of septic as well as aseptic necrosis and may also be seen with

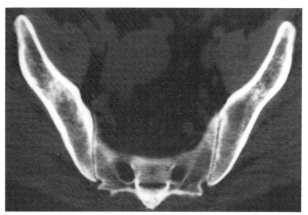

Figure 2.82 *Sclerosing sarcoid. Focal areas of high attenuation or sclerosis are demonstrated in both iliac blades.*

rapidly growing tumours, but still represents devascularized bone. Cortical splitting is a prominent feature of infection, sickle-cell and Gaucher's diseases.

SARCOIDOSIS

Osteosclerosis is seen in a widespread or focal form in the axial skeleton—ribs, spine (Figure 2.81) and pelvis (Figure 2.82)—resembling malignant deposits.

BIBLIOGRAPHY

Albers-Schönberg H (1904) Röntgenbilder einer seltenen Knochenerkrankung *Münchener Medinische Wochenschrift.* S1; 365.

Beltran J, Herman LJ, Buck JM et al (1988) Femoral head avascular necrosis. MR imaging with clinical-pathologic and radionuclide correlation. *Radiology* **166**: 215–20.

Galasko CSP (1986) *Skeletal Metastases.* London: Butterworths

Hamdy RC (1981) *Paget's Disease of Bone.* New York: Prager

Kanis JA (1991) *Pathophysiology and Treatment of Paget's Disease of Bone.* London: Martin Dunitz.

Kerr R, Resnick D, Sartoris DJ et al (1986) Computerized tomography of proximal femoral trabecular patterns. *J Orthop Res* **4**: 45–56.

Maroteaux P, Lamy M (1962) La Pycnodysostose. *Presse Médicale*, **70**: 999.

Mitchell MD, Kundel HL, Steinberg ME et al (1986) Avascular necrosis of the hip. Comparison of MR, CT and scintigraphy. *Am J Roentgenol* **147**: 67–71.

Roberts MC, Kressel HY, Fallon MD et al (1989) Paget disease: MR imaging findings. *Radiology* **173**: 341–5.

Chapter 3   **Localized lesions in bone**

Localized lesions in bone may be solitary or multiple, and their distribution may be assessed by radiological skeletal survey or isotope bone scans. Multiple lesions are often due to the spread of malignant disease, especially if the patient is over 45 years of age, in which case the assumption is that multiple lesions are malignant until proven otherwise. If a lesion is seen to

be solitary and has the radiological features of malignancy in a patient over 45 years of age, it is more likely to be a secondary deposit than a primary malignant tumour of bone as these are rare in middle and old age. It is most important to distinguish between benign and malignant lesions. Most bone lesions are distinctive in appearance but some cannot easily be diagnosed radiologically or even histologically (Table 3.1).

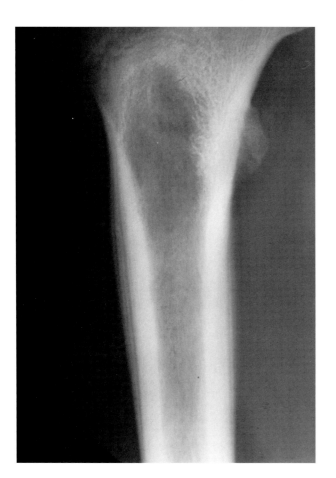

Figure 3.1 *In this patient with Ewing's sarcoma, the zone of transition between normal and abnormal bone is wide, particularly inferiorly. Permeation extends beyond the main mass of the lesion, as shown by the presence of a lamellar periostitis extending to the midshaft.*

RADIOLOGICAL DIFFERENTIATION BETWEEN BENIGN AND MALIGNANT LESIONS OF BONE

ZONE OF TRANSITION

This defines the nature of the interface between normal and abnormal bone. In general, malignant lesions are characterized by rapid growth which may be assessed on serial radiographs. Tumour permeation results in a wide and poorly defined zone of transition between normal and abnormal bone (Figure 3.1). Infection may give a similar appearance.

Benign lesions usually grow slowly and often do not alter on serial radiographs; aneurysmal bone cyst and giant-cell tumour are the exceptions to this rule. Their lack of local permeation results in a narrow zone of transition, so that the lesion is surrounded by normal bone (Figures 3.2 and 3.3). This may be altered by infection, fracture, surgery or healing. Malignant transformation of benign lesions occasionally occurs, for example, from chondroma to chondrosarcoma (Figure 3.4) or fibrosarcoma in fibrous dysplasia (Figure 3.5). This is associated with a change in the nature of the lesion, with rapid growth and loss of definition, resulting in a wide zone of transition, pathological fracture and pain.

ZONE OF REACTIVE SCLEROSIS

The slow growth of benign lesions enables the surrounding bone to form a shell of reactive sclerotic

Table 3.1 Classification of primary bone tumours and tumour-like lesions.

	Benign	*Malignant*
A Presumed to arise from skeletal connective tissue		
Tumours forming bone	Osteoma	Osteosarcoma*
	Exostosis	Parosteal osteosarcoma
	Osteoid osteoma	Periosteal osteosarcoma
	Benign osteoblastoma	Malignant osteoblastoma
	(Giant osteoid osteoma)	
Tumours forming cartilage	Enchondroma	Chondrosarcoma
	Solitary or multiple	
	Benign chondroblastoma	
	Chondromyxoid fibroma	
	Osteochondroma	
	(Cartilage-capped exostosis)	
	Solitary or multiple	
Tumours forming fibrous tissue	Non-ossifying fibroma	Fibrosarcoma
	Fibrous cortical defect	Malignant fibrous histiocytoma
	Metaphyseal fibrous defect	
	Fibrous dysplasia	
	Probably not neoplastic	
Tumours forming osteoclastic tissue	Giant-cell tumour	Malignant giant-cell tumour
B Tumours of unknown histogenesis		
	Simple bone cyst	Ewing's tumour
	Adamantinoma of long bones	Undifferentiated sarcomas
C Presumed to arise from other skeletal components		
Blood and lymph vessels	Haemangioma	Angiosarcoma
	Solitary or multiple	
	Haemangiomatosis	
	(Massive osteolysis)	
	(Gorham's disease)	
	(Vanishing bone disease)	
	Lymphangiomatosis	
	Aneurysmal bone cyst	
	Glomus tumour	
	Haemangiopericytoma	
Nerves	Neurofibroma	Neurosarcoma
	Neurilemmoma	
Fat	Lipoma	Liposarcoma
Notochord		Chordoma
		Locally malignant
Epithelium	Implantation dermoid cyst	
Dental epithelium	Ameloblastoma of jaw	
Lymphoid and haemopoietic tissues		Leukaemia
		Lymphadenoma
		(Hodgkin's disease)
		Lymphosarcoma
		Plasmacytoma
		Myelomatosis
		Malignant lymphoma of bone

*Paget's sarcoma is usually osteosarcomatous but may be a fibrosarcoma, a malignant lymphoma of bone or, rarely, a chondrosarcoma.

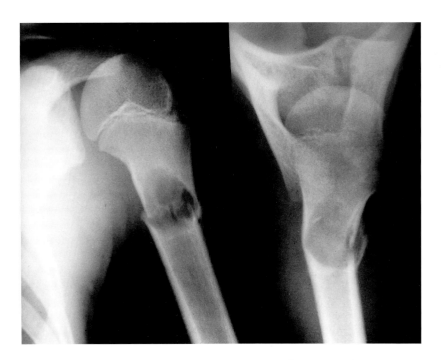

Figure 3.2 *This simple bone cyst is at a characteristic site, the proximal humerus, and shows endosteal scalloping. There is a narrow zone of transition between normal and abnormal bone with a thin zone of reactive sclerosis. A pathological fracture has occurred.*

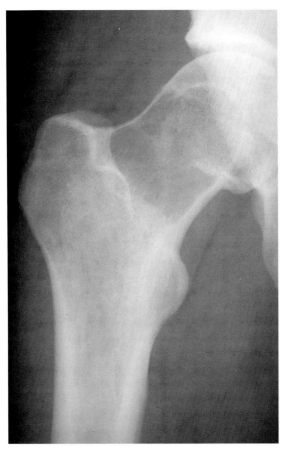

a

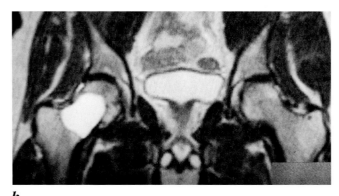

b

Figure 3.3 *Simple bone cyst, again, in a very common site for this lesion. (**a**) The plain film shows a slightly expansile cystic lesion with a narrow zone of transition and a thin rim of reactive sclerosis. There is no matrix mineralization. (**b**) The T$_2$-weighted MR scan confirms these appearances. The fluid nature of the cyst content gives the same bright signal as the bladder content. The lesion has a narrow zone of transition and a thin rim of low signal corresponding to the mineralized margin seen on the plain film.*

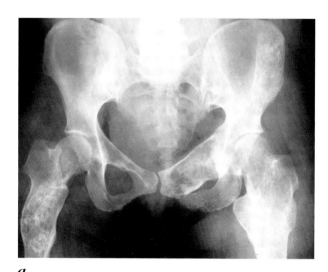

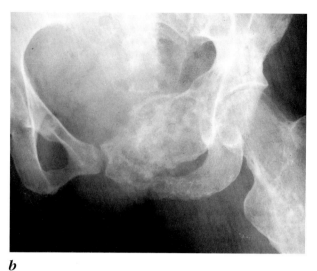

a   *b*

Figure 3.4 *Chondrosarcoma in multiple enchondromatosis. (**a**) Expansile lesions are present in the left iliac blade, left ischium and pubis and in the proximal femora. They are well defined and have narrow sclerotic margins. (Compare these appearances with those seen in hyperparathyroidism (see Figure 1.78), fibrous dysplasia (see Figure 3.47) and even hydatid disease (Figure 3.116).) The lesions show matrix mineralization. (**b**) The same patient showing transformation of the lesion in the left pubis into chondrosarcoma. The lesion has expanded, become poorly defined and is associated with a soft tissue mass. A pathological fracture has occurred.*

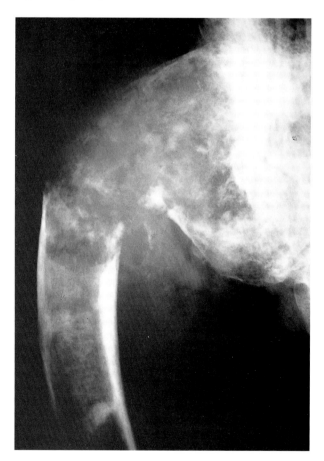

Figure 3.5 *Fibrosarcoma in fibrous dysplasia. There is a pathological fracture of the upper femur with resultant deformity and a soft tissue mass. Expansion is longstanding, as shown at the greater trochanter. The abnormal bone extends down the shaft of the femur, which is expanded and bowed; in places, a ground-glass appearance may be seen.*

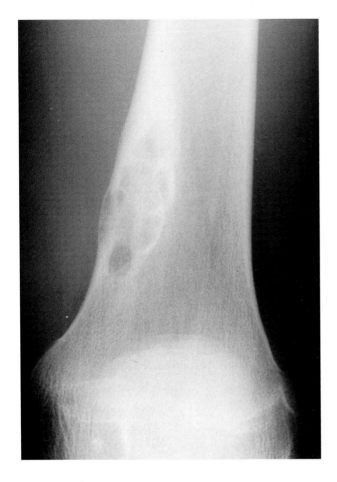

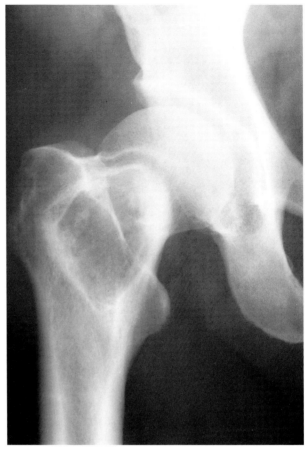

Figure 3.6 *Fibrous cortical defect. These lesions characteristically occur at the metaphyses around the knee, often posteriorly. They are characterized by their subcortical location and a narrow zone of reactive sclerosis.*

Figure 3.7 *In this patient with fibrous dysplasia, the lytic lesion in the pertrochanteric region of the upper femur is surrounded by a thick rind of reactive sclerosis. There is some matrix mineralization within it. The femoral neck is slightly expanded.*

new bone. In some conditions, such as fibrous cortical defect, this is thin and well defined (Figure 3.6). Fibrous dysplasia tends to have a fairly well defined zone of reactive sclerosis, 2–4 mm wide, whose appearance is similar to that of the rind of an orange, giving the so-called 'rind sign' (Figure 3.7). Osteoblastomas tend to be surrounded by gross reactive sclerosis (Figure 3.8), which is often poorly defined. Giant-cell tumours, although usually benign, are often surprisingly poorly defined on the plain film (Figure 3.9).

Malignant tumours are permeative and usually have little surrounding reactive sclerosis. An exception is the chondrosarcoma, because its growth is often slow (Figure 3.10).

THE NATURE AND SHAPE OF THE BONE LESION

Benign lesions arising in the medulla are often round or ovoid until they reach the cortex where their shape is modified. Endosteal scalloping may occur (Figure 3.11), and the resorption of cortex is smooth. Some malignant lesions, such as osteogenic sarcoma, expand centrifugally, breaking through the cortex into the soft tissues to form well defined masses (Figure 3.12), whereas other malignant lesions, such as Ewing's tumour and fibrosarcoma, tend to infiltrate along the shaft of the bone, irregularly permeating cortices before invading soft tissues. Infection can be difficult to distinguish from Ewing's sarcoma. The

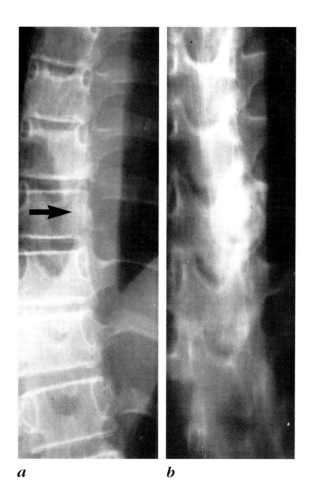

a   *b*

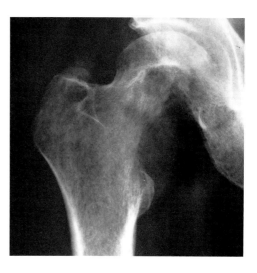

Figure 3.9 *Giant-cell tumour. Superiorly, the lesion has a fairly well demarcated rim of reactive sclerosis but inferiorly and medially, where the calcar has been destroyed, the tumour is poorly defined. It may be diagnosed as a giant-cell tumour because it reaches the articular surface of the femoral head, although only marginally.*

Figure 3.8 *Osteoblastoma. (**a**) A scoliosis is associated with expansion of the left pedicle of the ninth thoracic vertebra (arrow) at the apex of the curve. On the concavity, an expansile lesion, shown on tomography (**b**), is seen as a very densely ossifying nidus surrounded by laminar sclerosis. These appearances are characteristic of osteoid osteoma and osteoblastoma in the spine; the latter is the larger lesion.*

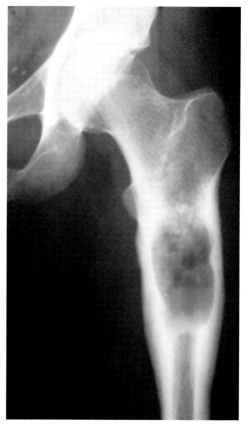

Figure 3.10 *Chondrosarcoma. Despite the medullary bone destruction and endosteal cortical scalloping, smooth periosteal new bone is laid down on the outside of the cortex. The centre of the lesion shows punctate calcification. The zone of transition inferiorly is narrow with a well demarcated zone of sclerosis, but superiorly the lesion is permeative.*

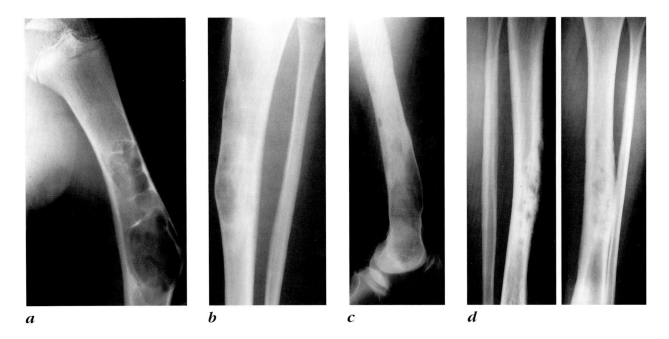

a   b   c   d

Figure 3.11 (*a*) *Simple bone cyst. The multilocular expansile lesion lies at the midshaft, having been left behind by bone apposition at the epiphyseal plate. There is a narrow zone of transition with a thin rim of reactive sclerosis. The cortex shows endosteal scalloping but is not breached.* (***b***) *Osteofibrous dysplasia—so-called because it bears a strong resemblance pathologically and radiologically to fibrous dysplasia. Most cases affect the tibia, usually in its middle third. The patients generally present in infancy and early childhood, often with deformity or pathological fractures, which regress spontaneously.* (***c***) *Hydatid disease. An expansile unilocular cyst is demonstrated at the distal femur. There is cortical thinning.* (***d***) *Adamantinoma. A multilocular, expansile, anterior tibial lesion is associated with cortical thickening.*

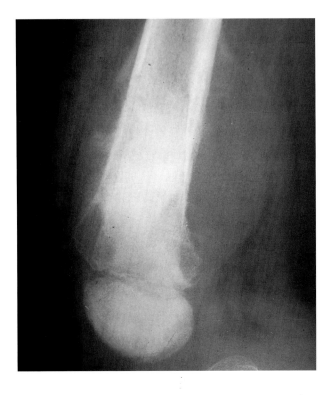

Figure 3.12 *Osteogenic sarcoma. There is a well defined soft tissue mass around the distal femur. The periphery of the tumour is marked by a Codman's triangle and the tumour extends to the distal epiphyseal plate. The epiphysis is also dense, possibly because of invasion by tumour or avascular necrosis. There is perpendicular sunray spiculation.*

history will be shorter and the child febrile. Radiological change is more rapid with infective lesions (see also page 199).

In general, bone replacement in benign lesions is total, within the confines of the circumscribed tumour. Malignant lesions tend to be permeative, patchy and infiltrative so that destruction and replacement is not always uniform. Tumours are not uniformly radiolucent; their appearance depends upon their nature and subsequent behaviour.

CORTICAL AND PERIOSTEAL CHANGES

Benign lesions can cause such endosteal cortical scalloping, thinning and displacement that the displaced cortex is no longer radiologically visible. This unusual sequence occurs, for example, with aneurysmal bone cysts (Figures 2.18 and 3.13).

Generally, malignant lesions rapidly breach the cortex, elevating the periosteum, beneath which new bone is laid down. Primary malignant tumours of bone often result in large, well defined, soft tissue masses which are visualized because of the displacement of overlying and intact fat planes (Figure 3.12).

Expansion is also a feature of some secondary malignant tumours originating in renal and thyroid primary lesions, as well as in myeloma, but most secondary deposits are not associated with significant bone expansion or soft tissue masses. Following the collapse of thoracic vertebral bodies, displacement of the paraspinal lines is seen against radiolucent lung. Infective soft tissue masses are poorly defined because oedema infiltrates local fat planes which are therefore no longer visible.

Where a tumour mass breaks centrally through the elevated layers of periosteal new bone, a Codman's triangle is formed at the margins of the extracortical lesion. This can also be seen in infections. A similar appearance with marginal buttressing occurs with rapidly growing benign lesions, such as aneurysmal bone cyst and giant-cell tumour.

MATRIX AND SOFT TISSUE CALCIFICATION

Table 3.1 classifies tumours according to their cell of origin and benignity or malignancy. Usually, tumours are of osteoid, chondroid, fibrous, lipoid or angioma-

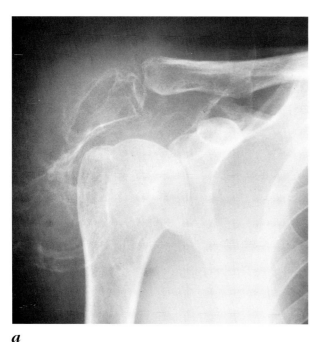

a

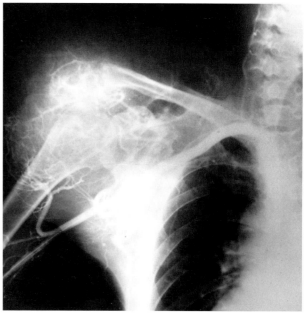

b

Figure 3.13 *Aneurysmal bone cyst. (**a**) These lesions can grow faster than any other tumour. They characteristically enlarge the bone, giving a balloon-like appearance. The cortex may become so thinned that it is invisible, but will re-appear after radiotherapy. (**b**) The arteriogram shows the highly vascular nature of the lesion and its extent.*

tous origin and may be benign or malignant. Each of these basic matrices may mineralize both in bone and soft tissue, usually in a fairly typical diagnostic manner. For example, progressive ossification occurs centrally in osteoid osteomas, and punctate ossification in chondral tumours. Classically, fibrous dysplasia ossifies producing a speckled or a ground-glass appearance. The osteoid matrix in osteosarcoma is heavily and irregularly ossified, both in bone and soft tissues (Figure 3.14).

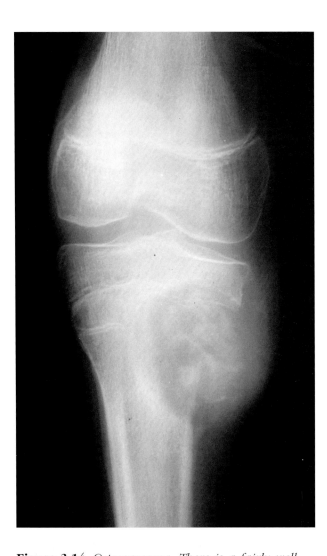

Figure 3.14 *Osteosarcoma. There is a fairly well defined metaphyseal area of bone destruction which has breached the cortex. A large soft tissue mass contains amorphous mineralization and there is a minor Codman's triangle. Elsewhere, quite marked osteoporosis is shown by loss of medullary trabeculation and thinning of the cortices.*

AGE OF INCIDENCE OF BENIGN AND MALIGNANT LESIONS

The patient's age is invaluable for the correct diagnosis of bone tumours. Osteogenic sarcoma should not be diagnosed below the age of 5 years, and giant-cell tumours below the age of local epiphyseal fusion. Giant-cell tumours can arise in children and also in the seventh decade, but these lesions are rare exceptions to the rule. Simple bone cysts and non-ossifying fibromas are not generally seen after skeletal fusion, although exceptions occasionally occur. Most primary tumours of bone present before or around skeletal maturity (Tables 3.2, 3.3 and 3.4).

Table 3.2 Age of incidence of benign lesions.

Lesion type	Age (years)
Eosinophilic granuloma	2–30
Simple bone cyst	5–20
Non-ossifying fibroma	5–20
Aneurysmal bone cyst	5–20
Osteochondroma	5+
Enchondroma	10+
Chondroblastoma	10–20
Fibrous dysplasia	10–30
Osteoblastoma	10–30
Chondromyxoid fibroma	10–30
Giant-cell tumour	20–45

Table 3.3 Age of incidence of malignant lesions.

Lesion type	Age (years)
Leukaemia	0–5
Neuroblastoma	0–5
Ewing's sarcoma	5–25
Osteogenic sarcoma	10–25; 60–80
Periosteal osteosarcoma	20–30
Fibrosarcoma	20–40
Parosteal osteosarcoma	25–35
Malignant lymphoma of bone	25–60
Chondrosarcoma	30–60
Malignant fibrous histiocytoma	40+
Secondary lesions and myeloma	45–80

Table 3.4 Solitary lesions of bone.

	Calcifies	Expands	Before skeletal fusion
Enchondroma	C	E	B
Non-ossifying fibroma	—	E	B
Fibrous dysplasia	C	E	B
Aneurysmal bone cyst	—	E	B
Hyperparathyroidism	—	E	—
Chondroblastoma	C	—	B
Chondromyxoid fibroma	C	—	—
Cystic infection, particularly tuberculosis	C	—	—
Eosinophilic granuloma	—	—	B
Giant-cell tumour	—	E	—
Hydatid	—	E	—
Haemophilic pseudotumour	—	E	B
Metastasis from carcinoma of kidney and thyroid	—	E	—
Plasmacytoma	—	E	—
Simple bone cyst	—	—	B
Osteoid osteoma	C	—	B
Osteoblastoma	C	E	B
Vascular lesions	C	E	—
Malignant fibrous histiocytoma	—	E	—

SITES

The site of a tumour before skeletal fusion may be epiphyseal, metaphyseal or diaphyseal (Tables 3.5–3.8), and is often specific. Thus, chondroblastoma occurs before fusion in the epiphysis, simple bone cyst in the metaphysis and fibrous dysplasia in the diametaphysis. After fusion, giant-cell tumours occur in previous epiphyses or apophyses and should not be diagnosed elsewhere. Ewing's sarcomas are classically diaphyseal and osteogenic sarcomas metaphyseal.

Table 3.5 Tumours and tumour-like lesions appearing in epiphyses or apophyses.

Chondroblastoma (in the immature skeleton)

Fibrous dysplasia ⎤ After skeletal
Giant-cell tumour ⎦ maturity

Malignant fibrous histiocytoma (late adult life)

Cysts or geodes associated with ⎤
   arthritides   Usually on
Synovial tumours   both sides
Osteomyelitis, especially cystic of a joint
   tuberculosis ⎦

Secondary deposits after 45–50 years of age

Table 3.6 Tumours and tumour-like lesions of the metaphysis.

Aneurysmal bone cyst
Simple bone cyst
Non-ossifying fibroma, fibrous cortical defects
Malignant fibrous histiocytoma
Fibrous dysplasia
Enchondroma
Chondromyxoid fibroma
Eosinophilic granuloma
Simple and tuberculous infections
Osteogenic sarcoma
Parosteal osteosarcoma
Chondrosarcoma
Leukaemia
Neuroblastoma

Table 3.7 Tumours and tumour-like lesions occurring in the diaphysis.

Ewing's tumour, malignant lymphoma of bone
Less commonly, osteogenic sarcoma
Metastases
Myeloma
Simple bone cyst (late)
Enchondroma
Fibrous dysplasia
Brown tumour in hyperparathyroidism
Eosinophilic granuloma
Adamantinoma (of the tibia)

Calcification or ossification occurs in tumours originating in osteoid, chondroid and fibrous tissue, as well as in lipomatous or vascular tumours. Usually the appearance of each lesion is characteristic, enabling the diagnosis to be made (Table 3.9).

Table 3.9 Focal lucent area containing calcification surrounded by sclerosis.

Osteoid osteoma (<1.5 cm) Osteoblastoma (>1.5 cm) Brodie's abscess Chondrosarcoma	Generally solitary and painful
Lipoma of bone Enchondroma Fibrous dysplasia	Generally painless, solitary or multiple
Infarcts	Often painful, generally multiple

Table 3.8 Focal lesions occurring in specific sites.

Site	Lesion
Ribs	Metastases
	Myeloma
	Brown tumours in hyperparathyroidism
	Fibrous dysplasia
	Hydatid disease
	Angioma
	Paget's disease
Fingers	Enchondroma
	Cysts or geodes associated with arthritides
	Sarcoidosis ⎤
	Leprosy ⎦ Granuloma
	Tuberculosis ⎤
	Syphilis ⎦ Spina ventosa
	Enlarged nutrient foramina in Sarcoidosis
	Leprosy
	Haemolytic anaemia
	Implantation dermoid ⎤
	Subungual fibroma ⎥ Distal phalanx
	Tuberous sclerosis ⎦
	Glomus tumour
	Brown tumour in hyperparathyroidism
	Secondary deposit, usually pulmonary in origin
Sacrum	Anterior sacral meningocoele
	Myeloma
	Chordoma
	Neurofibroma
	Ependymoma
	Dermoid
	Invasion from rectal or ovarian cancer
Skull	Fibrous dysplasia
	Osteoporosis circumscripta (Paget's disease)
	Neurofibromatosis
	Eosinophilic granuloma
	Sarcoidosis
	Osteomyelitis, including tuberculosis
	Fungal infections (Madura skull)
	Developmental defects
	Hydatid
	Erosion from skull tumours
	Leptomeningeal cyst
	Brown tumour of hyperparathyroidism
	Arteriovenous malformation, haemangioma
	Metastasis, myeloma, occasionally tumours, e.g. osteoblastoma
	Meningioma
	Cholesteatoma
	Burr hole

SPECIFIC LESIONS

OSTEOID OSTEOMA

Incidence: In the Mayo Clinic series this accounts for 13.5% of benign bone tumours.
Sex: M:F = 2:1.
Age: 50% in the second decade.
Site: see Figure 3.15. More than 50% of cases arise in the femur and tibia and some 15% in the vertebral

column, almost inevitably in the vertebral appendages. The lesions are also found in the talus (around the neck), but rarely in the face or jaws.

This is a small (<1.5 cm) lesion found in children and young adults, producing pain characteristically at night. Radiologically, it has a lucent nidus consisting of vascular osteoid which undergoes progressive ossification, starting with a small central fleck of density (Figure 3.16). Most cases of osteoid osteoma can be diagnosed on the plain film alone, or in combination with linear or computed tomography. The surrounding reactive sclerosis may be so marked that it obscures the tumour, particularly if the lesion is related to the cortex (Figure 3.17). This classically occurs in the region of the lesser trochanter of the femur (Figure 3.18), when tomography may be helpful. Alternatively, if the lesion is in a bone which has little or no periosteum, it may not be visualized because of a lack of surrounding sclerosis, although it may be seen on tomography (Figure 3.19). In the talus the entire tumour is often extruded from the neck into the local soft tissues, resembling an osteochondroma (Figure 3.20). An osteoid osteoma is characteristically well visualized on isotope bone scans, both on the early and delayed images (Figure 3.21). The lesion often cannot be distinguished from a Brodie's abscess in chronic osteomyelitis, which may be seen in areas atypical for osteoid osteoma, for example, the skull. Brodie's abscess is often metaphyseal since, in child-

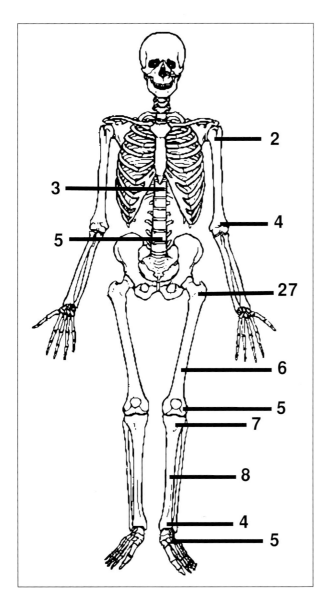

Figure 3.15 *Osteoid osteoma: percentage distribution at major sites only. (After Unni, 1996, with permission.)*

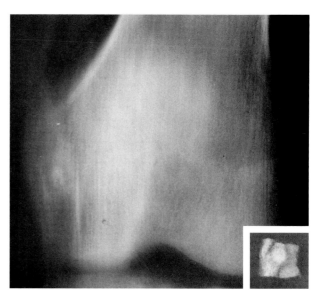

Figure 3.16 *Ossification of an osteoid osteoma in the femoral condyle. Insert: surgical specimen.*

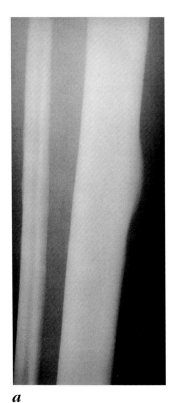

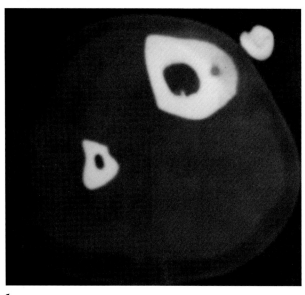

a

b

Figure 3.17 *Osteoid osteoma.* (*a*) *There is a smooth exostosis lying on the tibial shaft. It is uniformly dense and incorporates into the underlying cortex. No central lucency is seen.* (*b*) *In the CT scan the tibia shows cortical thickening within which lies the nidus. This shows early central mineralization.*

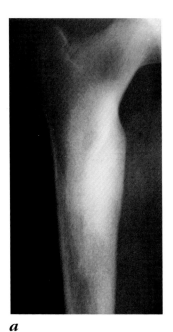

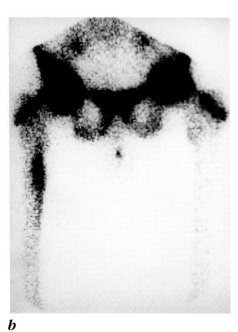

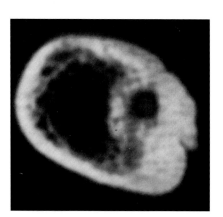

a　　　　*b*　　　　*c*

Figure 3.18 (*a*) *An osteoid osteoma in the region of the lesser trochanter presents as a sclerotic mound of cortical bone, often without visualization of the causative lesion.* (*b*) *Radioisotope bone scan showing focus of increase in uptake locally.* (*c*) *The CT scan through an area of bone sclerosis shows cortical thickening encroaching upon the medulla with a central mineralized nidus.*

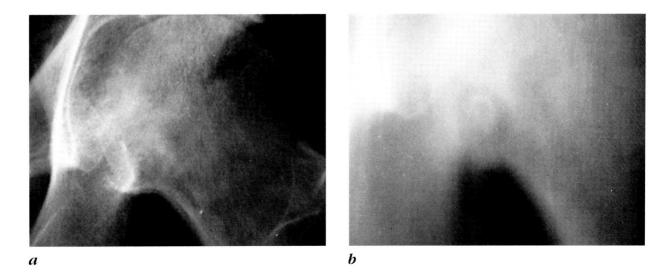

a

b

Figure 3.19 *Osteoid osteoma.* (*a*) *The radiograph shows osteoporosis but, at the medial aspect of the femoral head, there is patchy sclerosis with buttressing periostitis on the calcar.* (*b*) *The tomogram clearly reveals the radiolucent osteoid osteoma with central density. Osteoid osteomas excite little reactive sclerosis in the absence of local periosteum.*

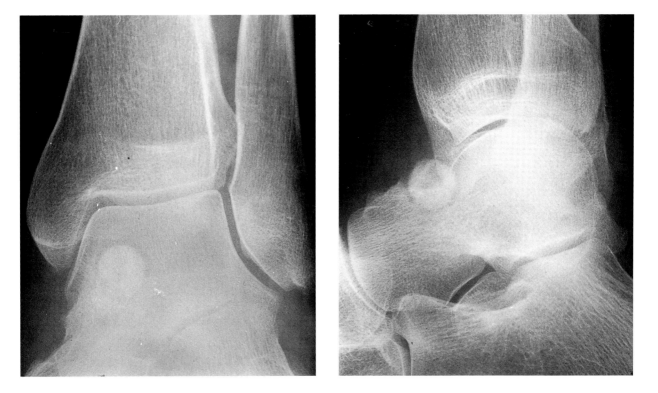

Figure 3.20 *Osteoid osteoma of the neck of talus. In this situation there is little surrounding sclerosis because of the lack of local periosteum. The lesion protrudes from the underlying bone into the adjacent soft tissues.*

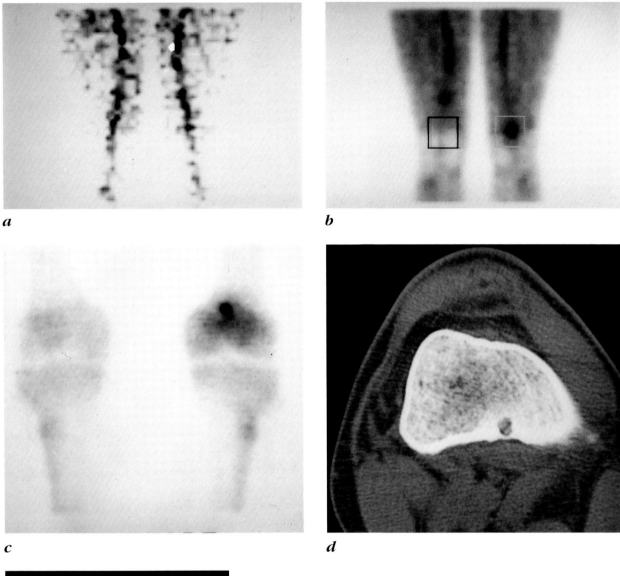

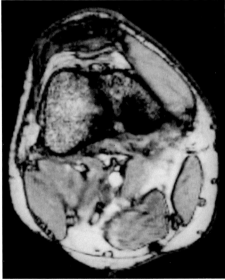

Figure 3.21 *Osteoid osteoma. (**a**) Radionuclide bone scan—vascular phase. There is no significant difference between the two sides. (**b**) On the blood pool image there is substantial accumulation of isotope in the vascular lesion. (**c**) The delayed scan confirms the local focus of increase in uptake in the osteoid osteoma. (**d**) The CT scan shows a well defined area of low attenuation with a little central mineralization. (**e**) The gradient-echo MR sequence shows the subcortical lesion of the distal femur posteriorly and some surrounding reactive new bone formation. It is not significantly mineralized. The area of reactive sclerosis seen on the CT scan is reflected in the low signal change around the vascular lesion on the MR scan.*

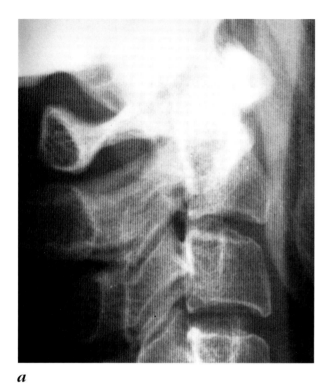

a

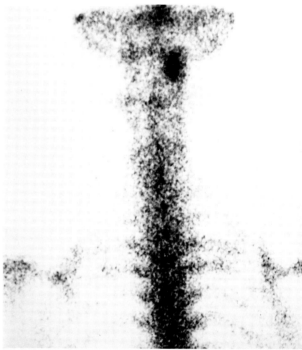

b

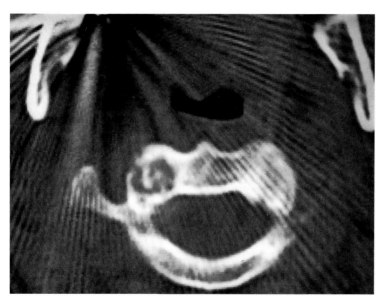

c

Figure 3.22 *Brodie's abscess. (**a**) The plain films show sclerosis in C2. (**b**) The posterior radionuclide bone scan shows increase in uptake around the lesion. (**c**) The CT scan demonstrates the lesion in the lateral mass with a sclerotic rim and a low attenuation centre within which sequestration is shown.*

hood, the metaphysis is commonly the site of infection. Dystrophic calcification occurs in the centre of the destructive infective lesion, which is surrounded by reactive sclerosis (Figure 3.22), and there may be an overlying periostitis as occurs with osteoid osteoma. The osteoid osteoma is more vascular and so shows up strongly on the blood pool isotope scan, while the centre of the Brodie's abscess is avascular. Similar changes are demonstrated at angiography; the

nidus enhances in the arterial phase, whereas a Brodie's abscess remains unenhanced.

Because the margin and the nidus are often heavily mineralized (only one-third having a purely lytic nidus), CT scanning of the osteoid osteoma is the imaging modality of choice after the plain radiograph (Figure 3.23). Areas of cortical sclerosis are particularly well shown at CT scanning and, on bone windows, the central nidus hidden on plain films may

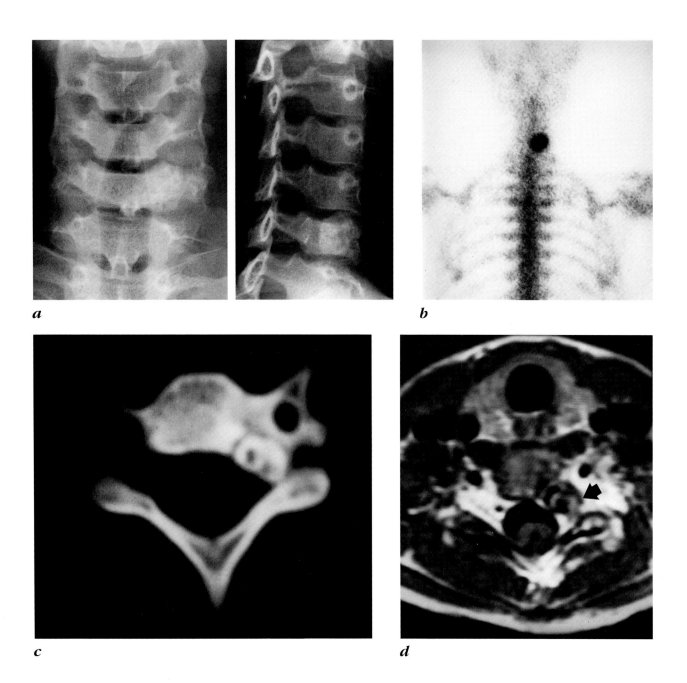

Figure 3.23 *Osteoid osteoma. (**a**) The plain films show intense sclerosis and expansion of the left pedicle of C6. (**b**) The radionuclide bone scan shows a solitary large focus of increase in uptake. (**c**) The CT scan shows bilobular ossification of the nidus. (**d**) The T₁-weighted MR image does not demonstrate the lesion as well as CT, but it does show a low signal cortical rim within which lies the vascular osteoid, itself showing central low signal mineralization (arrow).*

be revealed. Occasionally, the lesion may be bilobular (Figure 3.23). Osteoid osteoma may be excised directly under CT guidance.

At MR imaging, the changes shown are predictable. The cortical margin is of low signal and the nidus bright on T_2-weighted and fat suppression sequences, enhancing on T_1-weighting after administration of gadolinium. Nidal mineralization is seen as an area of central low signal intensity. The surrounding soft tissues are often oedematous (Figure 3.24).

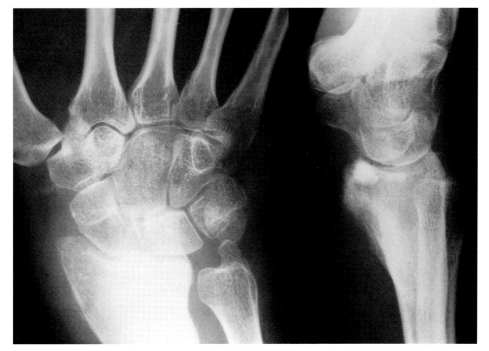

a

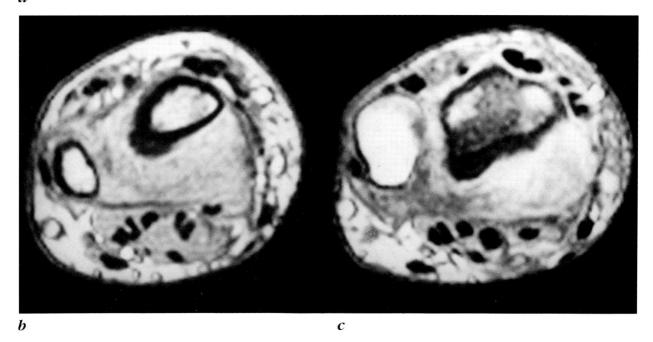

b   *c*

Figure 3.24 *Osteoid osteoma with oedema. (**a**) The plain films show an almost totally ossified nidus associated with irregular periostitis on the palmar surface of the distal radius. There is marked reactive sclerosis beneath the elevated periosteum. The carpus is demineralized. (**b**, **c**) The T₁-weighted MR images at different levels show cortical thickening and the nidus lying within this. The surrounding soft tissues are oedematous. (Reproduced from Burnett SJD, Stoker DJ (1995) Practical limitations of magnetic resonance imaging in orthopaedics. Curr Orth* **9***: 253–9, by kind permission of the authors and publishers.)*

OSTEOBLASTOMA

Incidence: 3.5% of benign bone tumours.
Sex: M:F = 3:1.
Age: 45% in the second decade, 30% in the third decade.
Site: see Figure 3.25. Some 40% of these lesions are seen in the spine, usually in the appendages (Figure 3.26) and, on occasion, *additionally* affecting the adjacent vertebral body, but generally not the body in isolation. Around 25% occur in long bones and, as

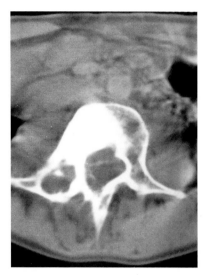

a

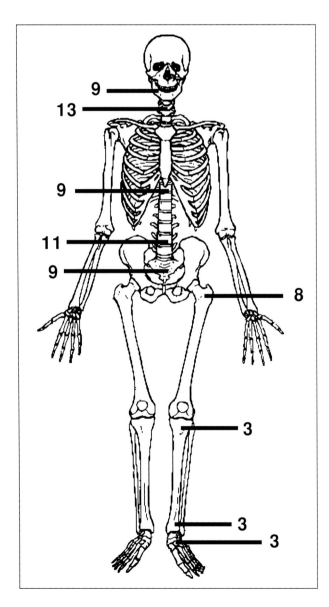

Figure 3.25 *Osteoblastoma: percentage distribution at major sites only. (After Unni, 1996, with permission.)*

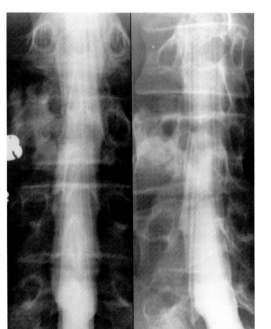

b

Figure 3.26 *Osteoblastoma in the right pedicle of the third lumbar vertebra. This 17-year-old male patient was referred for chronic back pain. A previous radiculogram had been negative. (**a**) The CT scan demonstrates marked sclerosis of the pedicle and transverse process, which is expanded and contains a lytic nidus with a central density. The adjacent part of the vertebral body also shows reactive sclerosis and enlargement. (**b**) The radiculogram shows the expanded, sclerotic vertebral appendage compressing the local nerve root. Referred pain was present.*

with osteoid osteoma (see page 118), the neck of the talus may be affected.

The lesion resembles osteoid osteoma radiologically and histologically, but may be painful by day as well as by night. They are larger than osteoid osteomas—over 1.5 cm in diameter, often with substantial reactive sclerosis (Figures 3.27 and 3.28).

The rare entity of *malignant osteoblastoma* is

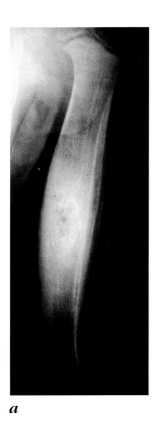 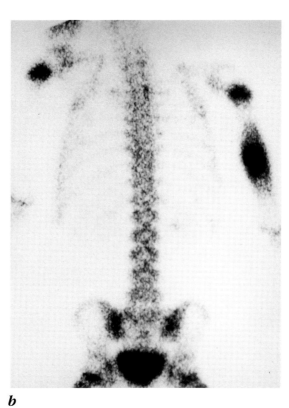

a   *b*

Figure 3.27 *Osteoblastoma. (**a**) There is a large, mainly mineralized lesion in the mid-shaft of the humerus associated with substantial reactive sclerosis and much cortical thickening. An extensive periostitis is demonstrated. The lesion is much larger than an osteoid osteoma would be. (**b**) The radionuclide bone scan shows a considerable area of increase in uptake comparable with the sclerotic area on the radiograph.*

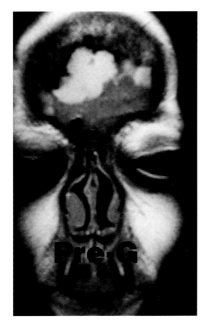 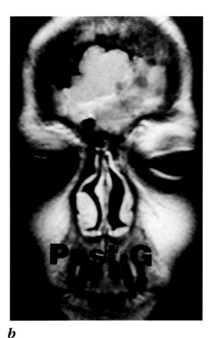

a   *b*

Figure 3.28 *Osteoblastoma of the frontal sinuses. These lesions are not common in the skull or mandible. (**a**) On the coronal T$_1$-weighted MR (pre-gadolinium) image, the lesion is lobulated and well demarcated. The inferior portion of the lesion is of soft tissue signal before enhancement, but shows substantial peripheral enhancement after gadolinium (**b**).*

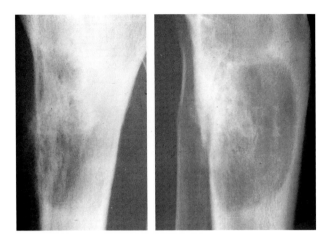

Figure 3.29 *Malignant osteoblastoma. A lytic lesion of the proximal tibia is well demarcated in parts but has broken through the cortex posteromedially and looks aggressive. There is ossification of soft tissues and within the large lesion, which is indistinguishable in many ways from an osteosarcoma.*

described; it may metastasize and this too is osteoblastic (Figure 3.29). These few cases however may represent osteosarcomas ab initio. The diagnosis rests on the histologist.

ENCHONDROMA

Incidence: 13% of benign bone tumours, though this probably underestimates the true incidence of these lesions which are often asymptomatic.
Sex: For solitary lesions, M:F = 1:1. For multiple lesions and in Maffucci's syndrome, males predominate; these patients present earlier in life.
Age: Seen at all ages from 10 years onwards.
Site: see Figure 3.30. 30–40% or more are seen in the hands, the majority in the phalanges, especially the proximal. Enchondromas are far less commonly seen in the feet. Some 10–20% are seen around the knee, mainly in the distal femur, but also in the proximal tibia and fibula. Statistically, therefore, a lucent phalangeal tumour is likely to be chondral in origin. It may be discovered incidentally, and pain is usually the result of fracture or malignant degeneration.

A solitary enchondroma is often metaphyseal in a small bone but extends to the bone end after skeletal fusion. With growth of the lesion, or in a small

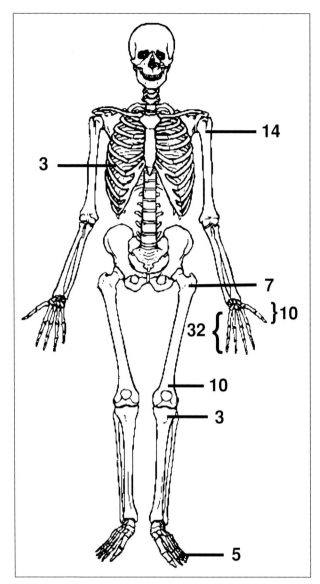

Figure 3.30 *Enchondroma: percentage distribution at major sites only. (After Unni, 1996, with permission.)*

bone, the cortex is scalloped and thinned, and the bone expanded. The zone of reactive sclerosis is always narrow, and calcific densities within the tumour may be multiple. The lesions can vary greatly in size so that soft tissue deformities result (Figure 3.31). Distinction from an infarct may be difficult (see page 147). Infarcts do not expand bone and are not associated with lucency. Their calcification tends to be peripheral rather than central, as in an enchondroma.

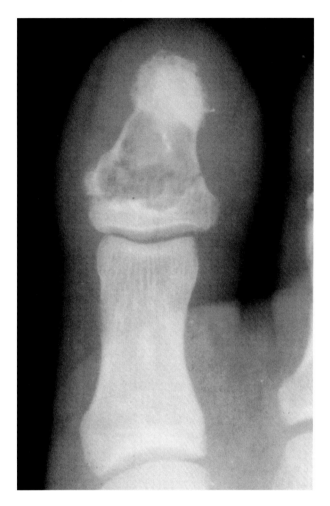

Figure 3.31 *Enchondroma. A pathological fracture has occurred, associated with soft tissue swelling. The lesion expands bone, thins the cortex endosteally and contains a few specks of calcification.*

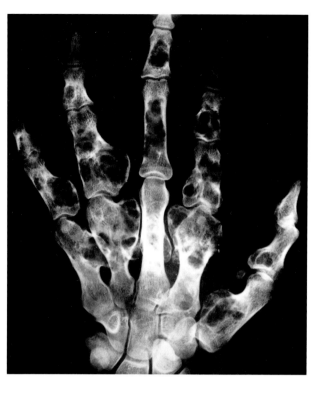

Figure 3.32 *Abnormalities of growth are seen in this patient with multiple enchondromas. There is quite marked metacarpal shortening. The lesions have caused gross deformity. They are well corticated, expansile and some contain punctate calcification.*

Multiple enchondromas are found mainly in the hands (Figure 3.32) and, to a lesser extent, the feet, and are dominant on one side of the body, as is often the case with fibrous dysplasia (see page 135). A linear type of cartilage deposition streaks proximally from the metaphysis (Figure 2.39).

Most lesions are small; larger tumours are more likely to fracture or to undergo malignant change. Pain, enlargement and loss of definition of central and marginal calcification suggest malignant transformation (Figure 3.4). A single enchondroma in a phalanx is not likely to become sarcomatous, but the incidence of sarcoma in multiple enchondromatosis and Maffucci's

syndrome is around 30% (see page 345).

CT demonstrates enchondromas well as they are corticated and centrally mineralized. At MRI, a lobulated, essentially homogeneous mass is demonstrated, containing low signal mineralized or calcified areas. This appearance is of course non-specific and a diagnosis should not be made on the basis of the MR appearances alone (Figure 3.33). Chondrosarcoma gives an inhomogeneous signal because of a fibrous stroma. Cortical breakthrough, soft tissue extension and a broad zone of transition are seen (for features of malignancy at MRI, see page 179).

Radionuclide bone scanning may reveal multiple lesions.

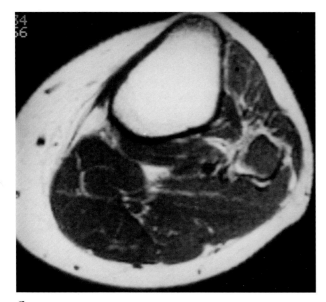

a

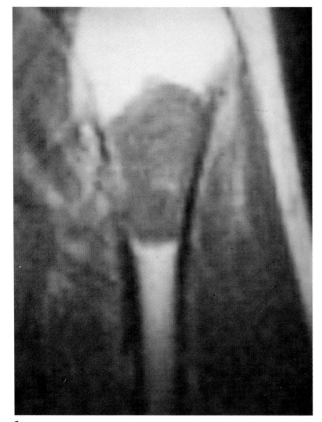

b

Figure 3.33 *Enchondroma of the fibula. On the axial and radial T$_1$-weighted MR images the appearances are non-specific. A soft tissue tumour replaces marrow fat. The lesion is well demarcated and not particularly mineralized.*

OSTEOCHONDROMA (see also Chapter 7)

(Synonyms: cartilage-capped exostosis; diaphyseal aclasia.)

Incidence: Osteochondromas constitute 35% of benign bone tumours. Most (90%) are solitary.

Sex: M:F = 3:2.

Age: 60% in the first two decades.

Site: see Figure 3.34. Generally in the metaphyseal regions of long bones, especially around the knee,

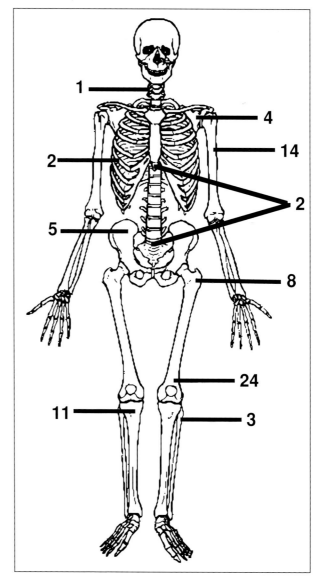

Figure 3.34 *Osteochondroma: percentage distribution at major sites only. (After Unni, 1996, with permission.)*

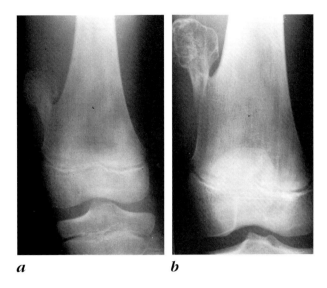

a   *b*

Figure 3.35 *Osteochondroma. (**a**) A well defined exostosis points away from the knee. There is undertubulation of the distal femoral metaphysis. (**b**) Its growth over 4 years is demonstrated.*

shoulder and iliac blade, as well as the scapula. Though not common, the lesion on the anterior scapular blade 'catches' on the thoracic musculature. Fusions occur at the joints around the tibia and fibula. Involvement of the spine leads to cord compression (see Chapter 8, page 402). Osteochondromas may be solitary or multiple.

The cortex of the lesion is contiguous with the adjacent cortex; similarly, the medulla is not separated from the underlying medulla but is contiguous with it, unlike as in bizarre parosteal osteochondromatous proliferation (BPOP) (see Chapter 5, page 302). The exostosis points away from maximum growth, for example, from the knee (Figure 3.35).

The cartilage cap ossifies progressively during the process of skeletal maturation. Eventually the entire cap shows mineralization. Pain and rapid growth may indicate malignant degeneration, as well as irregular mineralization and even resorption of previously mineralized areas (see page 197). The larger the cap, the more likely malignant degeneration, but growth of the cap usually ceases with skeletal maturity.

In patients with multiple exostoses, the metaphyses are undertubulated and growth anomalies result in deformity and shortening of long bones (see Chapters 5 and 7). The ulna is shortened and bulbous distally, and the radius overgrown.

Malignant degeneration is rare in a single osteochondroma and most cases of secondary chondrosarcoma arise in patients with multiple exostoses.

CHONDROBLASTOMA

Incidence: 4.8% of all benign lesions.
Sex: M:F = 2:1.
Age: Mainly (60%) in the second decade.
Site: see Figure 3.36. This is a rare, benign tumour of cartilaginous origin, which occurs before epiphyseal fusion and is a cause of local pain. Forty per cent occur around the knee, 20% around the shoulder,

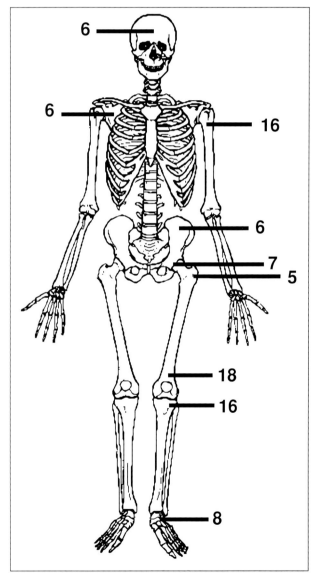

Figure 3.36 *Chondroblastoma: percentage distribution at major sites only. (After Unni, 1996, with permission.)*

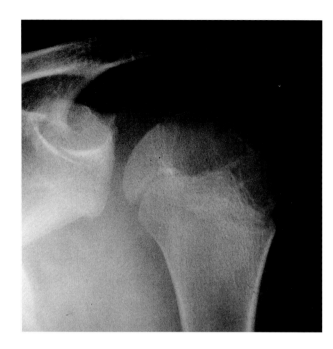

mainly in the upper humerus and greater tuberosity. Some 10% occur in the hindfoot.

The lesion is usually subarticular, but in the unfused skeleton (Figure 3.37). Giant-cell tumours occur at the same sites after skeletal fusion; the chondroblastoma however is usually smaller. It is typically surrounded by a well demarcated zone of reactive sclerosis and, therefore, is better defined than a typical giant-cell tumour. Approximately 50% of these lesions show central calcification. In the

Figure 3.37 *Chondroblastoma. A lytic lesion of the epiphysis before skeletal maturity is not due to a giant-cell tumour but is much more likely to be due to a chondroblastoma.*

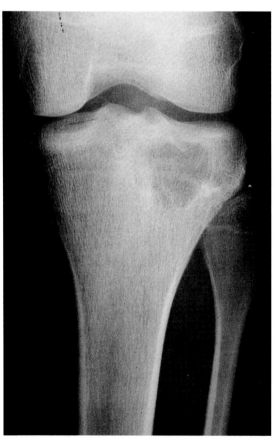

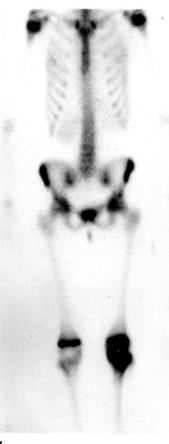

Figure 3.38 (a) *Chondroblastoma straddling the growth plate after epiphyseal fusion. There is no matrix mineralization. (b) The bone scan shows increase in uptake.*

a

b

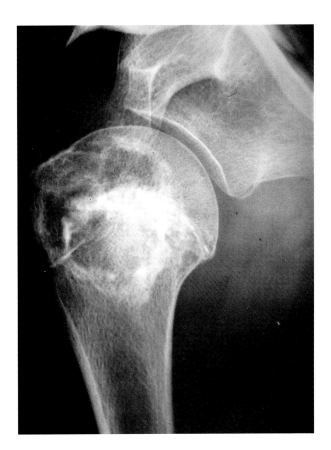

immature skeleton, both enchondroma and fibrous dysplasia are initially metaphyseal. Both lesions usually show matrix calcification, and reach the bone end only after fusion (Figure 3.38). The chondroblastoma can straddle the growth plate and extend into the metaphysis before fusion (Figure 3.39). CT confirms the nature of the lesion (Figure 3.40) and shows its benign nature. MR imaging is non-specific but confirms the benign nature of the lesion (Figure 3.41).

Figure 3.39 *Chondroblastoma. The growth plate is on the point of fusing and a lytic mineralizing lesion straddles it.*

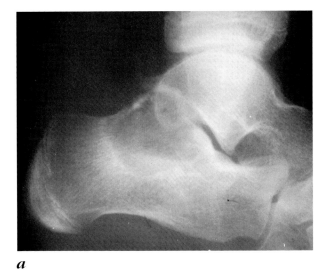

a

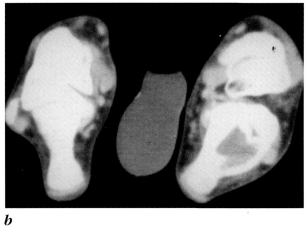

b

Figure 3.40 *Chondroblastoma (**a**, **b**). Ten per cent of these lesions occur at the heel. In this patient it is purely lytic and not mineralized. The skeleton is not yet mature (note the calcaneal apophysis). The tumour reaches the subtalar joint **in an immature skeleton**.*

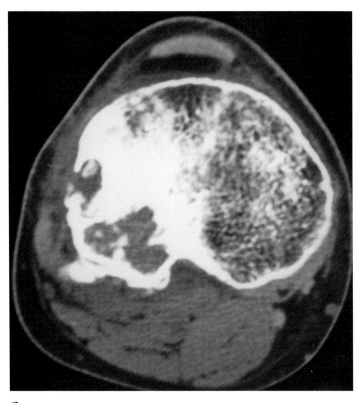

a

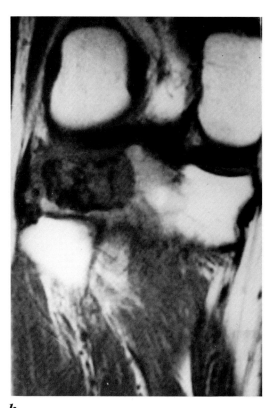

b

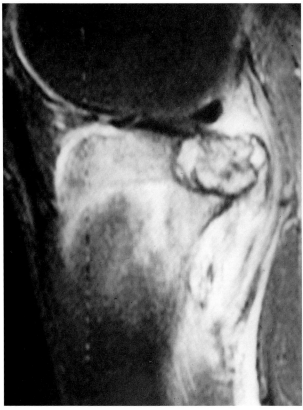

c

Figure 3.41 *Chondroblastoma.* (*a*) *The CT scan shows a destructive lesion of the proximal tibia with sparse central mineralization and quite marked, if ill defined, reactive new bone formation around the lesion. There is collapse of the cortex around the lesion.* (*b*) *Coronal* T$_1$-*weighted MR image shows the lesion extending to the articular cortex at the lateral tibial plateau. The articular cortex is thinned. The lesion is of soft tissue signal with interspersed areas of low signal corresponding to the mineralized matrix or trabeculae shown on the CT scan.* (*c*) *Sagittal fat suppression MR sequence demonstrating the intense vascularity of the surrounding bone and soft tissues, which is presumably related to a recent pathological fracture. The lesion itself is of mixed signal, varying from the hypervascular and bright to the low, presumably related again to the mineralized areas seen on the CT scan.*

CHONDROMYXOID FIBROMA

Incidence: 1.8% of benign neoplasms.
Sex: M:F = 1.6:1.
Age: 55% in the second and third decades.
Site: see Figure 3.42. Lesions typically occur at metaphyses, especially around the knee, with involvement of the tibia especially common (Figure 3.43). It is difficult to diagnose this lesion outside the tibia or the foot (Figure 3.44).

This rare, benign lesion is lytic, well demarcated with a few residual trabeculae. Matrix mineralization is not common. Lesions in the small bones of the foot come to occupy the bone and expand it (Figure 3.45). The diagnosis is made on the basis of age, site and appearance.

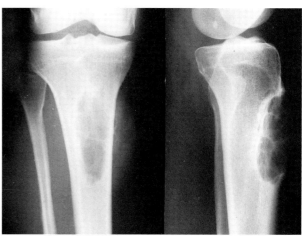

a

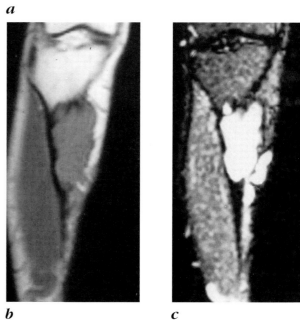

b   *c*

Figure 3.42 *Chondromyxoid fibroma: percentage distribution at major sites only. (After Unni, 1996, with permission.)*

Figure 3.43 *Chondromyxoid fibroma. (**a**) There is an anterior lesion at the proximal tibia. It is well defined and multiloculated. There is minimal matrix mineralization. It is associated with inferior cortical thickening. (**b**, **c**) The MR sequences show a well defined expansile lesion of soft tissue signal on the coronal T$_1$-weighted image (**b**), which is very bright on the fat suppression study (**c**).*

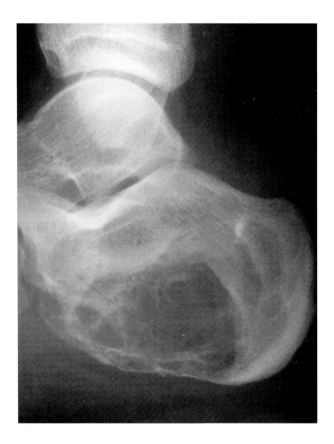

Figure 3.44 *Chondromyxoid fibroma of the calcaneus. The expansile, multilocular, osteolytic lesion resembles a giant-cell tumour or a very large aneurysmal bone cyst.*

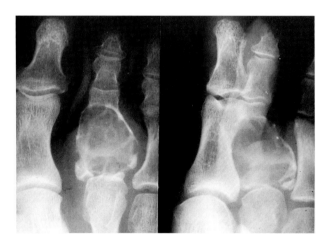

Figure 3.45 *Chondromyxoid fibroma of the proximal phalanx of the second toe. This is essentially undiagnosable. It resembles a solitary enchondroma but there is no matrix mineralization, merely residual trabeculation. A pathological fracture has been sustained.*

FIBROUS LESIONS

FIBROUS DYSPLASIA

Incidence: 80% of lesions are monostotic; 20% polyostotic. In Unni's series (Unni, 1996), there were 550 cases—an underestimate of the true total, as many are found incidentally. This would seem to represent around 12% of benign bone tumours.
Sex: Slight female predominance.

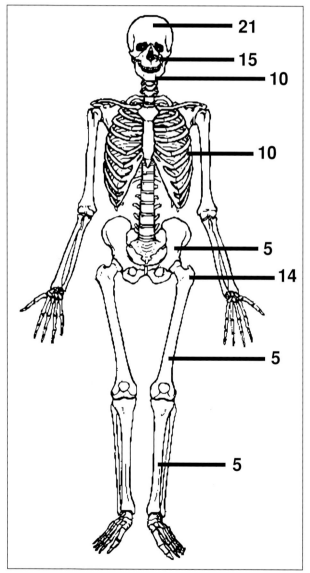

Figure 3.46 *Fibrous dysplasia: percentage distribution at major sites only. (After Unni, 1996, with permission.)*

Age: Mainly in the second and third decades.

Site: see Figure 3.46. After maturity, *monostotic* lesions are usually asymptomatic and present because of fracture which subsequently heals well. The lesions occur around the hip (Figure 2.72), in the jaws (Figure 2.73) and in the femoral (Figure 3.47) and tibial shafts (Figure 3.48). The maxilla is more often involved than the mandible (Figures 3.49 and 3.50). Rib lesions (Figure 3.51) are seen in an older age group than disease elsewhere.

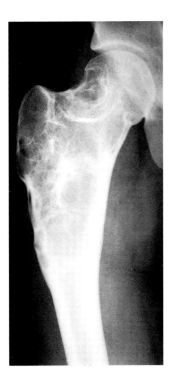

Figure 3.47
Fibrous dysplasia—expansion of the proximal femur. There is cortical thinning laterally with underlying cyst formation, but medially there is cortical buttressing. The bone is expanded. The lesion is well defined. It extends into the former epiphysis.

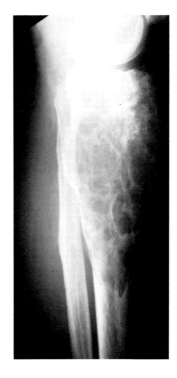

Figure 3.48
Fibrous dysplasia in the tibia extends to the proximal articular surface after epiphyseal fusion. Before fusion, lesions are metaphyseal.

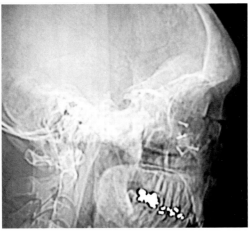

a

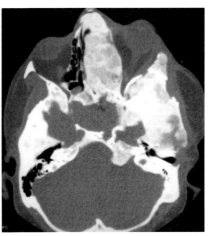

b

Figure 3.49 *Fibrous dysplasia. (**a**) There is thickening with sclerosis of the frontal bone, the floor of the anterior cranial fossa and the base of skull extending back to the sphenoid sinus, which is replaced by dense amorphous bone. (**b**) The CT scan shows expanded and abnormally mineralized bone occupying mainly the left side of the skull base. Considerable facial deformity is present.*

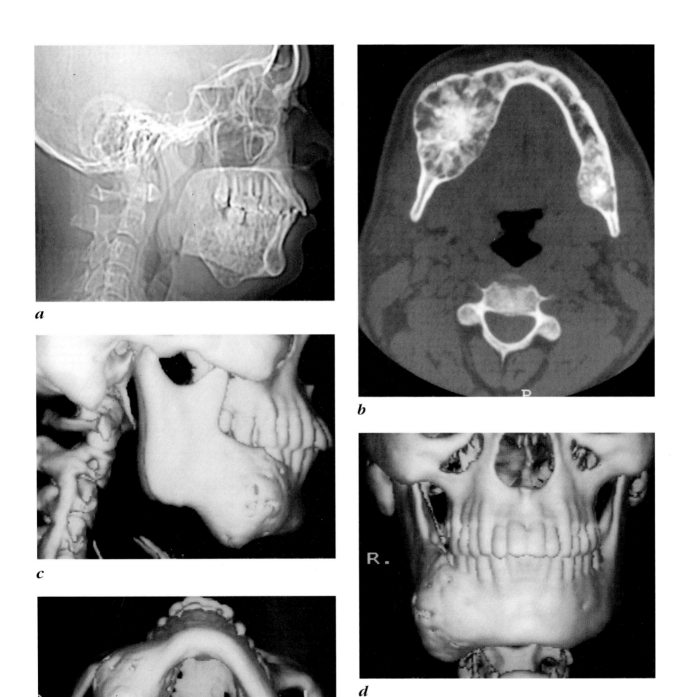

Figure 3.50 (*a*, *b*) *Fibrous dysplasia. There is quite marked expansion of the right body of the mandible and, to a lesser extent, the left. The cortex is displaced, thinned and shows endosteal scalloping. A variety of attenuation patterns are demonstrated, ranging from high, indicating mineralization, through ground-glass to low, indicating cyst formation. (c–e) A 3-D CT reconstruction of the patient's face prior to surgery.*

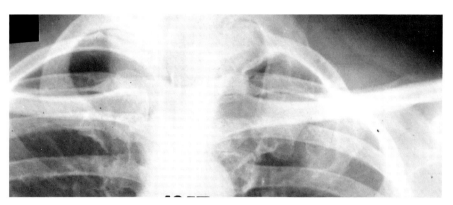

a

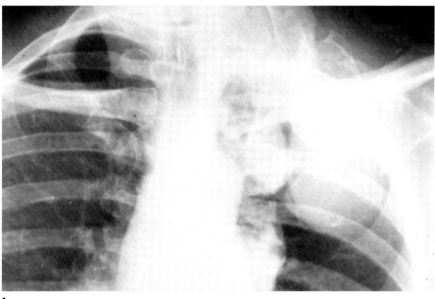

b

Figure 3.51 *(a, b) Fibrous dysplasia. Progressive expansion of the ribs over 11 years is shown in this patient with polyostotic disease. The enlargement of the ribs was progressive in this patient into the fifth decade. Rib changes occur in an older age group.*

Polyostotic disease presents in the first decade with pain and fractures, or with Albright's syndrome. Lesions affect the pelvis and lower limbs, metatarsals and phalanges in 70–90% of patients (Figure 3.52). Involvement of the skull and upper limbs is less common (Figure 3.52c,d). Malignant transformation is rare; osteosarcoma, fibrosarcoma (Figure 3.5), malignant fibrous histiocytoma and chondrosarcoma are seen.

In polyostotic disease, lesions, although widespread, have a predominance for one side of the body. There is a more random distribution to brown tumours in hyperparathyroidism and secondary deposits, where the lesions may have a similar appearance (Figure 1.76).

Patients with monostotic disease are often older. Pathologically, normal bone is very sharply demarcated from areas of fibrous tissue which may be multilocular and also contain cysts. The fibrous tissue undergoes ossification with horseshoe-shaped whorls of woven bone. The changes are usually diametaphyseal. Their growth often, but not inevitably, ceases with skeletal maturity. Occasionally they may progress in size, especially in the ribs, when the patients are often old, even in the sixth and seventh decades (Figure 3.51). After epiphyseal fusion, the tumours approach the articular surfaces and often expand bone (Figure 3.48).

Although initially radiolucent, the increasing ossification of the lesions in fibrous dysplasia gives them a mixed density, often with a very sclerotic margin or 'rind' (Figure 3.7). A ground-glass density may result (Figure 3.53). Expansion of bone occurs when the lesion reaches the cortex, which may be scalloped.

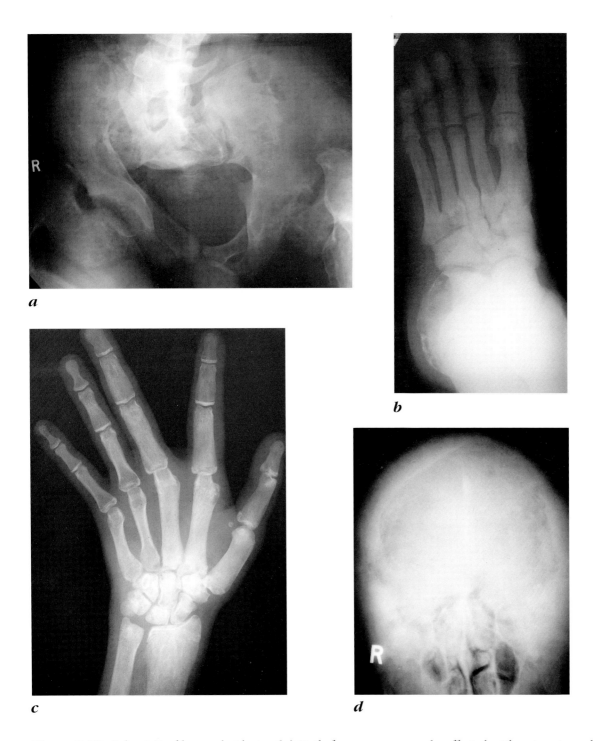

a

b

c

d

Figure 3.52 *Polyostotic fibrous dysplasia. (**a**) Both femora are severely affected with expansion, shepherd's crook deformities and an almost uniform ground-glass texture. The pelvis too is severely deformed, especially on the right, where the innominate bone is expanded, showing a ground-glass pattern. There is also involvement of the lowest lumbar vertebrae, which are expanded and show a ground-glass texture. (**b**) In the foot there is uniform expansion and almost total sclerosis with a ground-glass appearance. There is, however, cystic change in the calcaneus. (**c**) In the hand there is expansion of the first, second and third rays with a uniform ground-glass texture, also affecting the distal radius. (**d**) In this young man there is extensive involvement of the skull vault and base. There is gross thickening of the cranium which shows a uniform dense, highly mineralized pattern. (Professor C.E. Dent's case.)*

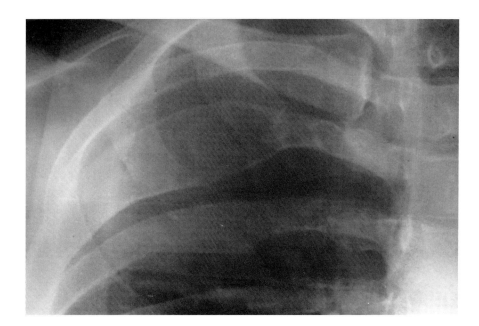

Figure 3.53 *Fibrous dysplasia. There is a cigar-shaped expansion of a rib which is typical of a benign lesion of bone. The cortex is thinned but preserved, and the lesion has a ground-glass texture.*

Since the lesions are soft, bowing and pathological fractures occur. In the femur, a 'shepherd's crook' deformity with expansion and bowing results (Figure 3.52a).

In the femoral neck the lesions may resemble bone islands. In the ribs, a cigar- or sausage-shaped lesion is common (Figure 3.53). Generally, benign tumours enlarge along the long axis of a bone rather than centrifugally as in malignant lesions (Figure 3.53). In the skull, a classic appearance of the vault is the blister lesion, a lenticular local expansion of bone of mixed or sclerotic density (Figure 3.54a). Paget's disease of the vault tends to be more widespread, crosses sutures and is less locally

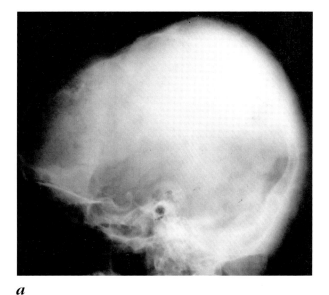

a

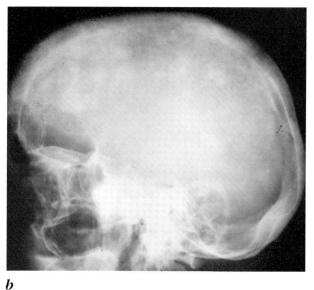

b

Figure 3.54 *(a) Fibrous dysplasia. Localized expansion and sclerosis of the skull vault results in a blister lesion. (b) In Paget's disease the texture may be identical but the patient is older and the distribution more widespread.*

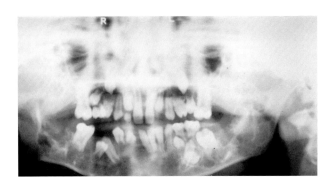

Figure 3.55 *Cherubism. Numerous cyst-like lesions are present in the mandible of this 14-year-old child, producing marked abnormality of dentition. Some of these lesions will be truly cystic but others have radiolucent fibrous tissue within them.*

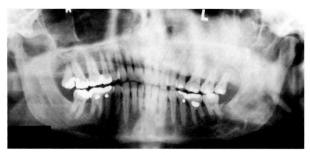

a

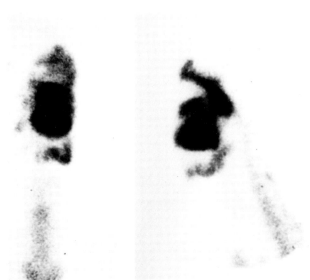

b

expansile, but the texture may be similar in both diseases (Figure 3.54b). Similarly, pseudo-Paget's disease of the skull in hyperparathyroidism (Figure 1.73b) is generally diffuse. Metastases too may be widespread and sclerotic in the absence of expansion.

The maxilla and the mandible of affected patients, usually children, show expansion, sclerosis and loss of normal bony markings, with obliteration of facial sinuses (Figures 2.73 and 3.52d).

A familial form, called *cherubism*, is localized to the maxilla and mandible and is unrelated to disease elsewhere (Figure 3.55). Here a predominantly cystic form of the disease is seen associated with maleruption and non-formation of teeth. The children have enlargement of the lower face and hence an angelic or cherubic look.

The spine is rarely involved in fibrous dysplasia (Figure 3.52a) or in enchondromatosis, but may be involved in diaphyseal aclasia. Cord compression may result (see Chapter 8, page 401).

Punctate ossification within fibrous lesions, with bone expansion, may cause the lesions to resemble enchondromas, but these may be more peripheral, commonly affecting the hands, feet, vertebral appendages and ribs. In enchondroma, a ground-glass texture is less usual than in fibrous dysplasia and the zone of reactive sclerosis around the lesions tends to be thinner and sharper (Figure 3.32).

Radionuclide bone scanning confirms the presence of an active lesion, and confirms or excludes lesions elsewhere (Figure 3.56). CT scans show the change

Figure 3.56 *Fibrous dysplasia. In this patient (**a**) the left antrum shows increased density and the left maxillary alveolus is enlarged by a sclerotic area of fibrous dysplasia. In the left side of the mandible, the expansile lesion is more radiolucent. (**b**) On the radioisotope bone scan, the anterior and lateral scans show a gross increase in uptake in the left maxillary antral region. Expansion is also confirmed. The abnormality extends to the base of the skull at the anterior cranial fossa. The lytic mandibular lesion seen on the plain radiograph is also seen as an area of increased uptake but, as expected, is not as prominent.*

because of matrix mineralization but also show cystic change within the lesions (Figures 3.57 and 3.58).

At MRI, fibrous tissue is heterogeneous and of low to intermediate signal on T_1-weighted images. Calcified areas exhibit lower signal. Cystic areas are bright on T_2-weighted and fat suppression sequences

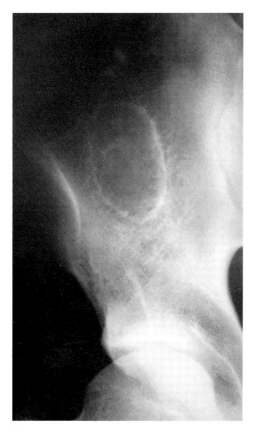

a

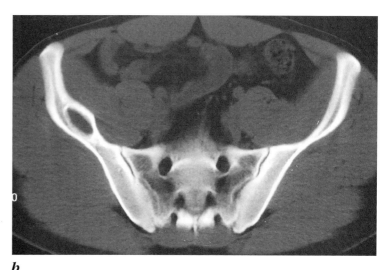

b

Figure 3.57 *Fibrous dysplasia. (**a**) An anterior view radiograph of the pelvis shows a well defined spherical lesion. There is a sclerotic margin and the centre of the lesion seems to show mineralization. The site is typical for this disease. (**b**) The CT scan demonstrates that the lesion is purely cystic, expansile and obviously benign. The mineralization seen on the plain film lies in the anterior thickened cortex and the lesion is truly cystic. These appearances may be due to a simple bone cyst, which infrequently occurs here.*

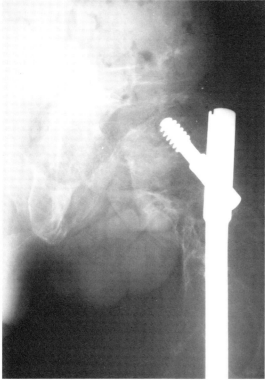

a

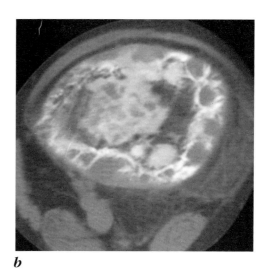

b

Figure 3.58 *Fibrous dysplasia. (**a**) The plain film in this much more severe polyostotic case shows marked enlargement and deformity of the pelvis and proximal femur. There is marked bony expansion with extensive cyst formation. The shepherd's crook deformity has been stabilized. (**b**) The CT scan shows the mixed pattern of tissues seen in fibrous dysplasia, ranging from cystic through ground-glass to heavily mineralized tissue.*

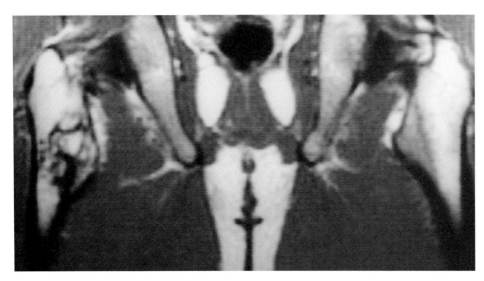

a

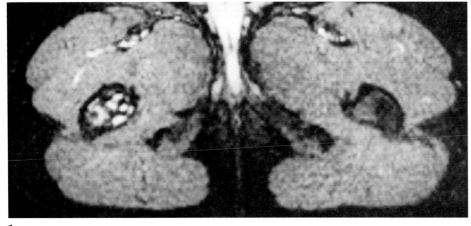

b

Figure 3.59 *Fibrous dysplasia. (**a**) On the coronal* T$_1$*-weighted and (**b**) axial fat suppression MR sequences, the well defined expansile lesion is seen to be multilocular with interspersed areas of mineralized bone or fibrous tissue.*

(Figure 3.59). Secondary malignant degeneration and aneurysmal bone cyst formation are well demonstrated at CT and MRI (Figure 3.60). Plain film, CT and MR changes in the skull are shown in Figure 3.61.

OSTEOFIBROUS DYSPLASIA

Osteofibrous dysplasia occurs in young patients, usually in the first decade of life and usually affects the middle third of the tibia, less often the fibula. Local swelling and deformity are the presenting symptoms, but pathological fracture may occur in the youngest patients, just after birth.

A large unicystic lesion occupies much of the midshaft of the bone. Subsequently, in older children, an anterior, multilocular, often well defined lesion is present (Figure 3.62). Bowing, fracture and pseudarthrosis may occur, as in neurofibromatosis, but no stigmata of neurofibromatosis are seen with osteofibrous dysplasia.

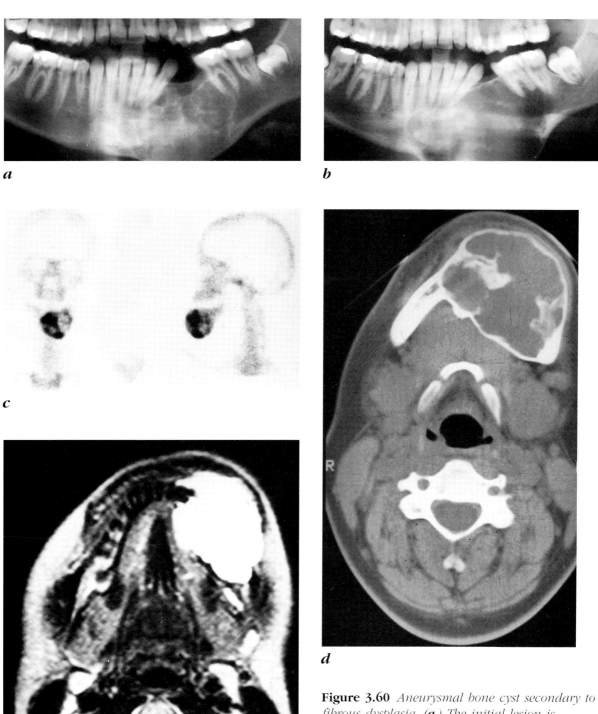

a

b

c

d

e

Figure 3.60 *Aneurysmal bone cyst secondary to fibrous dysplasia.* (*a*) *The initial lesion is moderately expansile.* (*b*) *Progressive expansion takes place inferiorly.* (*c*) *On the radionuclide bone scan there is a mixture of rim uptake and central uptake in this lesion.* (*d*) *The CT scan demonstrates a hugely expansile lesion with a thinned, but preserved cortex. The lesion is mainly of intermediate attenuation but there is some residual trabeculation.* (*e*) *The T$_2$-weighted MR sequence shows a large cystic lesion.*

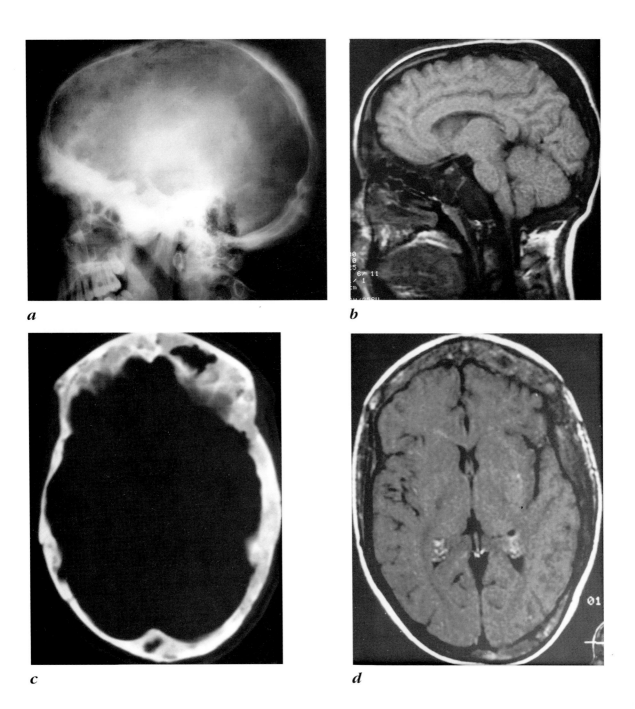

a

b

c

d

Figure 3.61 *Polyostotic fibrous dysplasia. (**a**) The plain film shows extensive involvement of the skull base which is sclerotic and thickened, but a rather more patchy and diffuse involvement of the vault, which shows areas of normal bone interspersed with areas of thickened bone. (**b**) On the sagittal T$_1$-weighted MR sequence the appearances exactly mirror the changes seen on the plain film. The skull base is thickened and shows extensive low signal with loss of marrow. Marrow is only to be seen in part of the frontal bone. The region of the frontal sinus, which is obliterated, shows a mixture of low and intermediate signal. The low signal indicates mineralization, the intermediate fibrous tissue, and the subcutaneous fat shows uniform bright signal. (**c**) An axial CT scan through the vault shows a typical mixed pattern of fibrous tissue which is partially mineralized. Cysts are also shown. (**d**) The same skull at MR imaging. On the T$_1$-weighted sequence the bright outer band represents fat beneath the skin; the thickened skull vault is seen as a mainly low signal area anteriorly.*

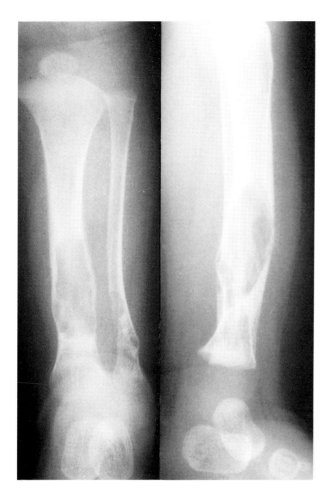

Figure 3.62 *Osteofibrous dysplasia in an infant. Changes are seen both in the tibia and the fibula. The expansile lesion of the tibia is associated with cortical thinning and minimal mineralization.*

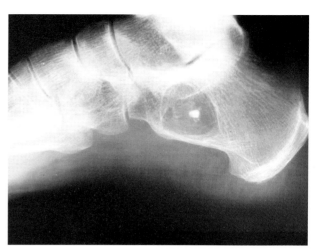

Figure 3.63 *Intraosseous lipoma. A characteristic site for this lesion, which is generally well defined with a thin zone of reactive sclerosis and contains a central fleck of calcium.*

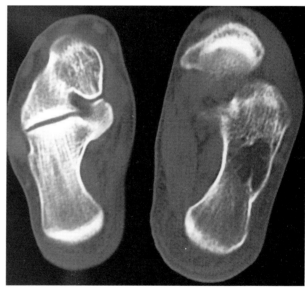

Figure 3.64 *Intraosseous lipoma at the calcaneus. At CT scanning the attenuation is that of fat.*

Anterior femoral lesions may resemble monostotic fibrous dysplasia and adamantinoma. Osteofibrous dysplasia generally occurs in significantly younger patients and the lesions often regress, unlike neurofibromatosis and fibrous dysplasia.

INTRAOSSEOUS LIPOMA

Matrix calcification is seen in this rather rare condition, which is slightly expansile and often seen in the calcaneus. The central calcification is extremely dense and the zone of reactive sclerosis narrow (Figure 3.63). Change at CT scanning is characteristic, as the bulk of the tumour is of fat attenuation, around −80 to −100 Hounsfield units (Figure 3.64). Similarly, at MRI, bright signal is obtained from fat on T_1-weighted sequences, which is suppressed on fat suppression sequences (Figure 3.65).

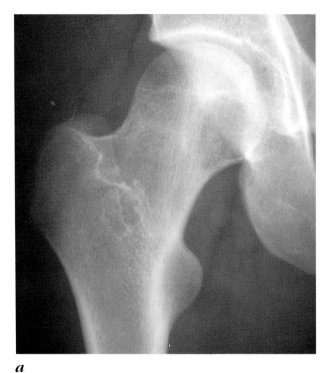

a

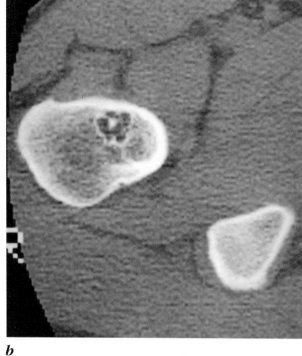

b

Figure 3.65 *Lipoma and chondroblastoma. (**a**) The plain film of the upper femur demonstrates two lesions. The proximal one straddles the growth plate, is fairly well defined and is a chondroblastoma. This is a totally tenable diagnosis at the age of 21. In the pertrochanteric region there is a multilocular radiolucent lesion with a narrow zone of transition and a thin rim of reactive sclerosis. (**b**) At CT scanning, the low attenuation of the central lipomatous lesion is confirmed and central mineralization is demonstrated. The overlying cortex is intact. (**c**) The MR scan shows bright signal within the lipoma on the T$_1$-weighted image. The chondroblastoma shows a non-specific appearance with a central low signal zone and a rather irregular zone of intermediate signal surrounding it, replacing marrow fat.*

c

INFARCTS

These result from deprivation of the blood supply to bone leading to death of its cellular elements with the trabecular framework initially remaining intact. The surrounding vital bone often loses density because of immobilization and hyperaemia, so that the infarcted area appears relatively sclerotic. Subsequent healing of the infarct involves peripheral revascularization, followed by laying down of a peripheral serpiginous

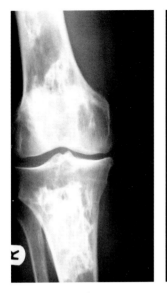
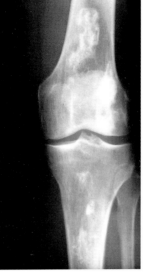
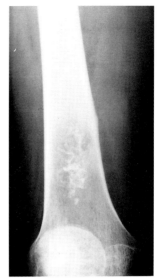
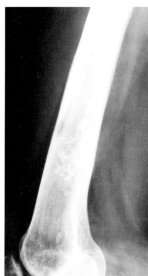

Figure 3.66 *Infarction in caisson disease. Areas of increased density are shown in all the bones around the knee joints. The densities are well defined, particularly peripherally, and although the increase in density is not uniform, there is no overt bone destruction surrounding them. The bones are not expanded, there is no endosteal scalloping and no periosteal reaction.*

Figure 3.68 *Chondrosarcoma. Many of the features of early chondrosarcoma are similar to those seen in the infarct due to caisson disease. There is distal femoral medullary stippling associated with proximal areas of radiolucency. In this patient, however, there is an early periosteal reaction with slight expansion of the bone which is maximal in the region of the bony lucency. The change is unifocal, unlike infarction when it may often be generalized at major joints.*

Figure 3.67 *Multifocal areas of subarticular infarction. On the coronal T_1-weighted (**a**) and sagittal fat suppression (**b**) MR sequences the appearances are symmetrically disposed around the joint. There is much cystic change in this chronic lesion, which contains fluid surrounding areas of necrotic bone, but there is also some intermediate signal change replacing marrow, presumably fibrous tissue.*

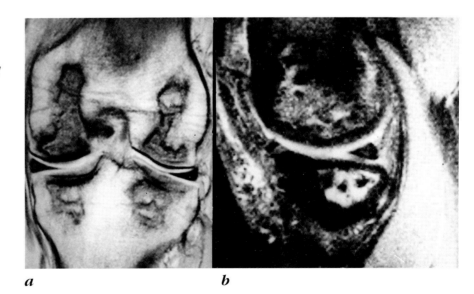

a   *b*

zone of sclerotic new bone at the margins of the infarct, which is referred to as the zone of creeping substitution. Centrally, fibrous tissue undergoes dystrophic calcification. An ovoid or circular sclerotic rim results, surrounding a central area of relative lucency which contains speckled densities.

These lesions are usually at epiphyseal and metaphyseal sites, are often multiple and symmetrical

Table 3.10 Causes of medullary infarction.

Old age, presumably due to atheroma
Sickle-cell anaemia
Gaucher's disease
Caisson disease
Infection
Radiation
Pancreatitis
Vasculitis
Chemotherapy

(Figures 3.66 and 3.67), but occasionally are solitary. Collapse results in epiphyses such as the hip. The local bone is never enlarged.

The lesions most closely resemble fibrous dysplasia, enchondroma, and chondrosarcoma (Figure 3.68); bowing or expansion are however not present. The zone of peripheral sclerosis around an infarct is serpiginous. A detailed patient history often elicits the cause of infarction (Table 3.10).

Fibrous dysplasia may be 'warm' (Figure 3.69) or 'hot' (Figure 3.56) on an isotope bone scan. Initially the infarcted area is 'cold' on the scan, may be hot during the phase of active repair, but is subsequently quiescent.

LYTIC LESIONS

GEODES—CYSTS IN THE ARTHRITIDES

Geodes usually present as cysts of varying size in the subarticular regions, in weight-bearing areas, such as hips, knees, and ankles, but are also seen in the wrists and elbows. Rheumatoid and osteoarthritis are the main causes of these lesions, and therefore they are usually associated with evidence of major joint disease, such as joint narrowing, deformity, erosions or osteophytosis.

These well defined cystic lesions normally reach the articular surface and are totally lucent (Figure 3.70). They vary in size, may be 5 or 6 cm in diameter, and multiple. The cyst may fill with contrast at arthrography. The thinned, overlying articular cortex is weakened and may collapse—so-called 'structural failure'. The aetiology of the cyst is usually determined on inspection of the local joint and any other joints involved, in rheumatoid or osteoarthritis, for example (Figure 3.71)

Patients may be middle-aged or elderly, but an identical lesion is found in young, often athletic, patients. The solitary traumatic subchondral cyst is probably the result of microfracture with synovial intravasation, so that the surrounding joint will be normal (Figures 3.72 and 3.73).

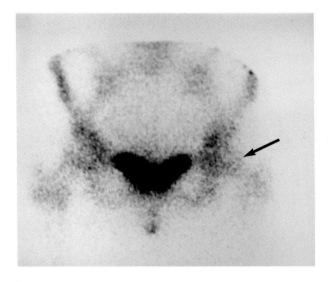

Figure 3.69 *Fibrous dysplasia. The radioisotope scan shows minimal increase in uptake in the region of the abnormal femoral neck (arrow).*

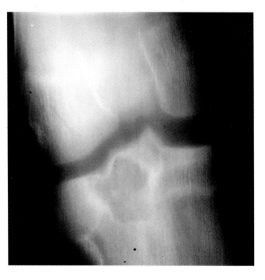

Figure 3.70 *This subarticular cyst was associated with local collapse of the weight-bearing surface of the joint (linear tomogram).*

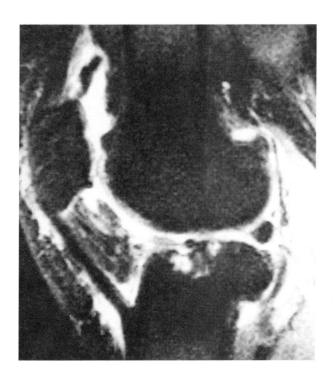

Figure 3.71 *Cystic change in osteoarthritis. On this sagittal fat suppression MR sequence pre-patellar oedema is shown together with oedema of the fat pad and a large effusion. Irregularity of articular surfaces is shown in this patient with chronic osteoarthritic change. There are at least two cysts filled with fluid in the proximal tibia.*

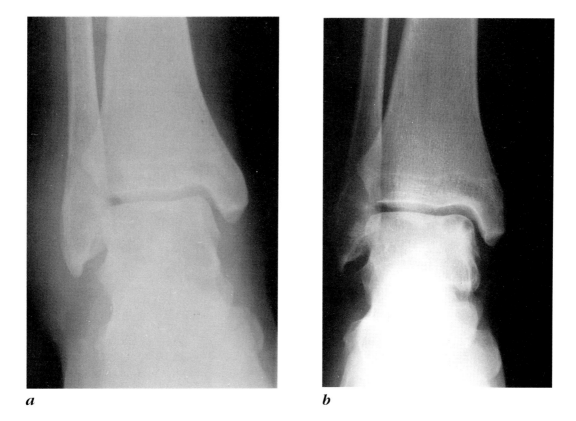

a *b*

Figure 3.72 *Post-traumatic subchondral cyst. (**a**) The initial radiograph shows soft tissue swelling around the ankle but no other abnormality. (**b**) Six months after trauma, a cyst is seen in the talus, but the joint is not narrowed.*

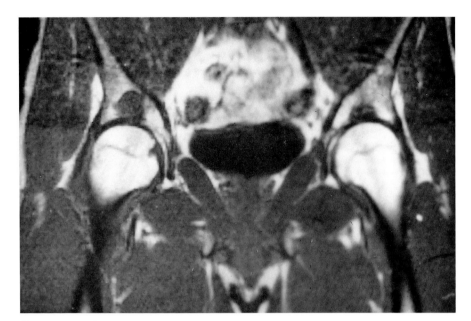

a

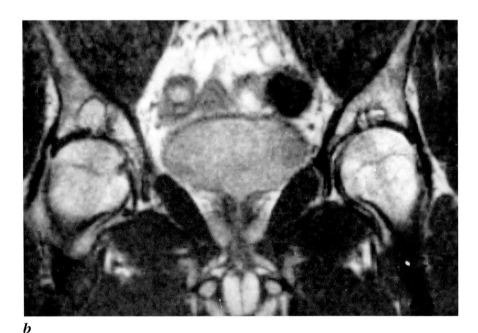

b

Figure 3.73 *Acetabular cysts in a 26-year-old male. The fluid-filled cysts are of low signal on T$_1$- (**a**) and bright on T$_2$-weighted MR images (**b**).*

CHRONIC OSTEOMYELITIS

This is occasionally the cause of a lytic lesion in the metaphysis before skeletal fusion (Figure 3.74), but reaching the joint line in the mature skeleton. One or many bones may be affected. If the lesions are multiple, the cause may be tuberculosis or chronic granulomatous disease. The surrounding bone may be expanded, there may be a periostitis, and the adjacent joint narrowed because of cartilage destruction by the inflammatory process (Figure 3.75).

Chronic osteomyelitis may also show a finger-like process of bone destruction—'tunnelling'—extending from the main lesion (Figures 3.76 and 3.77); this is pathognomonic of infection.

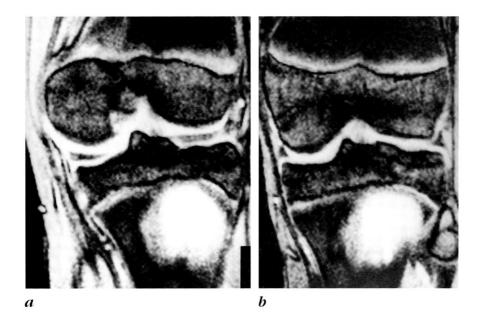

a   *b*

Figure 3.74 *(a, b)* Brodie's abscess. Radial T_1-weighted MR sequences demonstrate a well defined focus of increased signal at the metaphysis. Note also the increased signal at the distal metaphyses abutting the growth plate. This is normal and corresponds to the band-like zone of increase in uptake at the metaphysis seen on a radioisotope bone scan in the immature skeleton.

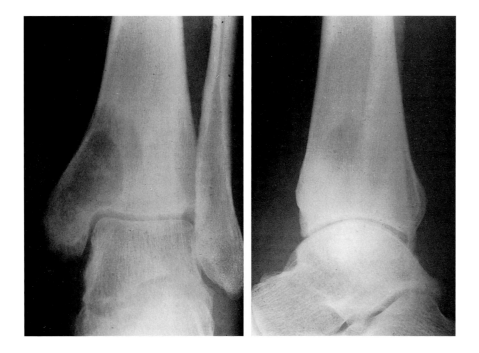

Figure 3.75 Chronic osteomyelitis. In this patient with an immune defect, expansion of the medial malleolus associated with a large cystic lesion can be seen, due to chronic infection.

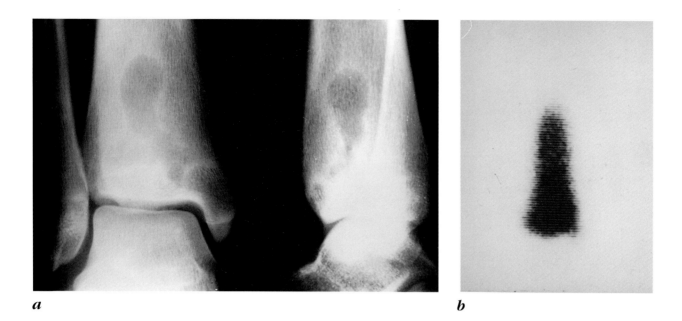

Figure 3.76 *Chronic osteomyelitis. (**a**) Cystic change and tunnelling with bone expansion are shown. (**b**) The radioisotope bone scan demonstrates substantial increase in uptake in the distal tibia.*

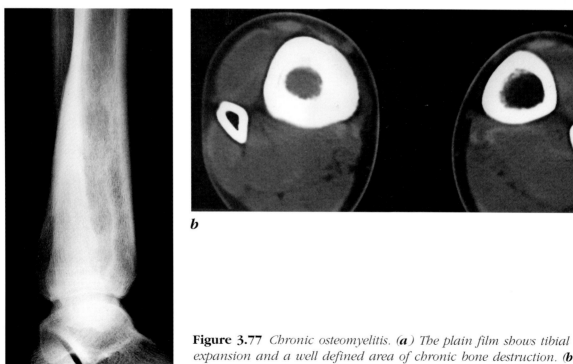

Figure 3.77 *Chronic osteomyelitis. (**a**) The plain film shows tibial expansion and a well defined area of chronic bone destruction. (**b**) The CT scan confirms cortical thickening with medullary encroachment.*

GIANT-CELL TUMOUR

Incidence: 20% of benign bone tumours.
Sex: M:F = 1:1.5.
Age: 35% in the third decade.
Site: see Figure 3.78.

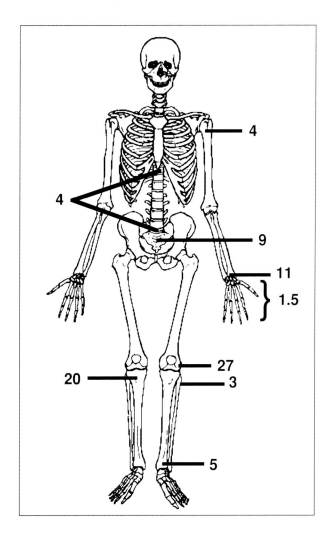

Figure 3.78 *Giant-cell tumour: percentage distribution at major sites only. (After Unni, 1996, with permission.)*

Figure 3.80 *Giant-cell tumour. A lytic lesion erodes the lesser trochanter which has been expanded and avulsed. This sequence is also seen with metastatic deposits in this region, but these usually occur over the age of 45 years. Between 20 and 40 years of age, a giant-cell tumour is perhaps more likely at this previous apophysis.*

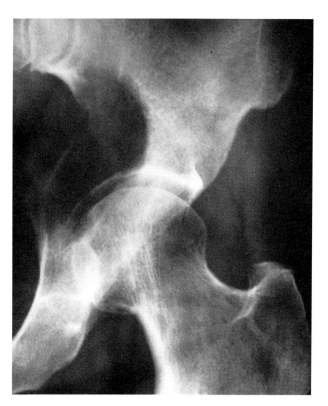

Figure 3.79 *Giant-cell tumour. A poorly defined lytic lesion extends to the acetabular surface of the hip joint.*

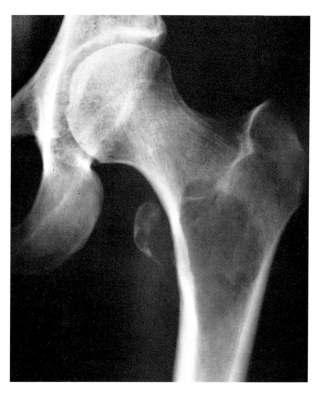

This is a relatively common, often highly expansile lesion lying at the joint surface of a mature bone (Figure 3.79). Both previous epiphyses and apophyses are affected (Figure 3.80). The most common sites are around the knee, the distal radius, shoulder and sacrum, but any bone may be affected (Figure 3.81). It is occasionally described in the metaphysis of an immature skeleton, but should not be diagnosed before epiphyseal fusion. Inevitably, the lesion extends to an articular surface, although this may not always be obvious. On the anteroposterior view of the knee, for instance, the tumour may appear not to extend to the distal femoral articular surface, but the lateral view shows that it extends to the femoral cortex anteriorly at the patello–femoral articulation (Figure 3.82).

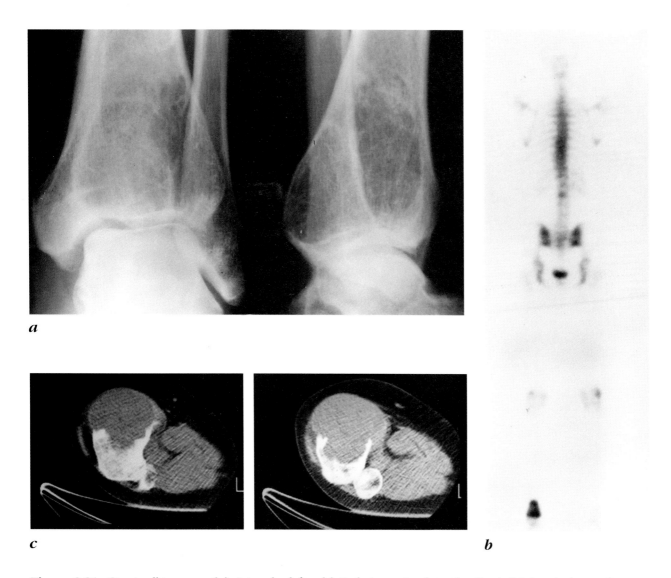

a

c

b

Figure 3.81 *Giant-cell tumour. (**a**) A poorly defined lytic lesion extends to the distal tibial articular surface. There is slight expansion of bone and residual septation. (**b**) The radioisotope bone scan shows this to be a solitary lesion. (**c**) The CT scan shows the expansile and destructive nature of the lesion, but a thin rim of bone remains at its periphery.*

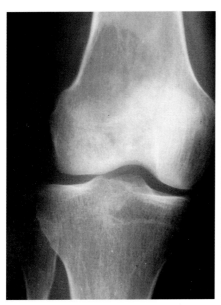 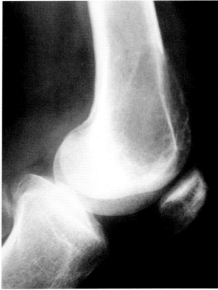

a

Figure 3.82 *Giant-cell tumour.* (*a*) *On the anteroposterior view the lesion does not seem to extend to an articular surface, but, on the lateral view, the patello–femoral joint is affected by a well defined lytic lesion in a mature skeleton.* (*b*) *The isotope scan confirms the highly vascular nature and cellularity of the tumour.*

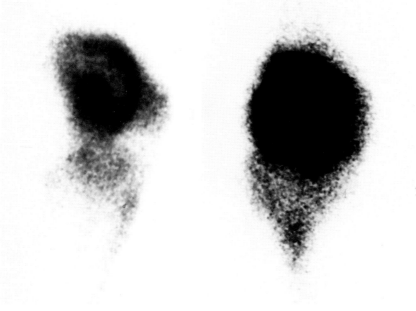

b

The lesion is generally lucent and may contain a few strands of residual trabecular bone. It is unusual to see the speckled, punctate calcification seen in fibrous and cartilaginous lesions. Fibrous lesions, such as fibrous dysplasia and malignant fibrous histiocytoma (see page 194), may be subarticular and have little or no matrix calcification and occasionally cannot be differentiated from giant-cell tumours (Figure 3.83). Cystic lesions may also have this appearance on plain films (Figure 3.3).

The margin of a giant-cell tumour is never very sclerotic and is often blurred. In places, there may be quite a wide zone of transition, suggesting local bone infiltration, which is also a feature of malignant fibrous histiocytoma.

Chondroblastomas occur in a subarticular situation prior to epiphyseal fusion but may persist beyond fusion. These are generally smaller, have a better visualized, more sclerotic margin and central calcification in 50–60% of cases. Giant-cell tumour rarely

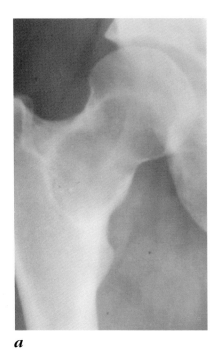

a

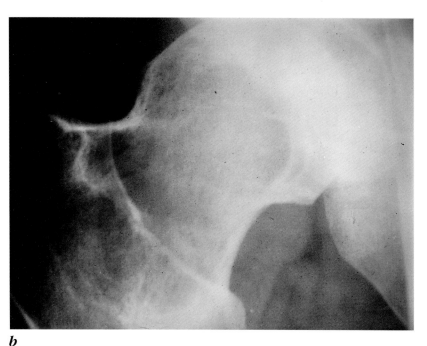

b

Figure 3.83 (*a*) *Fibrous dysplasia. A typical appearance in the upper femur is of an area of ground-glass bone texture surrounded by a thick rind of reactive sclerosis. The bone is expanded and the appearance resembles that of a giant-cell tumour reaching the margins of the articular surface but, in this case, the lesion is much better defined. (**b**) Giant-cell tumour. A lytic expansile lesion is shown in the neck of the femur which extends to the articular surface of the head. There is a fairly narrow zone of transition with a little reactive sclerosis.*

mineralizes. Some dystrophic calcification is occasionally and unusually seen, or reactive bone histologically.

The chondromyxoid fibroma also has a predilection for the tibia, may reach the articular margin and is indeed difficult to diagnose in an extra-tibial situation. It is rare, however.

The lesion that causes the greatest confusion, radiologically and pathologically, is the aneurysmal bone cyst. This is discussed elsewhere (see page 163), but is most commonly seen around the knee, as is the giant-cell tumour. It may reach the articular surface, and initially may be only minimally expansile, though eventually is larger. Again, it does not mineralize, but contains residual septation, often more than the giant-cell tumour (Figure 3.84). Both lesions are highly vascular and are strongly positive on a radionuclide bone scan. CT of both lesions shows expansion and cortical thinning (Figure 3.81). In a giant-cell tumour, fractures of the thinned and displaced cortex are seen in up to 40% and cortical breakthrough in up to 50%, in association with a soft tissue mass (Figure 3.85).

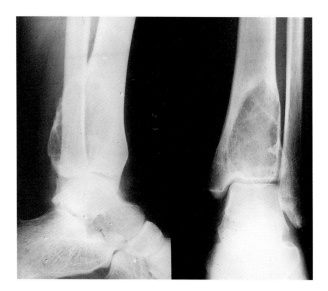

Figure 3.84 *Aneurysmal bone cyst. This is radiologically indistinguishable from Figure 3.81, which is a giant-cell tumour. The lesion is well demarcated and contains residual trabeculation. In this patient it also reaches the distal tibial articular surface.*

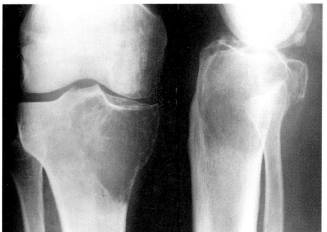

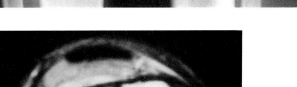

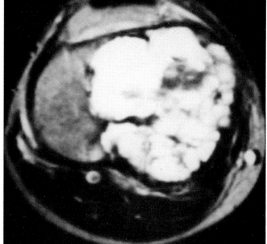

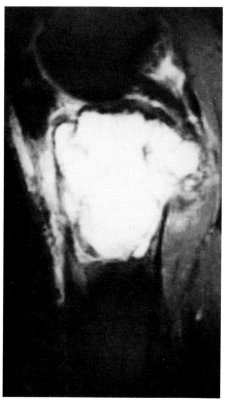

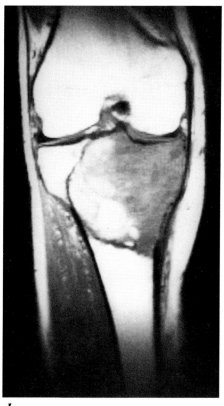

Figure 3.85 *Giant-cell tumour. (**a**) There is a slightly expansile osteolytic lesion of the tibia reaching the articular surface of the medial tibial plateau. Posteriorly there is substantial expansion with apparent cortical thinning and breakthrough. There is a very ill defined zone of transition and no reactive sclerosis. Residual septation is demonstrated within the lesion. (**b**) A sagittal fat suppression MR image confirms the changes seen on the lateral radiograph. There is, in addition, substantial oedema in the surrounding soft tissues. The posterior cortex of the proximal tibia is defective and the lesion is expansile. Distally the zone of transition appears much more narrowed than was apparent on the plain film, and residual septation is demonstrated in this highly vascular tumour. (**c**) An axial T$_2$-weighted MR image shows the hypervascularity of the lesion with interspersed low signal areas, perhaps due to fibrous septae or residual trabeculation. The margin of the lesion is lobulated. (**d**) The coronal T$_1$-weighted MR image shows a clear transition between tumour and marrow fat.*

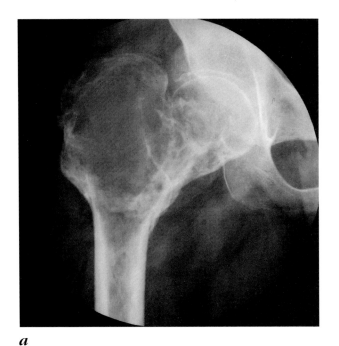

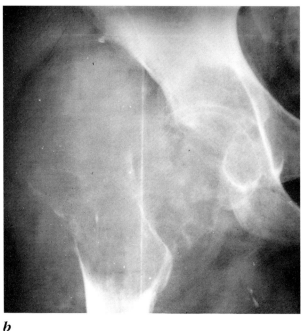

a   *b*

Figure 3.86 *Subarticular giant-cell tumour of the balloon type. (**a**) The tumour extends to the articular surface of the femoral head but there is no opportunity for expansion adjacent to the acetabulum. It also extends into the greater trochanter. It may have arisen here because this was an apophysis. Here, there is no obstruction to expansion, and the greater trochanter is hugely enlarged. (**b**) The subsequent film shows further expansion of the lesion. There is a well defined soft tissue mass, hugely expanding the greater trochanter. A few strands of cortex remain around the lesion. Aneurysmal bone cysts also cause balloon-like lesions, but these occur in younger patients. Large lesions of this type are rarely seen in the UK.*

At CT, if fluid–fluid levels are seen and the appearances are otherwise compatible with a giant-cell tumour, it is likely that secondary aneurysmal bone cyst formation has occurred in association with a primary giant-cell tumour. The fluid–fluid level is the result of (1) internal septation and (2) separation of serum above the degraded products of blood cells.

A giant-cell tumour may be eccentric in over 50% of cases, extending to the corner of the articular surface but, with growth, may occupy the entire subarticular zone. This is seen at the distal radius, proximal humerus and fibula. The cortex of the articular surface is often markedly thinned but remains faintly visible and the adjacent shaft often bulges aneurysmally (Figure 3.86). The junction between the bulging tumour and the normal adjacent shaft may be quite angular and buttressed with periosteal new bone, resembling a Codman's triangle. This is a feature of large, rapidly growing lesions such as the giant-cell tumour and aneurysmal bone cyst. It is not seen with a simple bone cyst. A renal or thyroid metastasis may also resemble a giant-cell tumour but the latter is solitary and usually seen between 18 and 45 years of age.

At MR imaging the uncomplicated giant-cell tumour is often of intermediate soft tissue signal on T_1-weighted studies, and bright with T_2-weighting; it may be heterogeneous. Generally, a better definition of the tumour margin is seen with MRI than on plain films (Figure 3.87), as is soft tissue extension following cortical breakthrough or fracture. The appearances at MRI are otherwise non-specific, allowing for the site and compatibility of signal with the lesion. Secondary aneurysmal bone cyst formation shows a rapidly expansile and highly vascular lesion.

Multifocal benign lesions are rarely seen. 'Benign' giant-cell tumours may also metastasize into lung, presumably by a vascular path, often in patients whose primary lesions show local recurrence after curettage. The metastases apparently have an ossified margin at CT scanning.

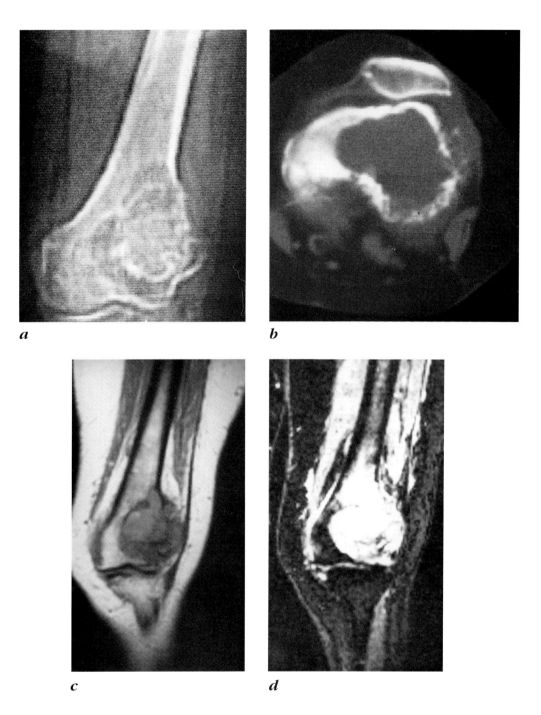

a *b*

c *d*

Figure 3.87 *Giant-cell tumour at the distal femur. (**a**) The scanogram shows an eccentric osteolytic lesion reaching the knee joint surface. There is lateral cortical breakthrough. (**b**) The CT scan confirms the presence of a lesion of soft tissue attenuation but which has no mineralization. The overlying cortex is expanded and irregular. There is local soft tissue swelling. (**c**) On the coronal T$_1$-weighted MR image a large non-homogeneous soft tissue mass breaks through the lateral femoral cortex and displaces the adjacent soft tissues. Its medullary aspect is well defined inferiorly but superiorly there is patchy loss of marrow signal. (**d**) The coronal fat suppression MR sequence shows the lesion to be well defined on its inferomedial aspect and of mixed signal. There are some low signal strands within it, possibly due to fibrous tissue. Superiorly, there is substantial marrow oedema; this is presumably related to the pathological fracture. There is also increase in signal in the adjacent soft tissues.*

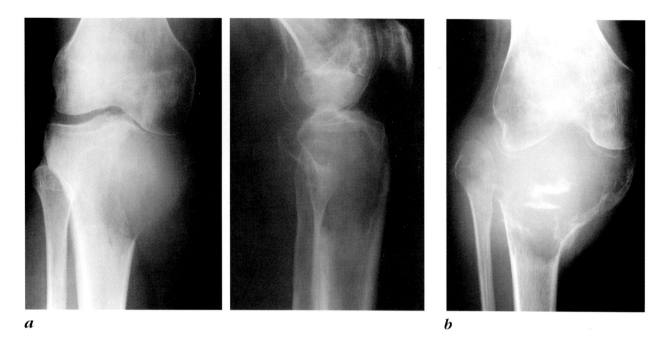

a   *b*

Figure 3.88 *(a) Another patient with giant-cell tumour has a typical lesion at the proximal tibia. (b) The lesion has been curetted and packed with bone chips but has recurred. Further expansion results in a balloon tumour.*

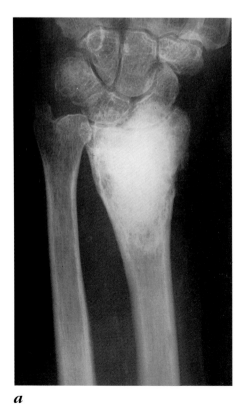

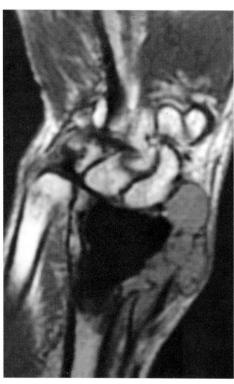

Figure 3.89 *Giant-cell tumour. (a) The initial radiograph shows curettage and cementing of a giant-cell tumour of the distal radius. (b) Coronal T$_1$-weighted MRI. A soft tissue recurrence is shown together with resorption of bone at the cement–marrow interface proximally. The cement gives a signal void.*

a   *b*

Local recurrence often takes place from the periphery of the lesion, with resorption of packed bone chips (Figure 3.88). Very aggressive looking margins may indicate malignant potential, but generally there is no correlation between the radiological appearance and the behaviour of the tumour. Recurrence also occurs after cement replacement (acrylic cementation). Bone resorption and soft tissue extension are seen (Figure 3.89).

The spine is rarely involved. The vertebral body is usually affected rather than the appendages, normal bone is completely replaced by the lucent tumour, and early expansion causes cord compression (Figure 3.90).

Malignant giant-cell tumour

These are rare and are often secondary to irradiation of a benign giant-cell tumour. The secondary malignancy may be an osteosarcoma or a malignant fibrous histiocytoma. The radiological changes are those of malignant bone disease. A primary malignant form is rarer still.

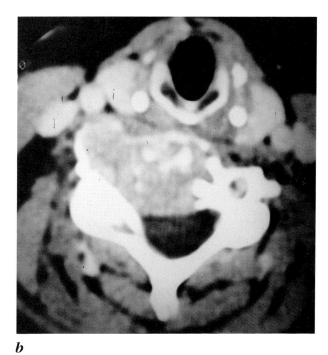

b

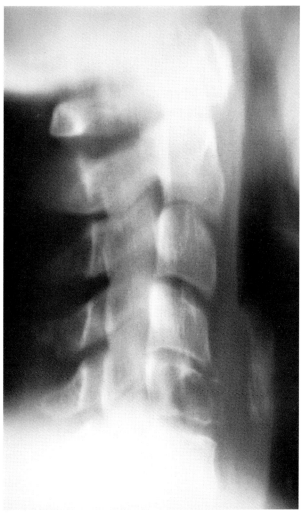

a

Figure 3.90 *Giant-cell tumour of C5. (**a**) An expansile osteolytic lesion of the body of C5 is demonstrated. (**b**) The CT scan shows osteolysis and expansion with cortical thinning. There is residual mineralization within the lesion, and early cord compression.*

ANEURYSMAL BONE CYST

Incidence: This is difficult to quantify as 28% are secondary. There were 289 cases in the Mayo Clinic series, and they saw 2469 benign tumours of bone, i.e. 10% were aneurysmal bone cysts but these lesions are not included in the neoplastic category.
Sex: A slight majority are female (56%).
Age: 76% in the first and second decades.
Site: see Figure 3.91. After the knee, the spine is a common site and generally the posterior elements are involved.

The lesion originates in the metaphysis of a long bone before skeletal fusion and, therefore, is totally unlike a giant-cell tumour in location, at least initially. After fusion, the aneurysmal bone cyst can extend to the articular surface and may be so expansile that occasionally the thinned and elevated cortex is not radiologically visible, and may often only reappear after radiotherapy (Figure 3.92). The angle between the cyst and the cortex is often filled with lamellar buttressing periostitis (Figures 3.93 and 3.94) as seen with giant-cell tumours. Its zone of transition may be sharp or poorly defined.

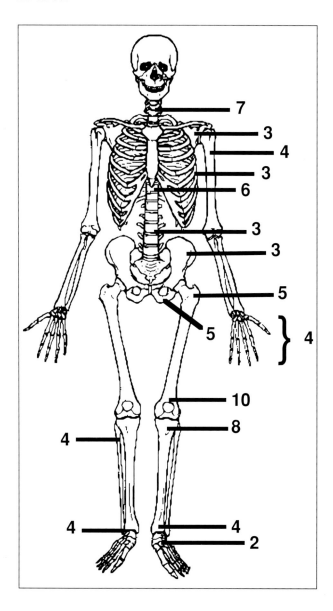

Figure 3.91 *Aneurysmal bone cyst: percentage distribution at major sites only. (After Unni, 1996, with permission.)*

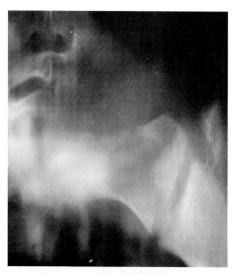

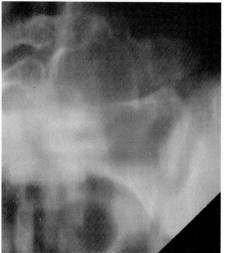

Figure 3.92 *Aneurysmal bone cyst. The initial linear tomogram (top) shows expansion and lysis of the vertebral appendages on the left with a large soft tissue mass. After radiotherapy (bottom) the cortex is visualized and the expansile nature of the lesion can be seen.*

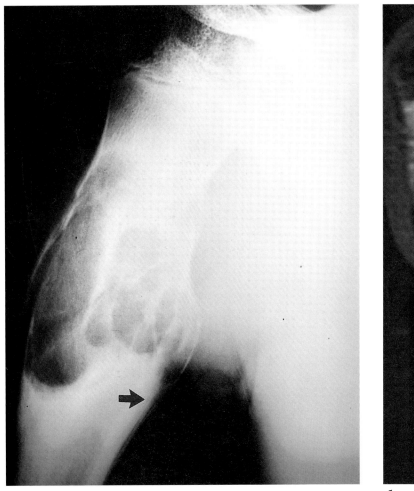

a

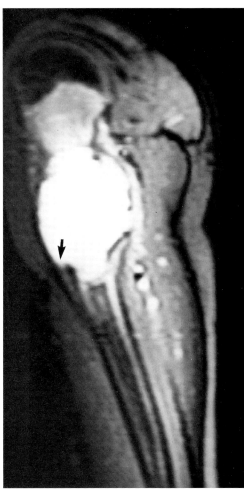

b

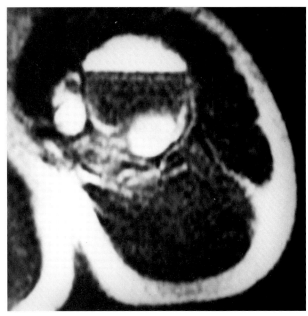

c

Figure 3.93 *Aneurysmal bone cyst. (**a**) The plain film shows an expansile multilocular lesion. Buttressing periostitis is seen at the angle between the normal cortex and the expanded bone (arrow). (**b**) Fat suppression MRI. The vascular nature of the lesion is shown by bright signal on this sequence. A Codman's triangle is demonstrated as an area of low signal cortical bone at the tumour–bone interface (arrow). (**c**) The axial T$_2$-weighted MR sequence of the proximal humerus, demonstrates fluid–fluid levels within the lesion.*

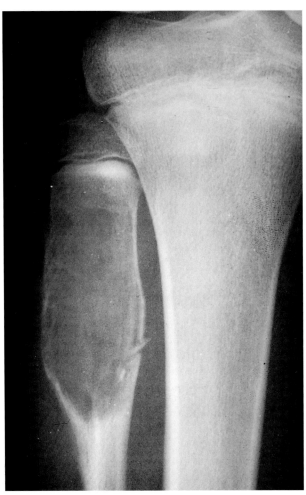

a

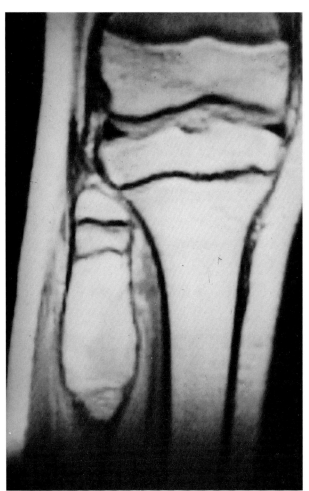

b

Figure 3.94 *Aneurysmal bone cyst with a pathological fracture. (**a**) An expansile lesion is demonstrated at the proximal fibular metaphysis. A Codman's triangle is shown. Pathological fracture has occurred. (**b**) The coronal T$_1$-weighted MR sequence demonstrates an expansile lesion. (**c**) On the axial T$_2$-weighted MR image the cortex is thin and fractured medially. Fluid–fluid levels are seen. There is substantial haemorrhage in the soft tissues.*

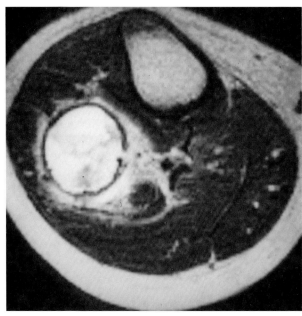

c

A feature of this lesion (Figure 3.95) is rapid growth under observation which often is faster than in malignant lesions such as renal or thyroid metastases. These usually occur after the age at which the aneurysmal bone cyst or giant-cell tumour is seen. Aneurysmal bone cysts are lightly trabeculated and commonly occur in the femur and humerus. In the spinal appendages, they show expansion and lucency (Figure 3.92), unlike the similarly situated osteoblastomas and enchondromas which show density (Figure 3.8). In the spine, an aneurysmal bone cyst can occasionally cross posteriorly from one set of vertebral appendages to the next (Figure 2.18), as may other vascular lesions, vanishing bone disease, haemangiomata and myeloma. Many lesions are eccentric and metaphyseal. Aneurysmal bone cyst may present with a pathological fracture.

Radionuclide bone scanning shows a generalized or rim uptake (Figure 3.96). As well as expansion of the bone, linear tomography and CT scanning may show a thin cortical rim otherwise invisible on the plain film. At CT and MRI, fluid–fluid levels are seen. These changes at MRI are more complex than at CT as blood degradation may be at different stages (Figures 3.97 and 3.98). At MRI the fluid-filled lesion is clearly separated from medullary fat. Arteriography demonstrates the vascularity of the lesion (Figure 3.99).

Rarely, some lesions are *solid* (Figure 3.100). This occurs when soft tissue obliterates the cyst.

Histologically, an association between giant-cell and other tumours and aneurysmal bone cyst is found (Figure 3.101). Up to 28% of aneurysmal bone cysts arise as a secondary phenomenon in such various conditions as giant-cell tumour, chondroblastoma, fibrous dysplasia and telangiectatic osteosarcoma.

The simple bone cyst (see below) occurs at three typical sites—the proximal humerus, the proximal femur and the calcaneus—but is generally smaller than an aneurysmal bone cyst. Apart from a giant-cell tumour, a telangiectatic osteosarcoma (see page 184) may occasionally mimic an aneurysmal bone cyst.

SIMPLE BONE CYST

The incidence of simple bone cyst is difficult to quantify as it usually only presents after a pathological fracture. (This lesion is also not classified as a tumour in the Mayo Clinic series.)

These lesions occur in children before epiphyseal fusion, and usually before aneurysmal bone cysts. They occur in the proximal humeral and proximal femoral metaphyses, as well as in the calcaneum (Figure 3.102). The lesions are well demarcated, only minimally expansile (Figure 3.103), and contain little or no residual trabeculation with no marginal periosteal buttressing. With time, they are left behind by growth at the epiphyseal plate so that they appear to migrate to the mid-shaft of the bone (Figure 3.104). They are not usually seen in the mature skeleton. Presentation usually occurs because of a pathological fracture. Occasionally, there may be a 'falling leaf' sign of cortical fragments moving in the serous contents of the cyst (Figure 3.103). After fracture, the 'falling leaf' sign is shown at CT and MRI; fluid–fluid levels may also be present at CT and MRI. In the calcaneus, CT and MRI emphasize the difference between this lesion and a lipoma.

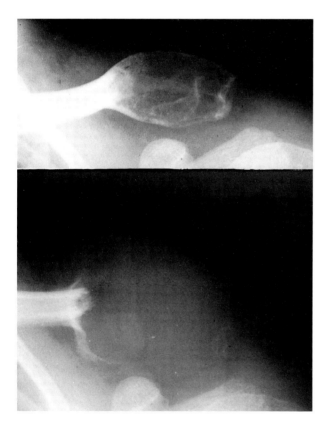

Figure 3.95 *The initial radiograph of an aneurysmal bone cyst of the clavicle shows a highly expansile lytic lesion resembling a giant-cell tumour of the distal end of the clavicle (top). Rapid growth produces a balloon tumour (bottom). Aneurysmal bone cysts tend to occur in a slightly younger age group but, occasionally, the lesions cannot be distinguished.*

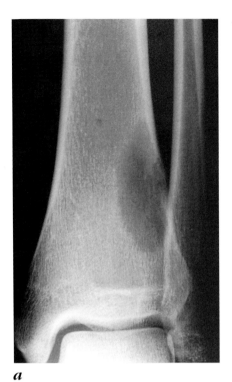

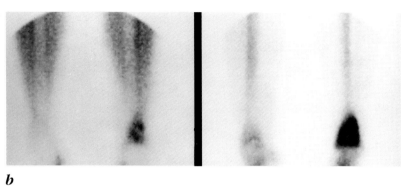

a

b

Figure 3.96 *Aneurysmal bone cyst. (**a**) The plain radiograph shows an eccentric osteolytic lesion with cortical thinning. (**b**) Extensive increase of uptake at radioisotope bone scanning.*

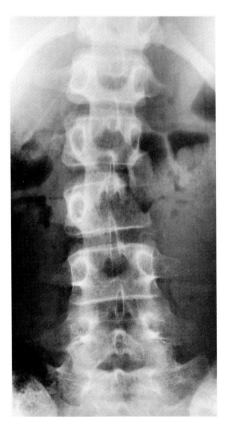

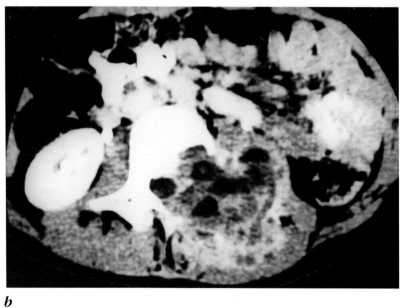

a

b

Figure 3.97 *Aneurysmal bone cyst to show fluid–fluid levels. (**a**) The plain film demonstrates a large aneurysmal bone cyst occupying the left aspect of the vertebral body and posterior elements of a mid-lumbar vertebral body. (**b**) The CT scan confirms the presence of a large expansile osteolytic lesion with multiple fluid–fluid levels.*

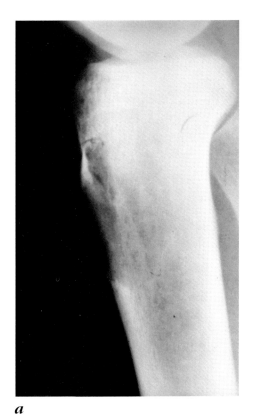

a

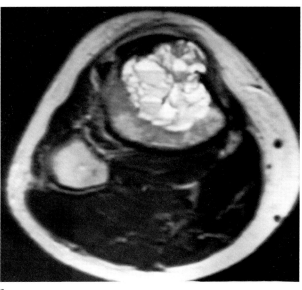

b

Figure 3.98 *Aneurysmal bone cyst. (**a**) The plain film shows an osteolytic lesion of the anterior tibia with cortical thinning and expansion of bone. (**b**) Complex multilocular fluid–fluid levels are demonstrated on the axial T₂-weighted MR sequence.*

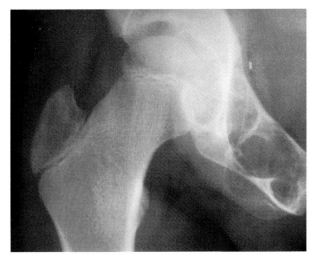

a

Figure 3.99 *Aneurysmal bone cyst. (**a**) In this young patient the pubis is the site of a multilocular expansile lesion. There is cortical thinning but not breakthrough. Residual trabeculation remains. (**b**) The angiogram shows the intense vascularity of the lesion.*

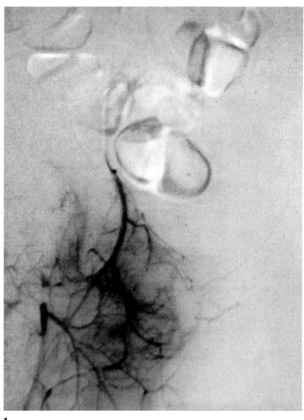

b

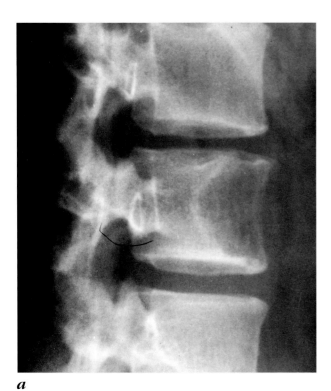

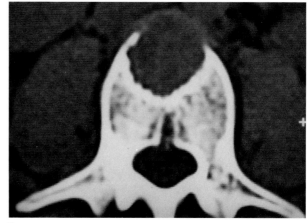

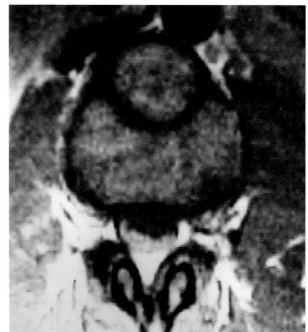

Figure 3.100 *'Solid' aneurysmal bone cyst. (a) The plain radiograph shows a well demarcated lytic defect of the anterior vertebral body of L3. (b) The CT scan confirms this change and shows an anteriorly displaced, thin cortical rim. (c) The axial T₁-weighted MR sequence shows the lesion to have signal identical to the marrow of the vertebral body. It is no longer cystic.*

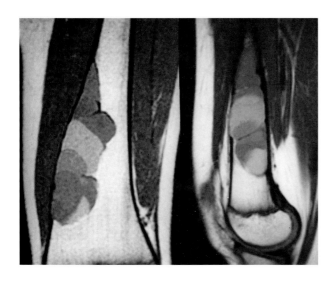

Figure 3.101 *Aneurysmal bone cyst secondary to non-ossifying fibroma. On these coronal and sagittal T₁-weighted MR images a complex and beautiful pattern of mixed signal is shown.*

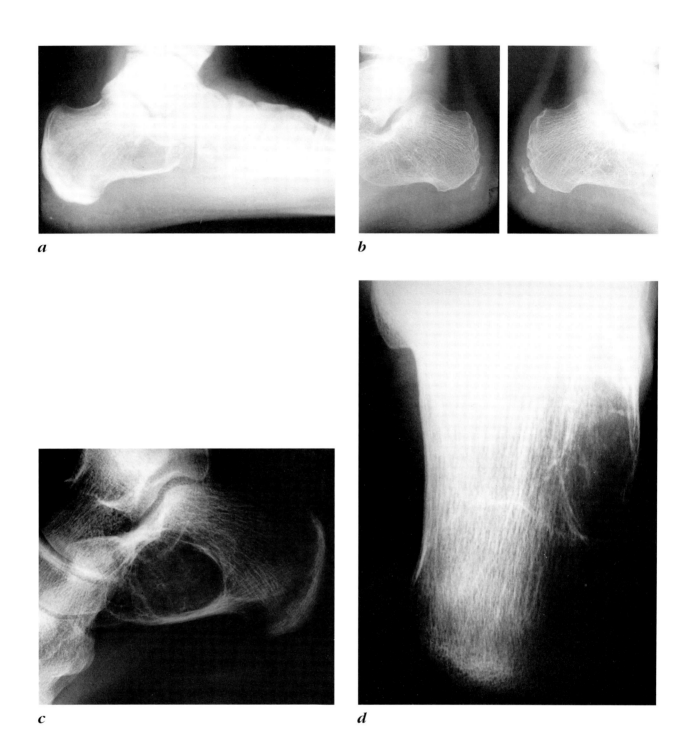

a

b

c

d

Figure 3.102 *(a) There is a well demarcated lucency representing a simple bone cyst in the anterior aspect of the calcaneus. This has no central calcification as typically seen with a lipoma (see Figure 3.63). It should also not be confused with a normal variant, the pseudocyst, which lies between the major groups of trabeculae. (b) Pseudocyst. Bilateral, rather poorly defined defects are seen as a normal variant. Note also the sclerosis and irregularity of the calcaneal apophyses and apparent thickening of the overlying soft tissues—in fact, a combination of tendo-Achillis and apophyseal cartilage. If pain is present, a diagnosis of Sever's disease can be made. (c, d) Fibrous dysplasia. An expansile osteolytic lesion of the calcaneus with minimal residual trabeculation is demonstrated. The appearances simulate those found in simple bone cyst, aneurysmal bone cyst and even a lipoma, but histology confirmed the diagnosis of fibrous dysplasia.*

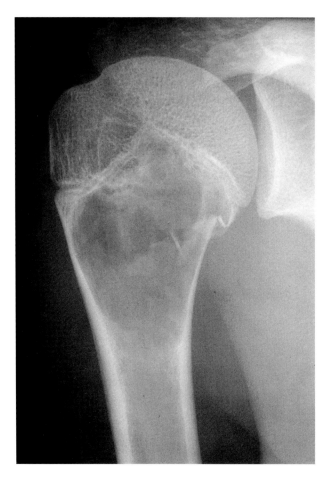

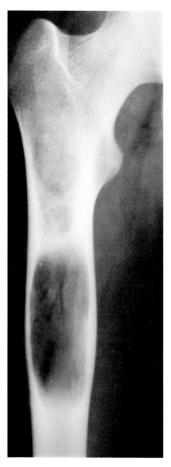

Figure 3.103 *Simple bone cyst. There is no expansion of the proximal humeral metaphysis. The lesion scallops the cortex endosteally, but the absence of aneurysmal dilatation and the site of the lesion indicates that this is not an aneurysmal bone cyst. A pathological fracture has occurred and a free-floating fragment of cortex is seen centrally within the lesion (the 'falling leaf' sign).*

Figure 3.104 *This simple bone cyst, in a mature skeleton, appears as a slightly expansile, monolocular lytic lesion situated in the midshaft of the femur and has sustained a pathological fracture. This lesion resembles a telangiectatic osteosarcoma (see Figure 3.129).*

FIBROUS CORTICAL DEFECT AND NON-OSSIFYING FIBROMA

The fibrous cortical defect is a small (<3 cm), lucent, fibrous lesion seen as an incidental finding in children. The lesion is metaphyseal in a long bone, usually the distal femur, oval in shape, thinning the cortex with a very narrow endosteal zone of reactive sclerosis. There may be slight cortical expansion (Figure 3.105a) and, occasionally, the lesion fractures. The majority ossify with age, leaving either normal or sclerotic bone (Figure 3.105b). Occasionally they enlarge and migrate to the centre of the bone, giving a multilocular, spherical or cigar-shaped lucency—a *non-ossifying fibroma*—which causes expansion and cortical thinning (Figure 3.106). These are diametaphyseal, well demarcated and multilocular, but are not as expansile as an aneurysmal bone cyst. They may be confused with simple bone cysts of the femur. These lesions also present because of pathological fracture.

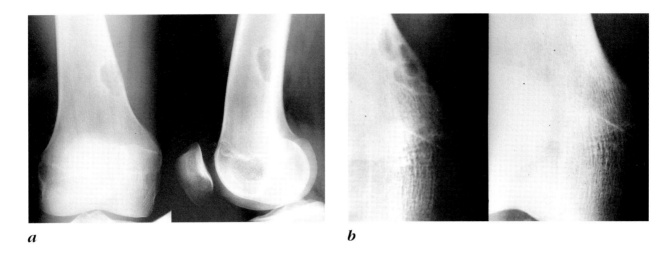

a   *b*

Figure 3.105 *Fibrous cortical defect. (**a**) This lesion is seen in young patients. There is slight expansion of the bone locally with thinning of the cortex. The lesion is multilocular and has a very narrow zone of transition with a thin rim of reactive sclerosis. They are normally asymptomatic but occasionally may fracture. (**b**) Fibrous cortical defects usually fill up with normal bone and vanish, but on occasion their healing is associated with filling of the lesion with sclerotic bone.*

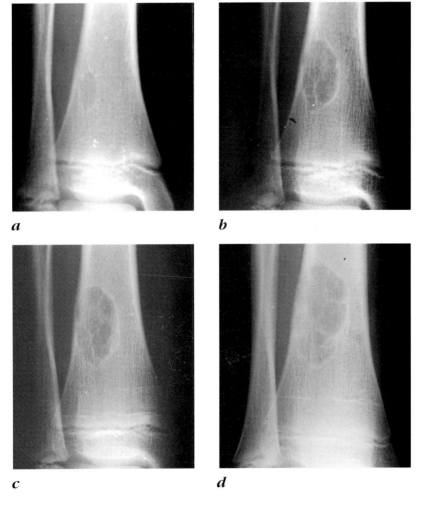

a   *b*

c   *d*

Figure 3.106 *(**a–d**) Growth and expansion of a non-ossifying fibroma. The initial lesion starts off at the periphery of the bone but enlarges and migrates towards its centre, though still cortically based. It is multilocular but otherwise not mineralized and shows a thin rim of reactive sclerosis.*

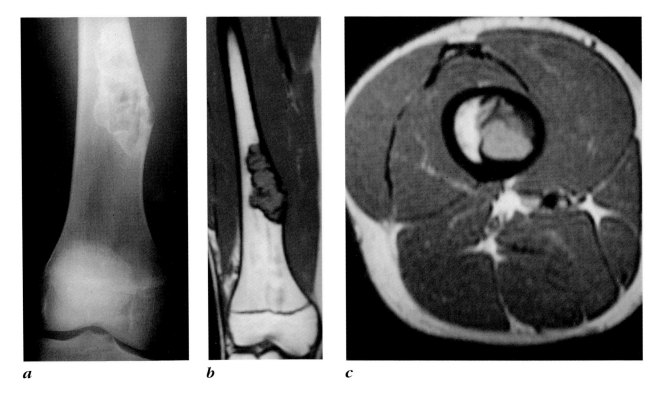

a　　　　　　*b*　　　　*c*

Figure 3.107 *Non-ossifying fibroma. (**a**) An expansile, multilocular and well defined lesion is demonstrated on the medial aspect of the midshaft of the femur. The cortex overlying it participates in the process and is superficially expanded and thinned over a rather more lucent area, beneath which there is cortical thickening and buttressing. (**b**) The equivalent coronal T$_1$-weighted MR image shows the anatomy displayed on the conventional film. The signal from the lesion is homogeneous and resembles that of the adjacent muscle. The mineralization in the lesion shown on the plain film is seen as low signal interspersed within soft tissue. (**c**) On the T$_1$-weighted MR sequence the marrow fat is bright within the femoral shaft laterally; the bulk of the lesion itself shows septation.*

The tumours are also found incidentally at MRI and can be diagnosed because of their location. Fibrous lesions generally have low soft tissue signal at T_1-weighting (Figure 3.107).

EOSINOPHILIC GRANULOMA

This is a disease of children and occasionally of young adults. Solitary or multiple lytic lesions occur preferentially in the axial skeleton and skull, and resemble those seen with chronic infections such as tuberculosis and occasionally chronic granulomatous disease. The areas of lysis are initially well defined (Figure 3.108), but in their healing phase the sharp margin is lost and they ossify from within (Figure 3.109). In a tubular bone, a periostitis may be seen and, in the skull, a 'bevelled edge' effect occurs (Figure 3.108). Unfortunately, bevelled edges can also be seen in tuberculosis, while the margin of an eosinophilic granuloma can be irregular. 'Tunnelling', however, is not a feature of eosinophilic granuloma but of infection (Figure 3.110).

Multiple lesions may cause alarm and may mimic leukaemia in children (Figure 3.111); however, they undergo spontaneous remission, only for further lesions to reappear. Eosinophilic granuloma and fibrous dysplasia should always be considered when solitary or multiple lytic lesions are seen in children (Figure 3.112). Some lesions may look extremely aggressive, simulating malignancy. In the mandible, resorption of bone gives one of the causes of 'floating teeth' (Figure 3.113).

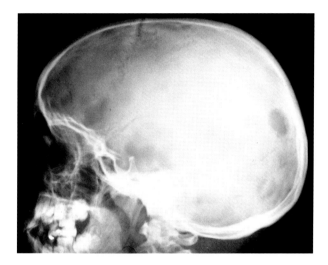

Figure 3.108 *Eosinophilic granuloma. A solitary, well defined lytic lesion with a bevelled edge in the posterior parietal region.*

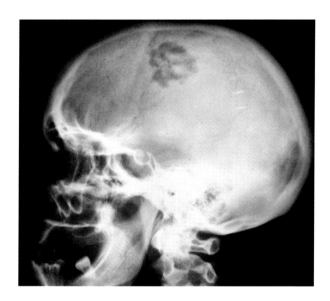

Figure 3.109 *Eosinophilic granuloma. The well defined margins seen in the previous patient have disappeared. This lesion is healing slowly with central ossification.*

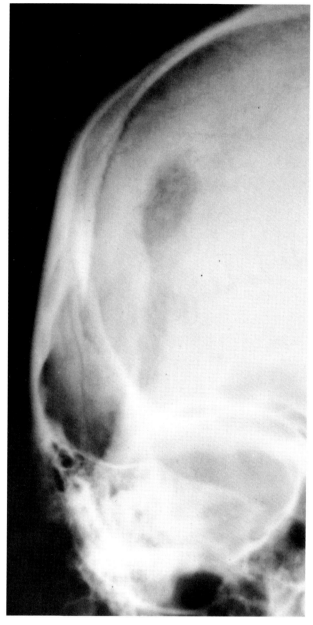

Figure 3.110 *In this patient with tuberculosis of the skull, the solitary osteolytic lesion is poorly defined, but this can be seen in a healing eosinophilic granuloma. However, the long finger-like process or tunnel leading from the lesion is a feature of infection.*

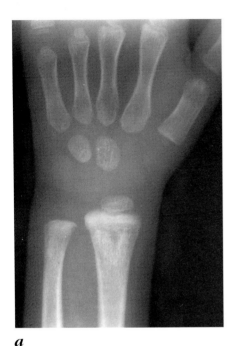

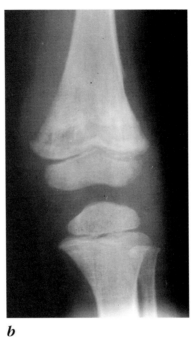

a

b

Figure 3.111 *Multicentric eosinophilic granuloma. Irregular medullary bands of bone destruction are seen at the distal radius (**a**) and distal femur (**b**), closely mimicking leukaemia in appearance.*

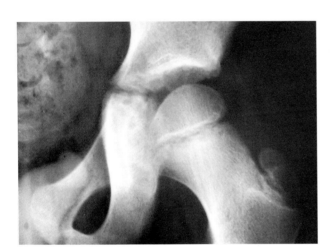

a

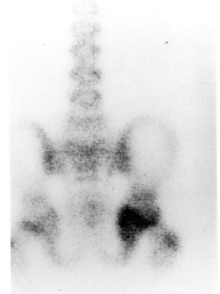

b

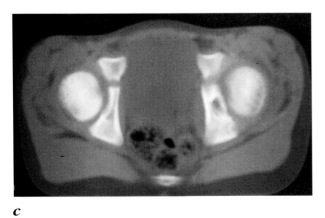

c

Figure 3.112 *Eosinophilic granuloma. (**a**) In this immature skeleton, the acetabulum is thickened and shows a generalized increase in density. (**b**) The radioisotope scan shows this region to be the site of increase in uptake. (**c**) The CT scan confirms the expansion of the acetabulum and shows an osteolytic lesion within it.*

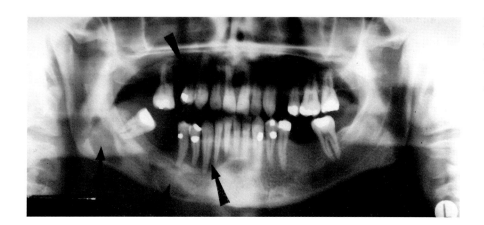

Figure 3.113 *Eosinophilic granuloma of the jaws. Multiple well defined osteolytic lesions are demonstrated (arrows).*

CYSTIC LESIONS IN HAEMOPHILIA

This disease is rare and will be diagnosed clinically before presentation to the radiologist. Large cysts due to subperiosteal or intraosseous bleeding, through which pathological fractures can occur, are found in the long bones or iliac blades (Figure 3.114). The patients have other bone changes; the epiphyses are overgrown due to hyperaemia and the joint spaces are narrow and irregular due to synovial proliferation (see Chapter 4, page 226).

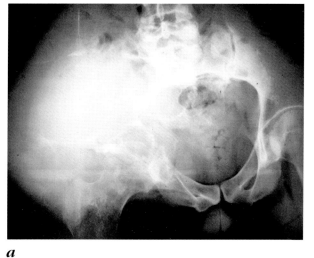

a

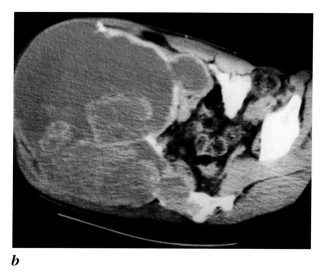

b

Figure 3.114 *Haemophilic pseudotumour. (a) There is a massive destructive lesion involving a whole wing of the right ilium and the hip joint, where a pathological fracture is shown. A few residual trabeculae remain. There is osteoporosis of the proximal femur. (b) The CT scan confirms the presence of a massive soft tissue lesion of different attenuations. The residual bone is shown to be mainly peripheral and centrally there is presumably clot and fluid. The lesion enters the neural canal. There is much displacement of gut. The swollen right leg results from vascular occlusion. The iliac wing is the commonest site for a haemophilic pseudotumour because of the large non-tendinous origin of iliacus. This allows haemorrhage to take place over a large area in and on bone.*

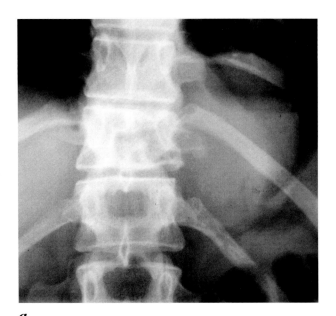

a

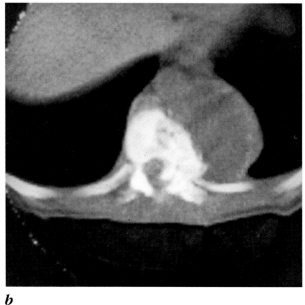

b

Figure 3.115 *Hydatid disease. (**a**) In this patient, an osteolytic lesion is present in the body of the eleventh thoracic vertebra, which is associated with a large paraspinal swelling and early collapse. (**b**) On the CT scan the soft tissue mass adjacent to the body of T11 is associated with vertebral destruction. There is a soft tissue capsule and the lesion is mainly fluid-filled.*

HYDATID DISEASE

This is common in sheep-farming regions, but bone lesions account for only 2% of total lesions. The cysts are occasionally single (Figure 3.115) but usually multiple (Figure 3.116) and are well defined, varying in size from small (1–2 mm) to very large. The cortices may be scalloped endosteally and the bone may be expanded with large cysts. Lesions occur around joints, and affect both sides similarly to other infections (see Chapter 4). In a long bone, the lesions can resemble fibrous dysplasia and brown tumours in hyperparathyroidism (Figure 3.117). They are obviously uncommon outside endemic areas but may be seen elsewhere because of population migration.

CT scans show cystic bony destruction and expansion of cystic lesions into adjacent soft tissue (Figure 3.115). MRI is particularly helpful in demonstrating the fluid-filled cysts, areas of bone destruction and sinuses through adjacent soft tissues (Figure 3.118).

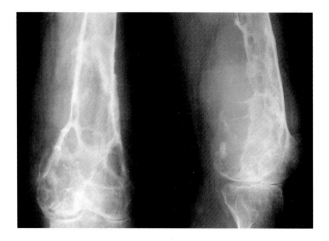

Figure 3.116 *Hydatid disease. Multiple cysts in the distal femur expand the bone and break through the cortex with the formation of soft tissue masses. The cysts within the bone are fairly well marginated and may occasionally resemble those seen in fibrous dysplasia, in which cortical breakthrough does not occur.*

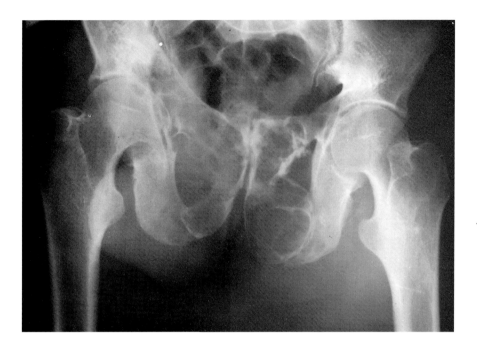

Figure 3.117 *Hydatid disease. Large, expansile, multicystic lesions associated with cortical thinning are seen affecting the pubic bones. The lesions have well defined margins with a narrow zone of transition and a thin rim of reactive sclerosis. The lesions mimic those seen in hyperparathyroidism and fibrous dysplasia. The right hip joint space is narrowed.*

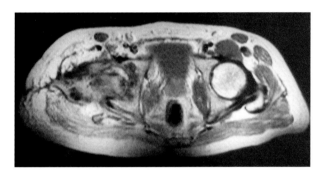

a

Figure 3.118 *Hydatid disease at MR imaging. The axial (**a**) and coronal (**b**) T₁-weighted sequences show extensive soft tissue wasting and muscle atrophy of the right lower limb. Bone destruction is especially demonstrated around the hip joint with a soft tissue mass distending the capsule. Cystic lesions are demonstrated in the femur.*

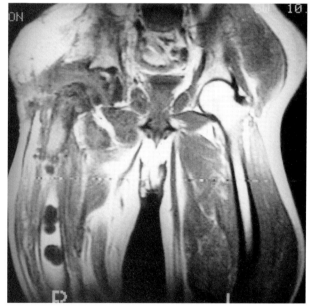

b

MALIGNANT LESIONS OF BONE

Solitary malignant lesions of bone have characteristics which usually enable them to be distinguished from benign lesions. These are:

- Rapid growth
- Wide zone of transition
- Ill defined or absent zone of reactive sclerosis
- Cortical breach
- Periostitis and possibly a Codman's triangle
- Soft tissue mass
- Matrix mineralization (see page 114)

RADIOLOGICAL INVESTIGATION OF MALIGNANT LESIONS OF BONE

The features listed above can be determined on the plain radiograph. In a long bone, the upper and lower margins of the lesion must be included on the film. Permeation may extend beyond the confines of major change and a distant periostitis may give a better indication of the extent of the lesion.

Radiographs demonstrate calcified structures well, and cortical breakthrough, periostitis and soft tissue swelling should be assessed. The soft tissue margin of a tumour was always said to be better defined than the margin of an infective mass because of a lack of local oedema, but MR imaging has shown oedema around tumours, apparently due to trauma to the overlying soft tissues.

Isotope scanning also gives a very accurate assessment of tumour size and shows 'skip' lesions, as well as metastases.

Ultrasound is of benefit in assessing soft tissues, tumour and blood vessels, and also in showing non-mineralized periosteal elevation.

CT scans are of great benefit in showing cortical and medullary destruction, and the attenuation of tumours in the medulla differs from that in the normal marrow on either side of the lesion. Periostitis and matrix mineralization are also well shown by this technique. Contrast enhancement will delineate the extent of the lesion, show changes of necrosis in tumour and neurovascular bundle involvement by the tumour.

CT scans of the lungs and mediastinum are an essential part of the diagnostic process. Metastases are seen smaller and earlier than on a chest X-ray. Biopsies may be performed under CT, ultrasound or fluoroscopic guidance.

MRI is now an essential part of the staging process to show the extent of the tumour, muscle and neurovascular involvement and the extent of medullary infiltration, as well as showing cortical and periosteal change. Tumour behaviour can also be assessed—margination, vascularity and necrosis and, indeed, tumour composition (Table 3.11). Giant-cell tumours in particular may be poorly defined at conventional imaging but are well defined at MRI (Figure 3.85). Many malignant tumours may also be sharply demarcated from surrounding fat (see page 186), just as the focus of uptake on a radionuclide bone scan may apparently be well localized. However, some malignant lesions will show peripheral permeation at MRI.

MRI should not be used in the *diagnosis* of the tumour type, however, as much of the change is non-specific. The plain film and biopsy are essential in making the diagnosis, but the extent, spread and aggression or otherwise of the lesion can be assessed at MRI scanning.

Table 3.11 Signal changes of malignant lesions at MR imaging.

	T_1-weighting	T_2-weighting	Fat suppression
Malignant lesions are heterogeneous because of:			
Pathological vascularity			
arterial	low	low	low
venous	intermediate	bright	bright
Cystic change	intermediate	bright	bright
Necrosis	low	low	low
Mineralization	low	low	low
Signal from basic stroma	intermediate	intermediate	low

Age incidence is often highly specific (Table 3.3), but the sex of the patient is less useful for diagnosis. The site is often characteristic, both generally, for example Ewing's tumours are diaphyseal, and specifically, that is, they often occur in ribs.

It is sometimes more difficult to make a distinction between malignancy and infection than between benign and malignant lesions. The common malignant tumours are listed in Table 3.1 and their sites in the skeleton and within a bone are shown in Tables 3.5–3.8. The nature of malignant periostitis is described in Chapter 6, page 139.

OSTEOGENIC SARCOMA

Incidence: 20% of sarcomas.
Sex: Slightly more common in males.
Age: This occurs as a primary lesion between 10 and 25 years of age, (45% in the second decade). In elderly patients, secondary lesions are often superimposed on Paget's disease and irradiated bone, and occur very rarely as a complication of fibrous dysplasia, bone infarcts and in areas of chronic osteomyelitis.
Site: See Figure 3.119. Lesions commonly arise around the knee, shoulder and pelvis, but any bone may be involved. In long bones, the tumours are typically metaphyseal. The resultant malignant osteoid destroys bone and undergoes irregular ossification.

The mandible is often involved in the third and fourth decades (Figure 3.120). Jaw lesions have a better prognosis.

A radiological spectrum exists. The commonest appearance is of gross central medullary destruction of bone in the metaphysis, with a broad zone of transition. Cortical breakthrough and a well defined soft tissue mass with a Codman's triangle are seen. Matrix ossification in bone and soft tissue is irregular and dense. The periostitis is coarse and may be lamellar or perpendicular (Figure 3.121). Occasionally, purely lytic or sclerotic metaphyseal tumours are encountered (Figures 3.122–3.125).

Tumours may contain not only malignant osteoid but also fibrosarcomatous and chondrosarcomatous elements, differing in appearance from that of the highly vascular and osteolytic telangiectatic form (see below).

Osteogenic sarcoma metastasizes to other bones and to the lungs. These secondary deposits are often osteoblastic and can be detected on isotope bone scans (Figure 3.126); CT scans are sensitive in the detection of pulmonary metastases (Figures 3.126–3.128).

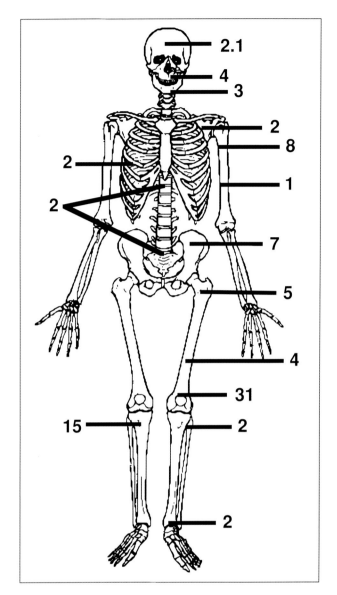

Figure 3.119 *Osteosarcoma: percentage distribution at major sites only. (After Unni, 1996, with permission.)*

Radionuclide bone scans show the extent of the tumour and 'skip' or metastatic lesions. CT scanning demonstrates cortical change and tumour new bone formation. MRI is of great value in staging marrow and soft tissue extension, and neurovascular bundle involvement.

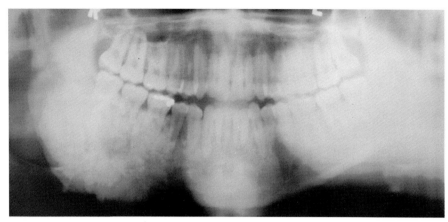

a

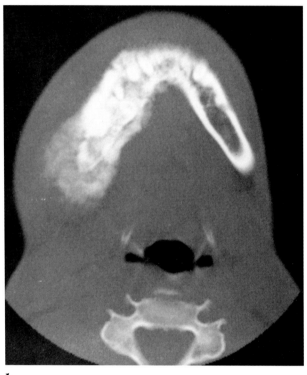

b

Figure 3.120 *Osteogenic sarcoma of the mandible.* *(a) The right side of the mandible shows expansion by a tumour which causes fairly well defined new bone formation. (b) The CT scan of the same patient shows extensive bone destruction with an ossifying soft tissue mass. (c) Radionuclide bone scan showing expansion and increased bone turnover. After radiotherapy the necrotic tumour was sloughed out through the skin. The 20-year-old patient survived.*

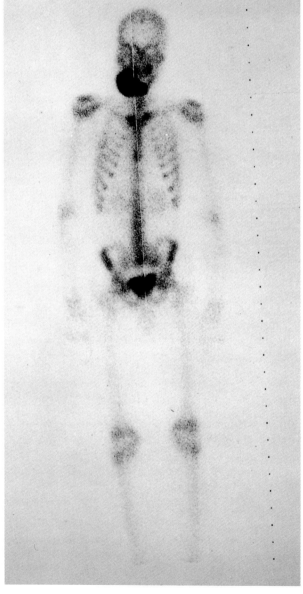

c

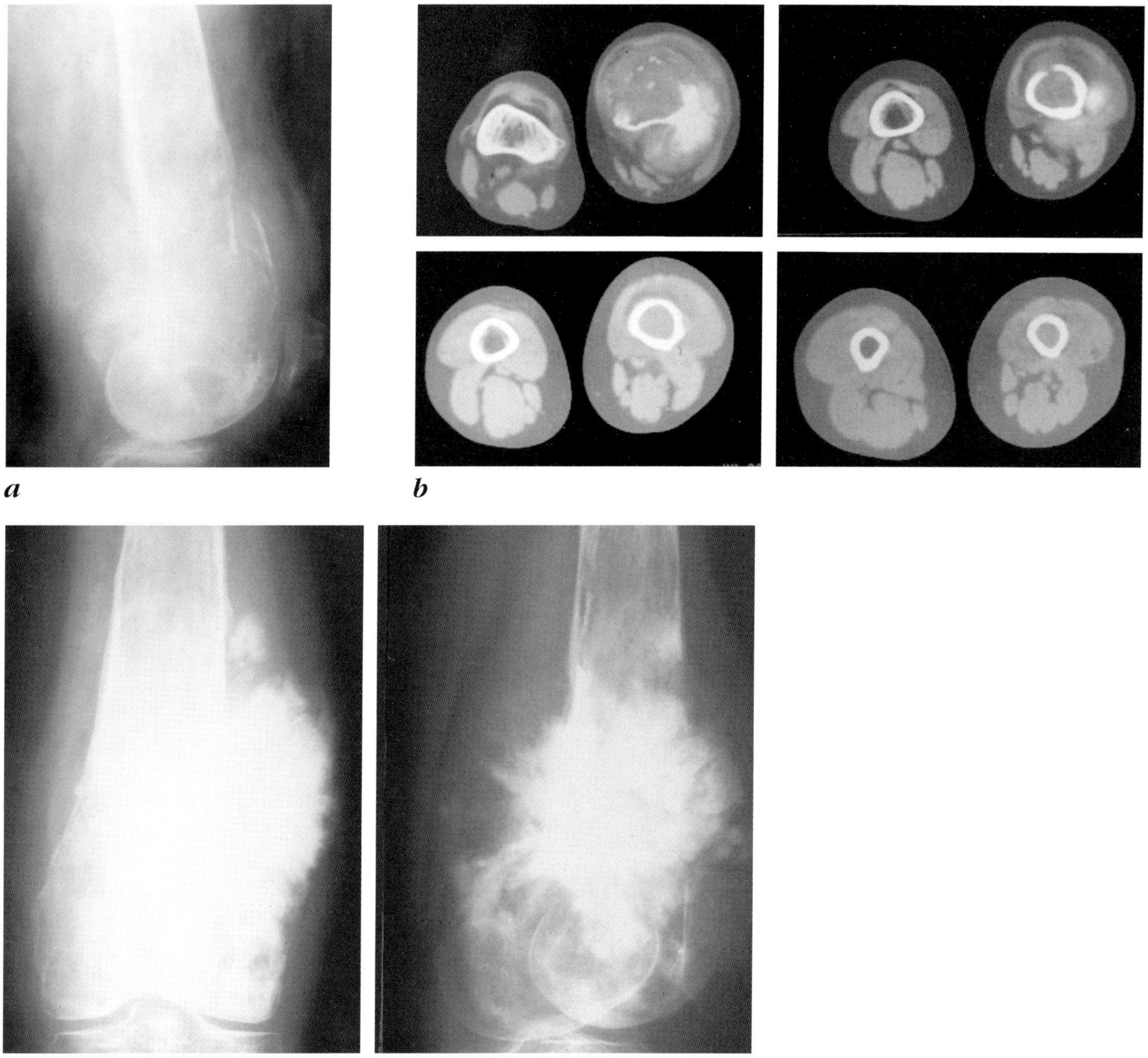

a

b

c

Figure 3.121 *Osteogenic sarcoma.* (***a***) *There is a large soft tissue mass at the distal femur. Remnants of dead cortex may be seen anteriorly, and the lesion is predominantly lytic posteriorly. There is some poorly defined tumour new bone and posterior 'saucerization' or erosion of the cortex, characteristic of malignant re-entry.* (***b***) *On the CT scan, the tumour permeates along the medulla, and eventually breaks through the cortex of the femur, with the formation of a large anterior soft tissue mass containing a few areas of ossification. The bulk of the tumour new bone lies postero-laterally and is associated with another large soft tissue mass.* (***c***) *Following radiotherapy, further ossification takes place within the tumour. This is coarse and shaggy, and is both amorphous and sunray in type.*

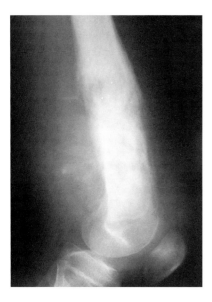

Figure 3.122 *Osteogenic sarcoma. A large soft tissue mass is associated with a metaphyseal destructive lesion. There is much new bone proliferation, both within the shaft of the femur and in the soft tissues. There is a 'sunray' or hair-on-end spiculation which is coarse, as well as periosteal elevation at the margin of the lesion with the formation of a Codman's triangle.*

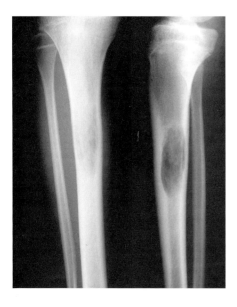

Figure 3.123 *Lytic osteogenic sarcoma. This lesion resembles a simple bone cyst, although the site might be unusual. It is poorly defined and causing endosteal scalloping, but as yet there is no significant expansion of the bone or obvious periostitis. The clinical findings might be helpful in such a patient.*

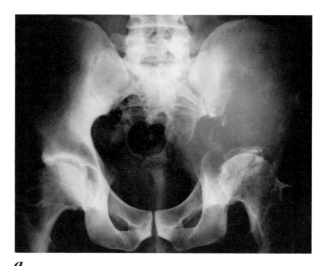

a

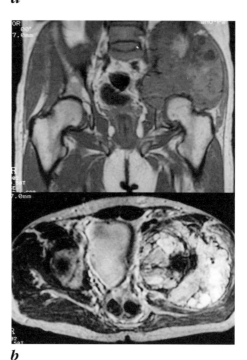

b

Figure 3.124 *Lytic osteosarcoma of the pelvis. (**a**) There is a predominantly lytic destructive lesion involving the left innominate bone. There is a pathological fracture of the acetabulum. A large soft tissue mass is demonstrated in the pelvis on the plain film. (**b**) The coronal T_1-weighted (top) and axial T_2-weighted (bottom) MR sequences confirm the presence of a large soft tissue mass arising in the pelvis on the left, which is not quite homogeneous. It is lobular, shows septation and some areas on the T_2-weighted image are very bright. The lesion seems well defined and separated from the overlying atrophic soft tissues which are partially oedematous.*

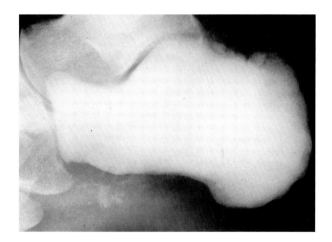

Figure 3.125 *Osteogenic sarcoma of the calcaneus. There is sclerosis of the entire calcaneus which is only slightly expanded. There is also some cortical irregularity and soft tissue ossification. The appearances may resemble Paget's disease but, in the latter, soft tissue swelling will not be evident, and there is usually no visible soft tissue ossification. The age of the patient is an important diagnostic tool. Paget's sarcoma occurs in a much older age group than primary osteosarcoma.*

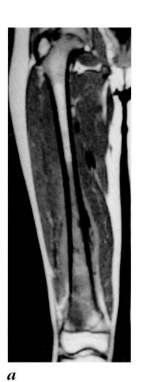

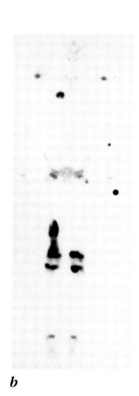

a   *b*

Figure 3.126 *Osteogenic sarcoma. A femoral diametaphyseal tumour is demonstrated similar in appearance to Figure 3.121.* (***a***) *The T$_1$-weighted MR image shows a permeative lesion in the mid and distal femur, replacing normal marrow fat, extending to the growth plate. The changes are heterogeneous with areas of low signal corresponding to matrix mineralization. The cortex is broken through. There is a soft tissue mass which has the same signal as the medullary lesion, a periostitis and a Codman's triangle.* (***b***) *The radioisotope bone scan shows an expansile lesion with increased uptake in the right femur, and also lesions around the left knee, deepening the image of the growth plate. A secondary deposit is noted in the lung.* (***c***) *The CT scan shows ossifying metastatic disease in the lungs.*

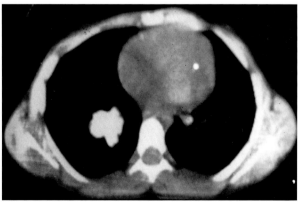

c

Telangiectatic osteosarcoma

The lytic or telangiectatic form may show little or no tumour new bone formation. MR imaging shows a large fluid-filled cavity with a few thin septa, which enhance with gadolinium (Figure 3.129). It is mainly seen in the femoral diaphysis. Fluid–fluid levels are seen, mimicking aneurysmal bone cyst.

For other forms of osteosarcoma, see Chapter 6.

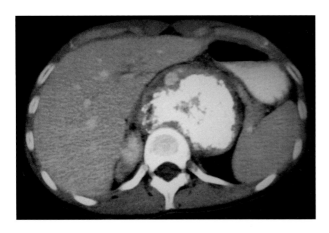

Figure 3.127 *Secondary deposit from an osteogenic sarcoma demonstrated by CT scanning. A large retroperitoneal mass is demonstrated which shows ossification (post-chemotherapy).*

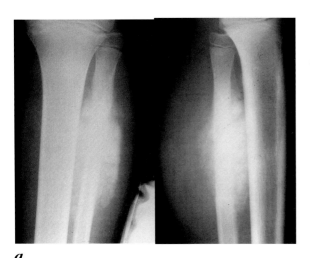

Figure 3.128 *In this patient with osteogenic sarcoma (**a**) a large ossifying tumour arises on the proximal fibula. (**b**) The lesion is seen on the radioisotope bone scan and there is quite marked increase in uptake throughout both lung fields and, particularly, at the hilum of the left lung. (**c**) The chest radiograph shows multiple pulmonary metastases which have added areas of density due to ossification. (**d**) A further radioisotope bone scan shows increase of uptake in both lungs and in the lymph nodes of the groin on the affected side.*

a

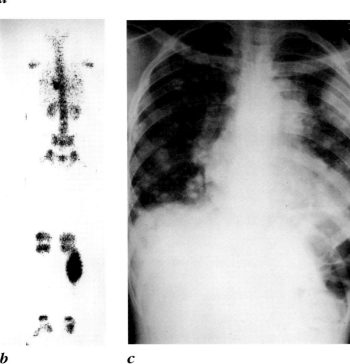

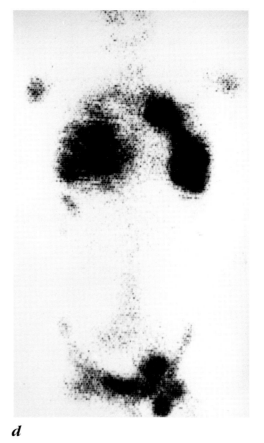

b   *c*   *d*

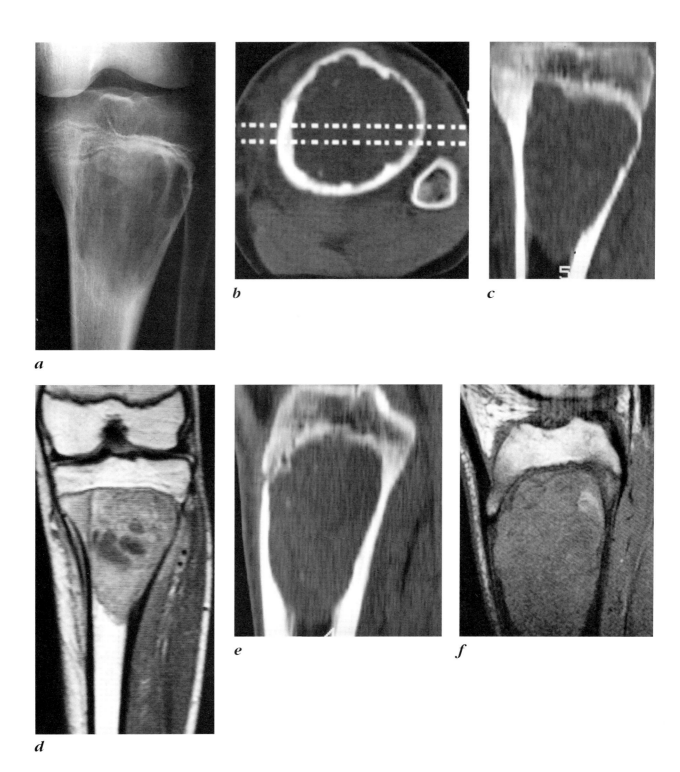

Figure 3.129 *Telangiectatic osteogenic sarcoma. (**a**) There is an extensive osteolytic lesion in the proximal tibial metaphysis with no evidence of new bone formation. (**b**) The axial CT scan confirms the absence of mineralization in this purely osteolytic lesion, as does the coronal CT reconstruction (**c**). (**d**) The coronal T₁-weighted MR image (post-gadolinium) shows enhancement of much of the lesion with some areas of necrosis. (**e**) Absence of mineralization is again confirmed on the sagittal CT reconstruction scan. (**f**) The sagittal T₁-weighted MR sequence (pre-gadolinium), at the corresponding level to (**e**), demonstrates a soft tissue mass occupying the marrow.*

EWING'S SARCOMA

Incidence: 9% of malignant bone tumours.
Sex: Marked male predominance.
Age: This is the other significant primary malignant tumour of bone which occurs between 5 and 25 years of age; 60% occur in the second decade.
Site: see Figure 3.130. Malignant round cells infiltrate the shaft of a long bone, or a flat bone. The diaphysis of a long bone is the usual site. The lower limbs and pelvis are especially involved.

The tumour produces a widespread 'moth-eaten', permeative and destructive lesion, aligned along the shaft of a bone, unlike the focal expansile lesion seen in osteogenic sarcoma. The central lesion is destructive and not osteogenic.

The periosteal reaction is often finer and more delicate than in osteogenic sarcoma, but is also associated with cortical breakthrough and a soft tissue mass (Figure 3.131).

In children, the ribs are frequently involved and extrapleural masses and effusions are formed (Figure

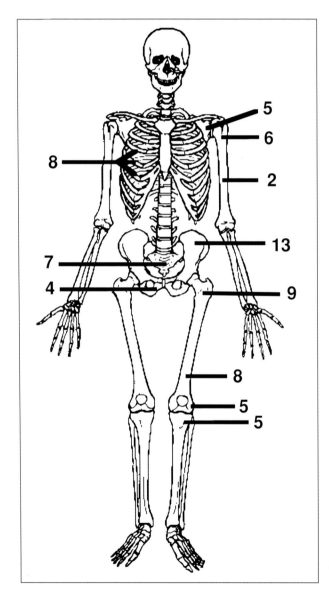

Figure 3.130 *Ewing's sarcoma: percentage distribution at major sites only. (After Unni, 1996, with permission.)*

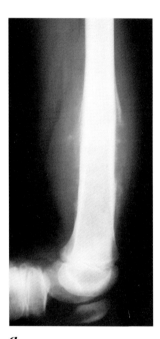

a

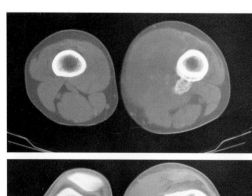

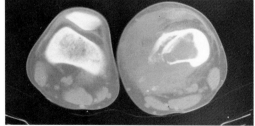

b

Figure 3.131 *(a)* In Ewing's sarcoma, a soft tissue mass is associated with a Codman's triangle and much finer sunray spiculation than is usually present in osteosarcoma. *(b)* The CT scan shows cortical breakthrough and a large soft tissue mass which is barely mineralized. The marrow shows replacement of normal trabeculation and fat by tumour.

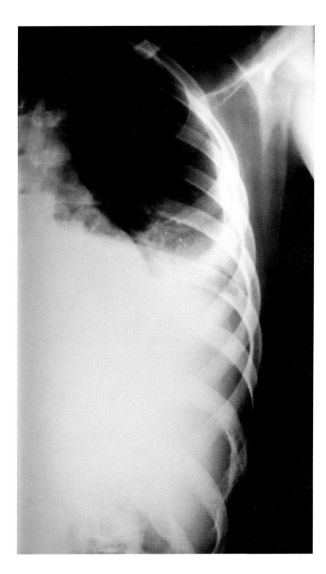

Figure 3.132 *The left ninth rib is irregular and increased in density. There is a large associated soft tissue swelling. This lesion in a child is strongly suggestive of Ewing's sarcoma.*

3.132). In flat bones, such as the pelvis and scapula, reactive sclerosis and lamellar periostitis cause bone expansion (Figure 3.133), which often obscures permeative destruction.

As with osteosarcoma, the radionuclide bone scan shows the extent of the lesion, CT assesses bone destruction and MRI assesses soft tissue change and vascularity (Figures 3.134 and 3.135). The MR images are only diagnostic in the sense that permeation of the diaphysis matches and improves upon the change seen on the plain film (Figure 3.136).

Metastases occur in the lungs and in bone.

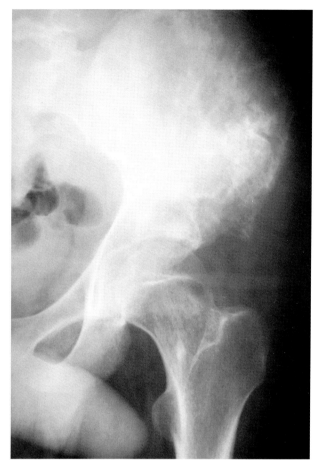

a

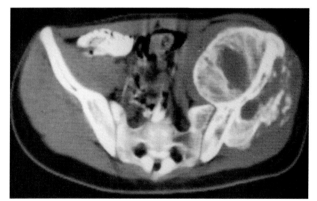

b

Figure 3.133 *Ewing's sarcoma. (**a**) An aggressive, expansile, destructive lesion of the left iliac blade is demonstrated associated with periosteal new bone formation and a soft tissue mass. (**b**) The CT scan shows a highly expansile destructive lesion. The soft tissue mass is mineralized. CT gives a better impression of the actual size of the lesion than the plain film.*

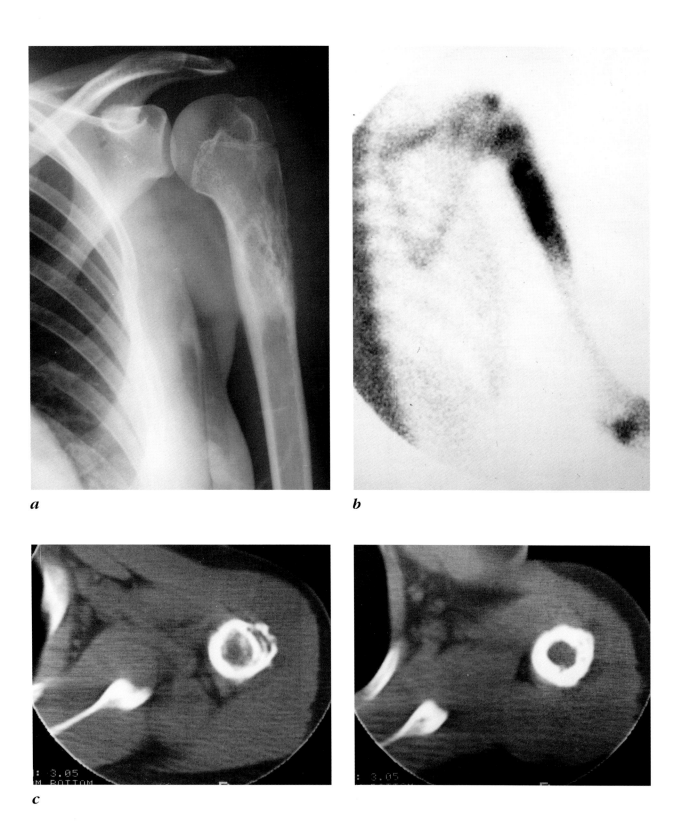

a

b

c

Figure 3.134 *Ewing's sarcoma. (**a**) There is a permeative destructive lesion of the proximal humeral metaphysis associated with cortical thickening. (**b**) The radionuclide bone scan shows expansion of the bone and local increase in uptake, which is ill defined inferiorly. (**c**) The CT scan shows permeation of the marrow, cortical thinning and a layer of periosteal new bone.*

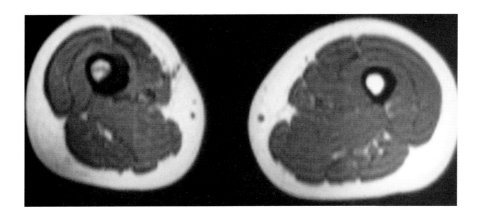

Figure 3.135 *Ewing's sarcoma. Diffuse infiltration of the marrow with decrease in signal is demonstrated on this axial T$_1$-weighted MR image. Periosteal elevation is also shown.*

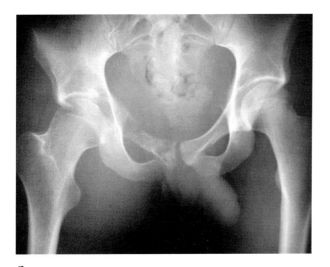

a

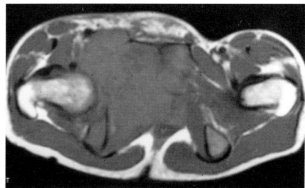

b

Figure 3.136 *Ewing's sarcoma. (**a**) A diffuse permeative lesion of the right ischium and pubis is demonstrated with a soft tissue mass, both of the upper thigh and of the lower pelvis. (**b**) On the axial T$_1$- (top) and coronal T$_2$-weighted (bottom) MR images an extensive soft tissue mass is shown which is essentially homogeneous. It is well defined, contains septation and is associated with substantial bone destruction, more than is evident on the plain film, with replacement of normal marrow by tumour. The thigh shows substantial oedema distal to the tumour. The tissue diagnosis cannot be made on the basis of the MR scan alone.*

PRIMITIVE (PRIMARY) NEUROECTODERMAL TUMOUR (PNET)

This rare entity has radiological features resembling Ewing's sarcoma, occurring mainly in the pelvis and lower limbs (Figure 3.137) and has a worse prognosis than Ewing's sarcoma. Its name derives from the fact that the cells have features resembling nerve cells at electron microscopy and immunohistochemistry.

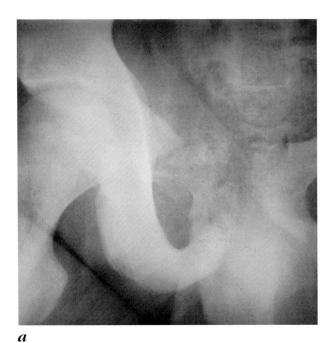

a

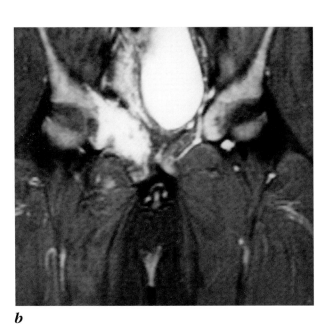

b

Figure 3.137 *Primitive neuroectodermal tumour (PNET). (a) The plain film shows an osteolytic defect with bone destruction involving the right pubis associated with pathological fractures and soft tissue swelling. (b) The coronal fat suppression MR sequence confirms the presence of bony abnormality and a large mass displacing the bladder. The lesion resembles a Ewing's sarcoma radiologically.*

MALIGNANT LYMPHOMA OF BONE (RETICULUM CELL SARCOMA)

Incidence: 8% of malignant lesions.
Sex: M:F = 4:3.
Age: This occurs between 25 and 60 years of age.
Site: see Figure 3.138.

The tumour causes diffuse malignant infiltration with cortical breakthrough, lamellar periostitis and a Codman's triangle. It resembles Ewing's sarcoma both microscopically and radiologically (Figure 3.139).

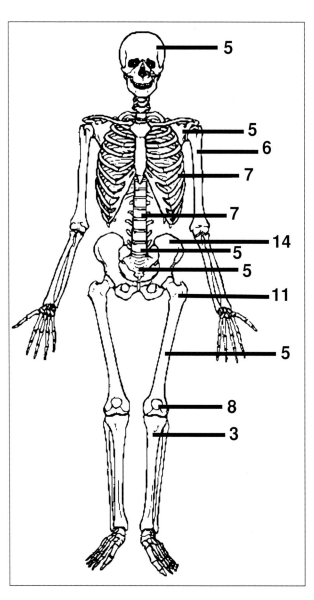

Figure 3.138 *Malignant lymphoma of bone: percentage distribution at major sites only. (After Unni, 1996, with permission.)*

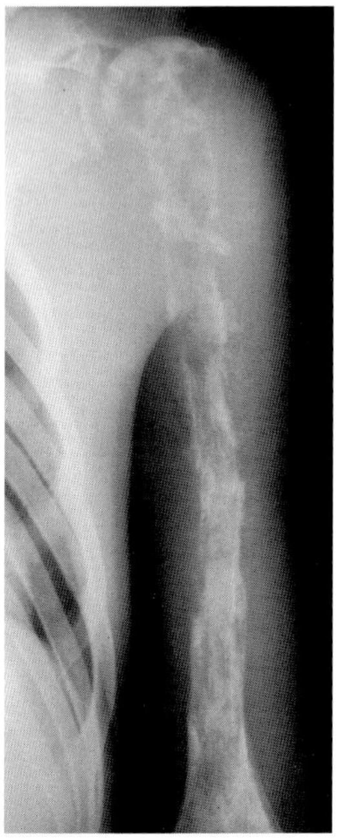

Figure 3.139 *Malignant lymphoma of bone. Diffuse infiltration along the shaft of the humerus causes lysis, although there is some reactive sclerosis. There is no new bone formation and very little evidence of a soft tissue mass, but cortical sequestration is present.*

LEUKAEMIA

Below five years of age, any malignant lesion which has the infiltrative features of a Ewing's sarcoma is likely to be due to leukaemia or neuroblastoma. These lesions are usually multiple and associated with metaphyseal bands of lucency and sutural widening in the skull. Lucent bands are also present beneath vertebral endplates, rib cortices and iliac crests (Figure 3.140).

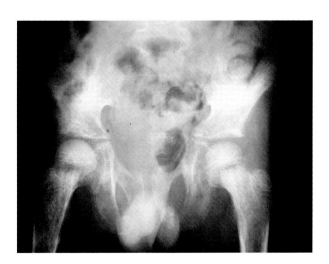

Figure 3.140 *In this patient with leukaemia, there is widespread demineralization of bone which is accentuated in subcortical and metaphyseal regions. The cortices are thinned.*

FIBROSARCOMA

Incidence: 2.3% of primary malignant bone tumours.
Sex: Probably more common in males.
Age: Third, fourth and fifth decades. Often discovered because of pathological fracture.
Site: see Figure 3.141. Distribution similar to osteosarcoma and malignant fibrous histiocytoma. Femur 40%; tibia 16%; humerus 10%; 33–80% of fibrosarcomas occur around the knee.

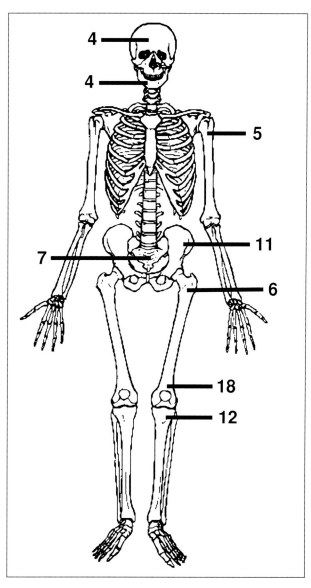

Figure 3.141 *Fibrosarcoma: percentage distribution at major sites only. (After Unni, 1996, with permission.)*

This is a rare primary malignant tumour of bone which also occasionally arises on pre-existing fibrous dysplasia, Paget's disease and bone infarcts. Fibrosarcoma is most commonly seen in the metaphyses around the knee and in flat bones. The tumour is highly destructive, breaking through the cortex, invading soft tissues, forming a mass, and causing diffuse and ill-defined destruction of the medulla within which residual bony sequestra may be seen (see Figure 3.5). The lesion may extend to an articular surface and the poorly marginated area of destruction may then resemble a giant-cell tumour (Figure 3.142). However, patients with fibrosarcoma are usually older than those with giant-cell tumour. Destruction of bone is probably more localized, but less permeative and moth-eaten than with malignant lymphoma of bone (Figure 3.143).

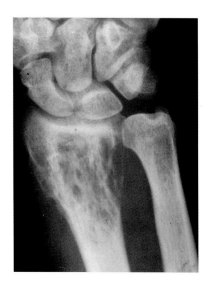

Figure 3.142
Fibrosarcoma. A diffuse, permeative, destructive lesion of the distal radius causes some local reactive sclerosis but minimal periostitis and no soft tissue mass.

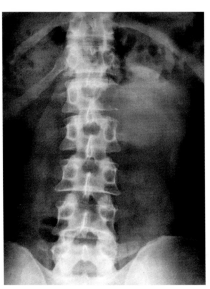

a

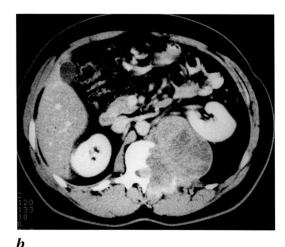

b

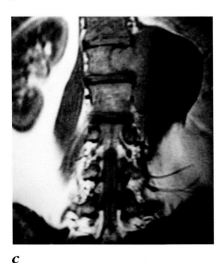

c

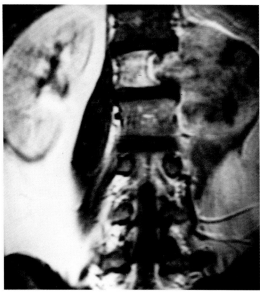

d

Figure 3.143
Fibrosarcoma. The lesion arises in the left half of the vertebral body of L1. (a) The plain film shows a destructive lesion of bone associated with a large soft tissue mass distorting the psoas shadow. (b) The CT scan confirms this appearance and shows the lesion is of mixed attenuation, presumably with necrosis, and enters the spinal canal. On the coronal T_1-weighted images, pre- (c) and post-gadolinium (d), the soft tissue mass extends from the vertebral body into the overlying psoas. Pre-gadolinium, it is rather homogeneous, but after gadolinium, enhancement occurs in and around the lesion.

There is little expansion, sclerosis or periostitis, unlike changes seen in osteosarcoma and chondrosarcoma. Sequestration may occur. Fibrosarcoma of bone has a worse prognosis than those occurring in the soft tissues.

MALIGNANT FIBROUS HISTIOCYTOMA

Incidence: 1% of primary bone tumours.
Sex: M:F = 3:2.
Age: The majority of patients are in the fifth and sixth decades, but occasionally adolescents are affected.
Site: see Figure 3.144. This lesion occurs in bone, the majority around the knee, but is more common in

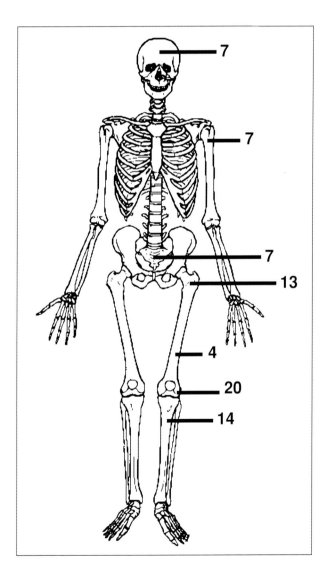

Figure 3.144 *Malignant fibrous histiocytoma: percentage distribution at major sites only. (After Unni, 1996, with permission.)*

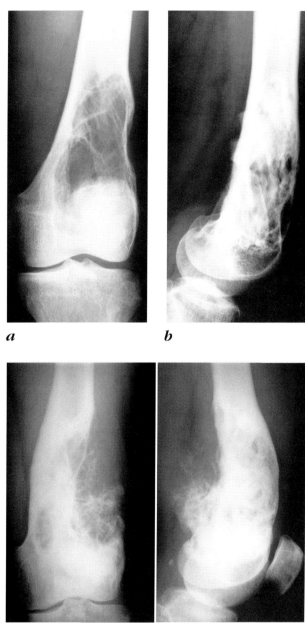

Figure 3.145 *Malignant fibrous histiocytoma. (**a**) The lesion is similar to, but perhaps more extensive proximally than, a giant-cell tumour. The cortex is scalloped endosteally and the bone marginally expanded by this eccentric lesion. Residual trabeculation remains. (**b**) Following surgery, the lesion has been curetted and packed with bone chips. (**c**) The bone chips have resorbed and the lesion has expanded. There is now quite obvious cortical breakthrough with the formation of a partially ossifying soft tissue mass, revealing the aggressive nature of this lesion.*

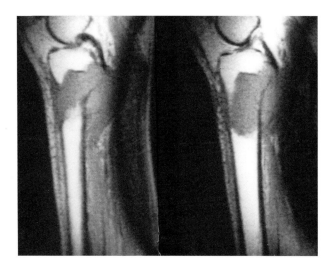

Figure 3.146 *Malignant fibrous histiocytoma. On the sagittal T₁-weighted MR image a large proximal tibial mass, exhibiting soft tissue characteristics, is demonstrated with anterior and posterior cortical breakthrough and the formation of a large posterior soft tissue mass.*

soft tissue. It is mainly metaphyseal, extending to the subarticular region. Malignant fibrous histiocytoma is commonest at the ends of the long bones, as is giant-cell tumour.

It is, however, an aggressive tumour which recurs and metastasizes. In behaviour, therefore, it is usually more like a fibrosarcoma, from which it has been pathologically differentiated, than a giant-cell tumour.

Radiologically, the lesion is centrally located with cortical destruction and a soft tissue mass (Figures 3.145 and 3.146). It is poorly defined and permeative. These appearances are also very similar to those seen with a giant-cell tumour (Figure 3.145). However, the soft tissue mass occasionally mineralizes and the lesion then resembles a fibrosarcoma rather than a giant-cell tumour.

CHONDROSARCOMA

Incidence: 10% of primary malignant bone tumours. They are half as common as osteosarcoma.
Sex: M:F = 1.5:1.
Age: The majority of patients are in the fourth, fifth and sixth decades. These presumably arise on a pre-existing chondral lesion, often in patients with a single exostosis (but only 1% of these turn malignant)

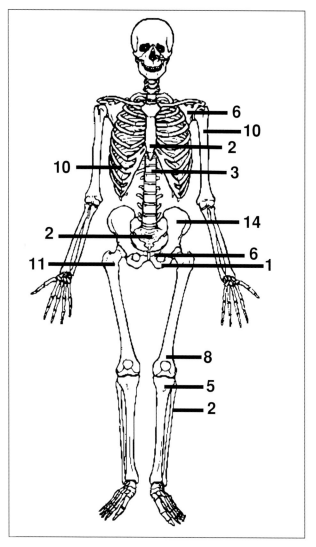

Figure 3.147 *Chondrosarcoma: percentage distribution at major sites only. (After Unni, 1996, with permission.)*

or multiple exostoses, Maffucci's syndrome (30% of which become malignant), or in those with multiple enchondromas. Solitary enchondromas rarely become malignant. Only a few patients develop chondrosarcoma in childhood.
Site: see Figure 3.147.

Chondrosarcomas arise in enchondromas, i.e. in the bone (Figures 3.4 and 3.148), or on exostoses (Figure 3.149), that is superficial to the cortex, or on the cortex on a cortical chondroma.

Loss of marginal definition, rapid growth and pain in a pre-existing lesion may all suggest malignant change (Figure 3.4).

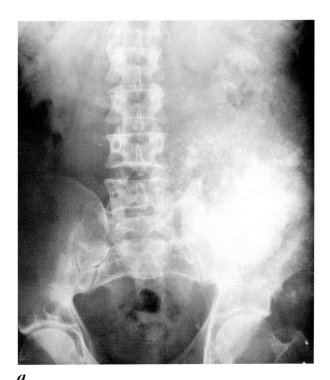

a

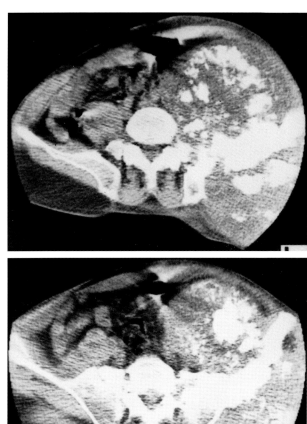

b

Figure 3.148 *Chondrosarcoma. (a) There is destruction of the left iliac blade associated with marked tumour new bone formation. (b) On the CT scan, soft tissue masses are seen anterior and posterior to the left iliac blade which is expanded, irregular and sclerotic. The soft tissue masses show new bone formation. The appearances are those of a highly aggressive malignant tumour of bone. Similar appearances may be seen with an osteogenic sarcoma at the same site.*

The typical appearance of a central chondrosarcoma is of an osteolytic lesion with a wide zone of transition, whose cartilaginous matrix undergoes patchy amorphous ossification. The cortex may be eroded and broken through, with the formation of a soft tissue mass (Figure 3.148), but often a typical tumour grows so slowly that it stimulates the overlying periosteum. The bone expanded by the tumour shows endosteal cortical scalloping, but external cortical thickening. Matrix ossification occurs *centrally* within the lesion rather than at its margin. (Infarcts do not expand bone and often show *marginal* sclerosis, the zone of creeping substitution. There should be no associated osteolysis.)

Radionuclide bone scanning may show minimal or peripheral enhancement only. CT shows features of medullary lysis, matrix mineralization and cortical thickening or breakthrough with a soft tissue mass. MRI, as always, shows the extent of medullary and soft tissue involvement, but is otherwise non-specific. Chondrosarcoma enhances little at MRI but may show a lobulated contour (Figure 3.150).

Malignant changes develop on the cartilage cap of the exostosis when the cartilage cap is large, i.e. over 2 cm thick. The large malignant cartilage mass is often only poorly mineralized (Figure 3.149), while the small benign cap (<5 mm thick) is totally or almost totally mineralized. Rapid growth of the cartilage cap is best assessed at MR imaging. The sarcoma may destroy the bony exostosis on which it arose.

Metastases to lung or bone will ossify (Figure 3.151).

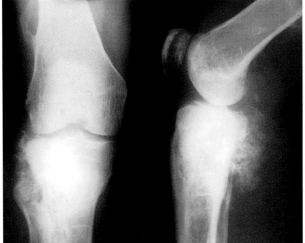

a

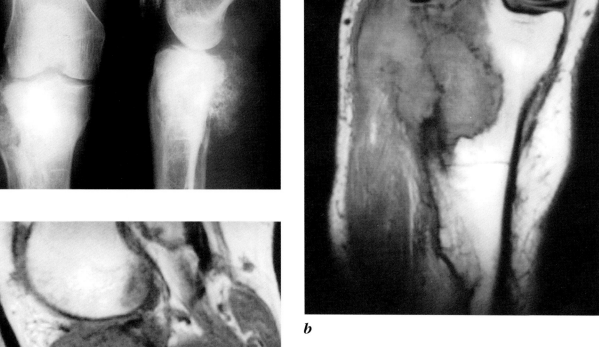

b

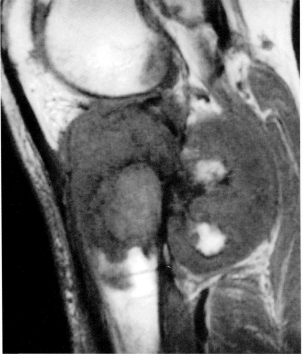

c

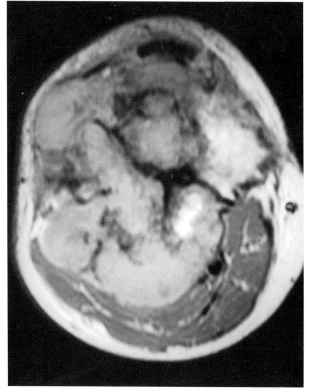

d

Figure 3.149 *Malignant degeneration of cartilage-capped exostosis. (**a**) The initial radiograph shows the exostosis with a large soft tissue mass lying peripheral to it; the margin of the exostosis is irregular. (**b**) Coronal T_1- and (**c**) sagittal T_1-weighted MR images demonstrate a large irregular soft tissue mass containing only a little mineralized bone. There is invasion of the underlying marrow by the tumour. (**d**) An axial T_1-weighted MR sequence showing very little mineralized bone within the large soft tissue mass.*

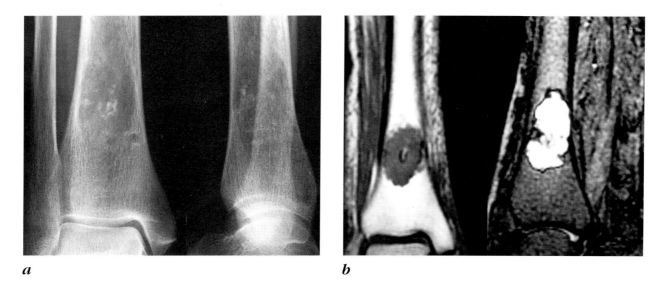

a   *b*

Figure 3.150 *Chondrosarcoma. (**a**) The plain film shows an osteolytic lesion of the distal tibia. It is poorly defined. There is early endosteal scalloping of the tibia on the lateral view. The lesion is mineralizing. (**b**) Coronal T$_1$-weighted (left) and sagittal fat suppression (right) MR sequences. Despite the biopsy-proven malignancy, the lesion is well defined, vascular and shows central mineralization.*

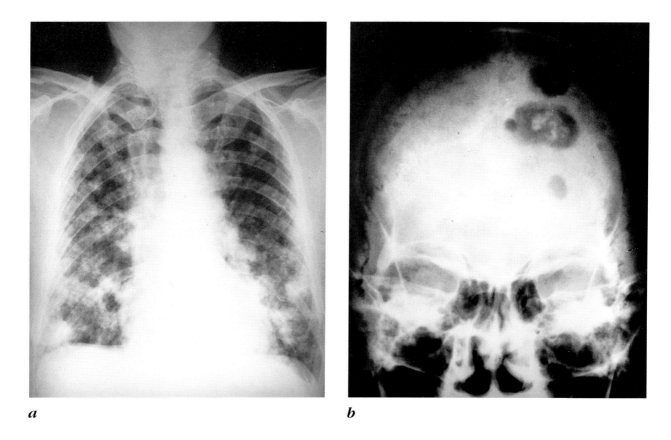

a   *b*

Figure 3.151 *Metastasizing chondrosarcoma. The metastases in both the lung (**a**) and skull vault (**b**) show mineralization.*

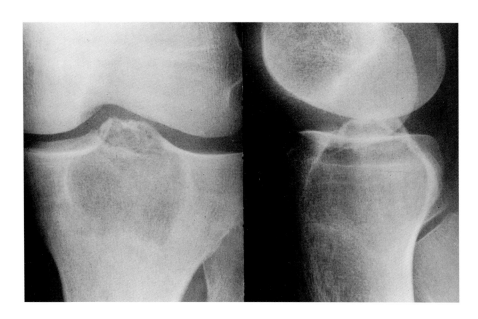

Figure 3.152 *Clear-cell chondrosarcoma. A rather nondescript, poorly defined lesion extends to the proximal tibia. The appearances resemble a giant-cell tumour, but the lesion is not particularly expansile. The patient was aged 61 years.*

Clear-cell chondrosarcoma

This is a rare lesion. Lytic change is seen at typical sites, the proximal femur, humerus and tibia. The lesions resemble giant-cell tumours in patients aged 30 to 50 years, being mainly lytic and minimally expansile (Figure 3.152).

DIFFERENTIATION BETWEEN INFECTION AND TUMOUR

CHRONIC OSTEOMYELITIS (BRODIE'S ABSCESS) AND OSTEOID OSTEOMA (OR OSTEOBLASTOMA)

Both of these lesions occur in children and young adults and are associated with pain, but night pain is a characteristic of osteoid osteoma. In both conditions, a central lucency surrounded by reactive sclerosis may contain foci of density, which are due to sequestra in granulation tissue in a Brodie's abscess or matrix ossification in the tumour (see Figure 3.23). Finger-like extensions of the destructive process called tunnelling only occur in infections (Figure 3.76).

The osteoid osteoma is a highly vascular tumour and therefore is well displayed at angiography and isotope scanning, whereas the central lucent area in

the Brodie's abscess is avascular. At MRI, the central vascular nidus is bright on T_2-weighted and fat suppression sequences, and enhances with gadolinium on T_1-weighted images.

ACUTE INFECTION AND MALIGNANT ROUND CELL TUMOURS (LEUKAEMIA, NEUROBLASTOMA AND EWING'S SARCOMA)

Both types of lesion may have similar clinical and laboratory features of pain, fever, local swelling and a raised erythrocyte sedimentation rate (ESR). Aggressive infiltration of bone causes a permeative lesion which destroys the cortex and elevates the periosteum, causing a periostitis with a soft tissue mass. Infections progress more rapidly than tumours and, although the initial radiological examination of the acutely painful limb may be normal, rapid progress usually confirms infection.

Sequestra are the hallmark of infection and are only occasionally seen with tumours (see Figure 3.121a), often in fibrosarcomas which usually occur in an older age group. Linear sequestration in infections is often very dense and should not be confused with matrix ossification in malignant tumours of bone such as osteogenic sarcoma. This tumour occurs in the same age group as infection and often at the same metaphyseal site. Dense sequestra can be seen with CT scans and as low signal structures on MRI, but will inevitably be less well seen with cross-sectional images unless the sequestrum lies in the plane of the scan.

On plain films, soft tissue masses in infection are generally poorly defined because of oedema of displaced fat planes, whereas in malignancy the fat planes are displaced, but not invaded, although MRI demonstrates substantial oedema around tumours. This oedema may cause some confusion with viable tumour around the margins of the lesion. Gadolinium may be helpful in enhancing vascular and viable tumour.

BIBLIOGRAPHY

Aisen AM, Martel W, Braunstein EM et al (1986) MRI and CT evaluation of primary bone and soft-tissue tumors. *Am J Roentgenol* **146**: 749–56.

Amstutz HC (1969) Multiple osteogenic sarcomata: metastatic or multicentric? Report of two cases and review of the literature. *Cancer* **24**: 923–31.

Beltran J, Simon DC, Katz W et al (1987) Increased MR signal intensity in skeletal muscle adjacent to malignant tumors: pathologic correlation and clinical relevance. *Radiology* **162**: 251–5.

Berquist TH, Ehman RL, King BF et al (1990) Value of MR imaging in differentiating benign from malignant soft tissue masses: study of 95 lesions. *Am J Roentgenol* **155**: 1251–5.

Bertoni F, Bacchini P, Capanna R et al (1993) Solid variant of aneurysmal bone cyst. *Cancer* **71**: 729–34.

Bertoni F, Present D, Sudanese A et al (1988) Giant cell tumor of bone with pulmonary metastases: six case reports and a review of the literature. *Clin Orthop* **237**: 275–85.

Bloem JL, Holscher HM, Taminiau AHM (1992) MRI and CT of primary musculoskeletal tumors. In: *MR Imaging and CT of the Musculoskeletal System: A Text Atlas* (eds, Bloem JL, Sartoris D), pp. 189–217. Baltimore: Williams & Wilkins.

Bloem JL, Mulder JD (1985) Chondroblastoma: a clinical and radiological study of 104 cases. *Skeletal Radiol* **14**: 1–9.

Bloem JL, Taminiau AHM, Eulderink F et al (1988) Radiologic staging of primary bone sarcoma: MR imaging, scintigraphy, angiography and CT correlated with pathologic examination. *Radiology* **169**: 805–10.

Bonakdarpour A, Levy WM, Aegerter E (1978) Primary and secondary aneurysmal bone cyst: a radiological study of 75 cases. *Radiology* **126**: 75–83.

Brady LW (1979) Radiation induced sarcomas of bone. *Skeletal Radiol* **41**: 72–8.

Brower AC, Culver JE Jr, Keats TE (1971) Histological nature of cortical irregularity of the medical posterior distal femoral metaphysis in children. *Radiology* **99**: 389–92.

Bufkin WJ (1971) The avulsive cortical irregularity. *Am J Roentgenol* **112**: 487–92.

Camilleri AE (1991) Craniofacial fibrous dysplasia. *J Laryngol Otol* **105**: 662–6.

Campanacci M (1976) Osteofibrous dysplasia of long bones. A new clinical entity. *It J Orthop Traumatol* **2**: 221–37.

Campanacci M, Baldini N, Boriani S, Sudanese A (1987) Giant-cell tumor of bone. *J Bone Joint Surg* **69A**: 106–14.

Campanacci M, Capanna R, Ricci P (1986) Unicameral and aneurysmal bone cysts. *Clin Orthop* **204**: 25–36.

Daffner RH, Kirks DR, Gehweiler JA Jr et al (1982) Computed tomography of fibrous dysplasia. *Am J Roentgenol* **139**: 943–8.

Dahlin DC (1978) Giant cell tumor (osteoclastoma). In: *Bone Tumors*, 3rd edn, pp 99–115, 228–95. Springfield: Charles C Thomas.

Dahlin DC (1985) Caldwell Lecture: Giant cell tumor of bone: highlights of 407 cases. *Am J Roentgenol* **144**: 955–60.

Dahlin DC, Coventry MB, Scanlon PW (1961) Ewing's sarcoma: a critical analysis of 165 cases. *J Bone Joint Surg* **43A**: 185.

Eyre-Brook AL, Price CHG (1969) Fibrosarcoma of bone: review of 50 consecutive cases from the Bristol Bone Tumour Registry. *J Bone Joint Surg* **51B**: 20–37.

Feldman F, Hecht HL, Johnson AD (1970) Chondromyxoid fibroma of bone. *Radiology* **94**: 249–60.

Greditzer HG III, McLeod RA, Unni KK et al (1983) Bone sarcomas in Paget disease. *Radiology* **146**: 327–33.

Harris WH, Dudley HR, Berry RV (1962) The natural history of fibrous dysplasia. *J Bone Joint Surg* **44A**: 207.

Henry A (1969) Monostotic fibrous dysplasia. *J Bone Joint Surg* **51B**: 300–6.

Herman SD, Mesgerzadeh M, Bonakdarpour A et al (1987) The role of magnetic resonance imaging in giant cell tumor of bone. *Skeletal Radiol* **16**: 635–43.

Hudson TM (1984) Fluid levels in aneurysmal bone cysts: a CT feature. *Am J Roentgenol* **142**: 1001–4.

Hudson TM (1984) Scintigraphy of aneurysmal bone cysts. *Am J Roentgenol* **142**: 761–5.

Hudson TM, Schiebler M, Springfield DS et al (1984) Radiology of giant-cell tumors of bone: computed tomography, arthro-tomography and scintigraphy. *Skeletal Radiol* **11**: 85–95.

Huvos AG, Higinbotham NL, Miller TR et al (1972) Bone sarcomas arising in fibrous dysplasia. *J Bone Joint Surg* **64A**: 1047–56.

Kattapuram SV, Phillips WC, Mankin HJ (1986) Giant cell tumor of bone: radiographic changes following local excision and allograft replacement. *Radiology* **161**: 493–8.

Klein MH, Shankman S (1992) Osteoid osteoma: radiologic and pathologic correlation. *Skeletal Radiol* **21**: 23–31.

Kroon HM, Schurmans J (1990) Osteoblastoma: clinical and radiologic findings in 98 new cases. *Radiology* **175**: 783–90.

Levine E, DeSmet AA, Neff JR et al (1984) Scintigraphic evaluation of giant cell tumor of bone. *Am J Roentgenol* **143**: 343–8.

Levy WM, Miller AS, Bonakdarpour A, Aegerter E (1975) Aneurysmal bone cyst secondary to other osseous lesions: report of 57 cases. *Am J Clin Pathol* **63**: 1–8.

Lichtenstein L (1953) Histiocytosis X: integration of eosinophilic granuloma of bone, Letterer-Siwe disease and Schuller-Christian disease as related to manifestations of a single nosologic entity. *Archives of Pathology* **56**: 84.

McLeod RA, Beabout JW (1973) The roentgenographic features of chondroblastoma. *Am J Roentgenol* **118**: 464–71.

Mainzer F, Minagi H, Steinbach HL (1971) The variable manifestations of multiple enchondromatosis. *Radiology* **97**: 377–88.

Matsuno T, Unni KK, McLeod RA et al (1976) Telangiectatic osteogenic sarcoma. *Cancer* **38**: 2538–47.

Mervak TR, Unni KK, Pritchard DJ, McLeod RA (1991) Telangiectatic osteosarcoma. *Clin Orthop* **270**: 135–9.

Munk PL, Helms CA, Hold RG et al (1989) MR imaging of aneurysmal bone cysts. *Am J Roentgenol* **153**: 99–101.

Murayama S, Numaguchi Y, Robinson AE et al (1988) Magnetic resonance imaging of calvarial eosinophilic granuloma. *J Comput Tomog* **12**: 251–2.

Murphy NB, Price CHG (1971) The radiological aspects of chondromyxoid fibroma of bone. *Clin Radiol* **22**: 261–9.

Onitsuka H (1977) Roentgenologic aspects of bone islands. *Radiology* **123**: 607–12.

Price CHG, Goldie W (1969) Paget sarcoma of bone. *J Bone Joint Surg* **51B**: 205.

Resnick D, Hemcek AA, Haghighi P (1983) Spinal enostoses (bone islands). *Radiology* **147**: 373–6.

Rosenthal DI, Schiller AL, Mankin HJ (1984) Chondrosarcoma: correlation of radiological and histological grade. *Radiology* **150**: 21–6.

Sanerkin NG (1980) Malignancy, aggressiveness and recurrence in giant cell tumor of bone. *Cancer* **46**: 1641–9.

Struhl S, Edelson C, Pritzker H et al (1989) Solitary (unicameral) bone cyst: the fallen fragment sign revisited. *Skeletal Radiol* **18**: 261–5.

Sun TC, Swee RG, Shives TC et al (1985) Chondrosarcoma in Maffucci's syndrome. *J Bone Joint Surg* **67A**: 1214–9.

Sundaram M, McLeod RA (1990) MR imaging of tumor and tumorlike lesions of bone and soft tissue. *Am J Roentgenol* **155**: 817–24.

Swee RG, McLeod RA, Beabout JW (1979) Osteoid osteoma: detection, diagnosis and localization. *Radiology* **130**: 117–23.

Taconis WK, Mulder JD (1984) Fibrosarcoma and malignant fibrous histiocytoma of long bones: radiographic features and grading. *Skeletal Radiol* **11**: 237–45.

Tehranzadeh J, Manymneh W, Ghavam C et al (1989) Comparison of CT and MR imaging in musculoskeletal neoplasms. *J Comput Assist Tomog* **13**: 466–72.

Tsai JC, Dalinka MK, Fallon MD et al (1990) Fluid-fluid level: a nonspecific finding in tumors of bone and soft tissue. *Radiology* **175**: 779–82.

Tubbs WS, Brown LR, Beabout JW et al (1992) Benign giant cell tumor of bone with pulmonary metastases: clinical findings and radiologic appearance of metastases in 13 cases. *Am J Roentgenol* **158**: 331–4.

Unni KK (1996) *Dahlin's Bone Tumors*, 5th edn. Philadelphia: Lippincott-Raven..

Utz JA, Kransdorf MJ, Jelinek JS et al (1989) MR appearance of fibrous dysplasia. *J Comput Assist Tomog* **13**: 845–51.

Wilson TW, Pugh DG (1955) Primary reticulum cell sarcoma of bone, with emphasis on roentgen aspects. *Radiology* **65**: 343.

Chapter 4   Lesions affecting the epiphyses; joint disease

John Poland, FRCS, Consultant Surgeon to the City Orthopaedic Hospital, London, the forerunner of the Royal National Orthopaedic Hospital, published his *Atlas of Skiagraphic Development of the Hand and Wrist* in 1898 (Figure 4.1). Standards for skeletal development have subsequently been established by Greulich and Pyle, and Tanner and Whitehouse (see Appendix). In particular, Pyle and co-workers have produced atlases of skeletal development for the hand and wrist, knee and foot.

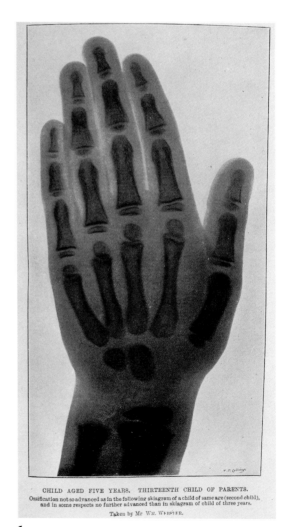

SKIAGRAPHIC ATLAS

SHOWING

THE DEVELOPMENT

OF THE

BONES OF THE WRIST AND HAND

FOR THE USE OF STUDENTS AND OTHERS

BY

JOHN POLAND, F.R.C.S.

LONDON
SMITH, ELDER, & CO., 15 WATERLOO PLACE
1898

All rights reserved

a

CHILD AGED FIVE YEARS, THIRTEENTH CHILD OF PARENTS.
Ossification not so advanced as in the following skiagram of a child of same age (second child), and in some respects no further advanced than in skiagram of child of three years.
Taken by Mr WM. WEBSTER.

b

Figure 4.1 (*a*) *The title page of* Atlas of Skiagraphic Development of the Hand and Wrist, *by John Poland, FRCS, published in 1898.* (*b*) *A specimen from the book assessing skeletal development.*

Table 4.1 Causes of delay in skeletal maturity.

Congenital heart disease
Hypothyroidism
Hypogonadism
Hypopituitarism
Diabetes
Severe generalized disease
  —renal failure, coeliac disease
Haemolytic anaemia
Malnutrition
Steroid therapy
Rickets
Skeletal dysplasias, eg the mucopolysaccharidoses

CAUSES OF DELAY IN SKELETAL MATURITY (Table 4.1)

HYPOTHYROIDISM

There is a delay in skeletal and dental maturation, accompanied by short stature (Figure 4.2). Epiphyses appear and fuse late, and are often abnormal in appearance, with increased density and fragmentation, particularly at the femoral and humeral heads (Figure 4.3). The changes are symmetrical, unlike in Perthes' disease, when the fragmentation of the ossific nucleus of the upper femoral epiphysis is almost inevitably asymmetrical, even if bilateral (Figure 4.4). In dysplasia epiphysealis multiplex, the femoral heads are also symmetrically flattened or fragmented, but there is no delay in fusion of the epiphyses (Figure 4.5).

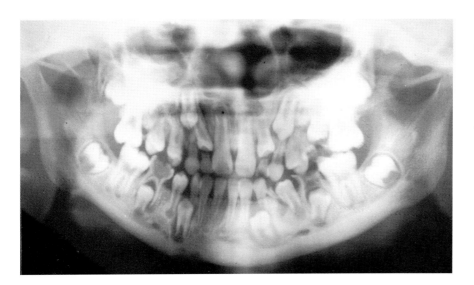

Figure 4.2 *This 17-year-old patient has hypothyroidism. There is gross retardation of dental age. The secondary dentition has failed to develop, and much of the primary dentition remains.*

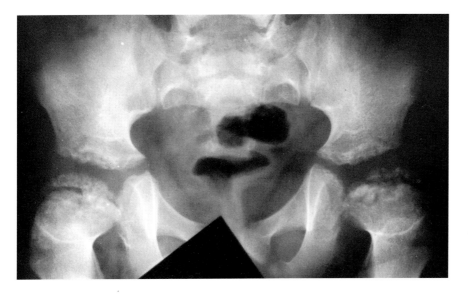

Figure 4.3 *Cretinism. Symmetrical fragmentation of the femoral heads resembles Perthes' disease in this 14-year-old boy; however, in the latter condition the changes are rarely symmetrical. There is associated broadening of the irregular femoral necks. The synchondrosis at the ischio-pubic ramus is still open. This is another feature of retarded skeletal maturity and is not to be confused with a Looser's zone.*

In hypothyroidism, a flattened or fragmented epiphysis may persist into adult life (Figure 4.6). In the shoulder, there may be humerus varus which has a 'telephone receiver' appearance (Figure 1.49c). Other radiological changes include Wormian bones and vertebral body hypoplasia, particularly at the thoraco-lumbar junction.

In the other diseases with Wormian bones, osseous density is *reduced* in osteogenesis imperfecta and hypophosphatasia, while pathological fractures and bony bowing are not a feature of cretinism. However, bone density is *normal* in cleidocranial dysplasia, in which skeletal maturity is slightly retarded, and is *increased* in pyknodysostosis (Table 4.2).

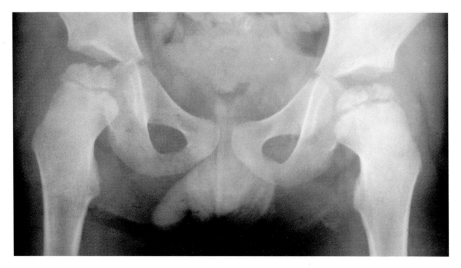

Figure 4.4 *Perthes' disease. In this patient the changes are seen at both femoral heads but there is asymmetry. Acetabular and supra-acetabular modelling are more normal.*

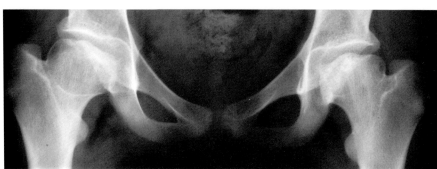

Figure 4.5 *Dysplasia epiphysealis multiplex. Both femoral heads are irregular and flattened, but not fragmented. Changes at the acetabular roof reflect this. In this patient abnormalities were also present at other large joints.*

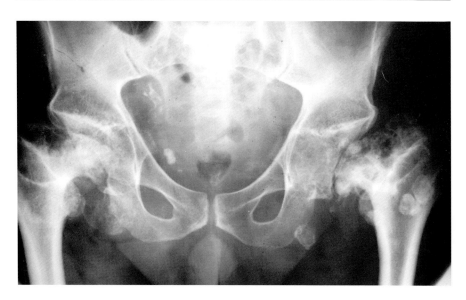

Figure 4.6 *Cretinism. The patient is an adult but irregularity and fragmentation of the femoral heads has persisted. The longstanding nature of the disease may be seen, particularly at the left acetabulum in which there is new bone medially, and loose bodies as a result of early fragmentation of the adjacent epiphysis.*

Table 4.2 Diseases occurring with Wormian bones.

Disease	Bone density	Pathological fractures; bowing	Skeletal maturity
Hypothyroidism	Normal	None	Delayed
Osteogenesis imperfecta	Reduced	Present	Normal
Hypophosphatasia	Reduced	Present	Delayed
Cleidocranial dysplasia	Normal	None	Slight retardation of growth
Pyknodysostosis	Increased	Present	Small stature

HYPOGONADISM AND HYPOPITUITARISM

In hypogonadism and hypopituitarism there is delay in skeletal maturation and fusion, which is associated with osteoporosis.

STEROID EXCESS

Steroid excess, whether iatrogenic or adrenal in origin, causes a delay in skeletal maturation, which is often gross. This is associated with osteoporosis and pathological fractures, vertebral collapse with callus formation (Figure 1.20) and avascular necrosis (Figure 4.7). There are no Wormian bones. Clinically the condition does not resemble osteogenesis imperfecta.

RICKETS

Rickets involves some delay in epiphyseal maturation, associated with an abnormal bone texture, metaphyseal irregularity and splaying, and widening of the growth plate (Figure 1.48b). Fusion of the ischio-pubic synchondrosis, which normally occurs at about 7 years of age, may be retarded in conditions where fusion in general is retarded, for example, cretinism. However, Looser's zones are commonly found at that site and should be diagnosed after 10 years of age if lucency persists there.

Skeletal maturity is often delayed in children with severe cardiac, renal or gastro-intestinal disease, or in those with malnutrition, and growth arrest lines may be seen. Severe haemolytic anaemias also retard maturation.

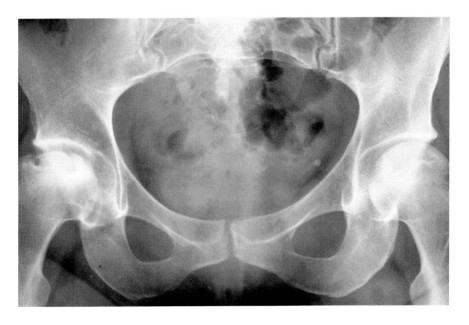

Figure 4.7 *In avascular necrosis following steroid therapy, structural failure is quite advanced at the right femoral head with collapse of sclerotic bone. In the left femoral head an avascular area is surrounded by a sclerotic zone of creeping substitution. Collapse will occur here too.*

CAUSES OF ACCELERATION IN SKELETAL MATURITY (Table 4.3)

HYPERTHYROIDISM

This is rare in children but is associated with accelerated skeletal maturation and osteoporosis.

HYPERPITUITARISM

This causes an excess of growth hormone, and produces gigantism before skeletal fusion, and acromegaly after it. An adult gigant has a different appearance to an acromegalic. Overgrowth in gigantism occurs when epiphyseal plates are open and leads to excessive longitudinal and transverse growth. Acromegalics cannot increase bone length, but soft tissues such as heel pads (Figure 4.8) and intervertebral discs are enlarged, as are joint cartilages, leading to an increase in the height of the

Table 4.3 Causes of accelerated skeletal maturity.

Hyperthyroidism
Hypergonadism
Hyperpituitarism—gigantism
Fibrous dysplasia
Adrenogenital syndrome
Homocystinuria
Neurofibromatosis
Juvenile chronic arthritis and other causes of
    increased blood flow, eg in infection (often
    localized)

patient. Bones also broaden, particularly at muscle insertions (Figure 4.9). Bone may be resorbed so that cortical thinning, osteoporosis and vertebral scalloping may result. (For other causes of vertebral scalloping, see Table 7.5, page 350.)

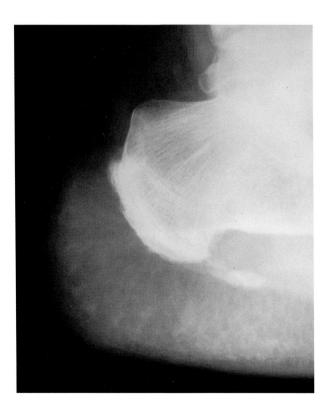

Figure 4.8 *Acromegaly. Much new bone is seen on the posterior aspect of the calcaneum and the heel pad thickness is increased.*

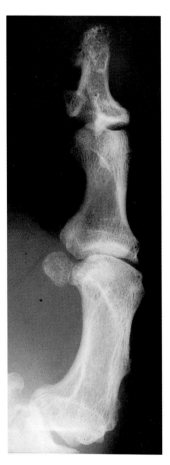

Figure 4.9 *In acromegaly, an increase in growth hormone thickens the cartilages so that the joint spaces appear widened. Muscle insertions become more prominent and secondary osteoarthritis often supervenes. The sesamoids are often enlarged and this can be measured (the sesamoid index).*

FIBROUS DYSPLASIA

This may be associated with endocrine abnormalities. Albright's syndrome associates fibrous dysplasia with skin pigmentation and precocious sexual development, usually in females. Growth discrepancy in fibrous dysplasia may be due to the fibrous lesion in a bone. Other endocrine anomalies associated with fibrous dysplasia—Cushing's syndrome, thyrotoxicosis and hyperpituitarism—can also result in altered skeletal maturity and growth.

Precocious sexual development occurs in neurofibromatosis, in which there is also skin pigmentation, although in a different form to that of fibrous dysplasia. Other endocrine abnormalities may also be found, but overgrowth of bones in neurofibromatosis is not usually endocrine in origin but part of the dysplasia and not confined to the epiphyses.

Large epiphyses are also found in homocystinuria, fibrodysplasia ossificans progressiva (see Chapter 9, page 451) and the Laurence–Moon–Biedl syndrome.

INCREASE IN EPIPHYSEAL MATURATION DUE TO LOCAL HYPERAEMIA

This occurs in any condition in which blood flow is increased locally. Epiphyseal growth is advanced and premature fusion may result, so that an initial gain in length is followed by eventual shortening.

PREMATURE FUSION

Premature fusion at epiphyses is rarely generalized but is more usually due to local disease. It usually

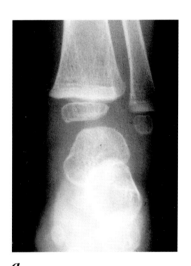

a

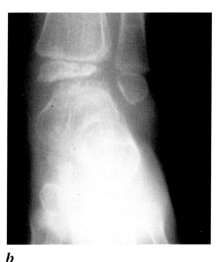

b

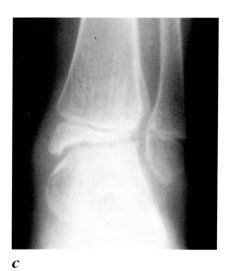

c

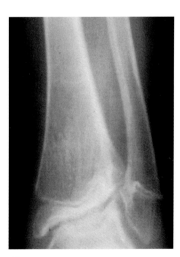

d

Figure 4.10 *Premature fusion in osteomyelitis. This series of radiographs was obtained over 3 years. (**a**) The initial radiograph shows diffuse soft tissue swelling around the ankle joint. (**b**) The second, after 1 year, shows irregularity of the head of the talus and of the adjacent distal tibial epiphysis. The joint space is narrowed, indicating cartilaginous destruction. (**c**) Subsequently, there is evidence of failure of growth of the lateral aspect of the distal tibial epiphysis which is associated with a parallel overgrowth of the adjacent talus. (**d**) The final radiograph, 3 years after the initial radiograph, shows premature fusion of the growth plate of the distal tibia laterally and of the adjacent fibula, with marked tibio-talar slant and a narrow and irregular joint line, which characterizes an infective aetiology.*

follows infection (Figure 4.10), trauma (Figure 4.11) or irradiation to the growth plate (Figure 4.12).

If the entire growth plate is destroyed, there will be growth arrest across the entire epiphysis. If only part of the growth plate is damaged, then growth around it moves away from the fused part, producing a deformed or V-shaped bone end known as the chevron sign. This appearance also occurs in achondroplasia (Figure 4.13), and in scurvy following fractures through the translucent metaphyseal zone at the knees.

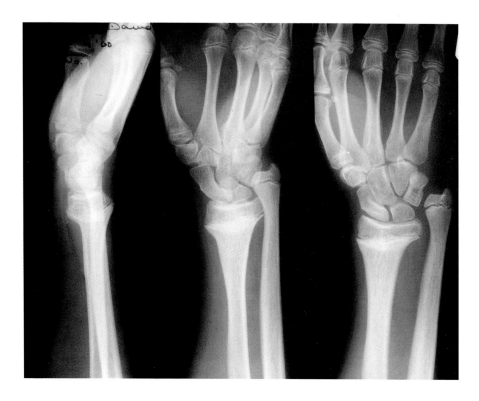

Figure 4.11 *Premature fusion secondary to trauma is relatively common and follows compression of the growth plate of the distal radius. The growth plate is fused centrally but is still open laterally, so that peripheral growth can still occur. A chevron deformity results.*

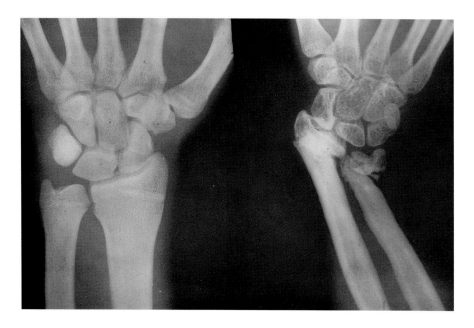

Figure 4.12 *Premature fusion following radiation. The left wrist is normal but on the right there is hypoplasia of the distal radius and ulna associated with premature fusion and sclerosis around the epiphyseal plate.*

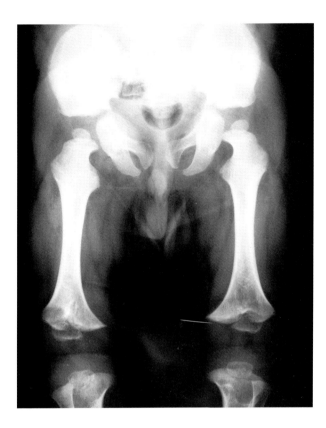

Figure 4.13 *Achondroplasia. A chevron deformity occurs as a normal phenomenon at the distal femur.*

GENERALIZED CHANGES AT EPIPHYSES—DISEASES OF JOINTS

Hyperaemia at epiphyses occurs in juvenile chronic arthritis and other collagen diseases, haemophilia, and occasionally with tumours. All these diseases have at least one common feature, that is, the joints are affected by changes at both articular surfaces within the confines of the joint capsule, and at the synovium (Tables 4.4 and 4.5). Identical appearances are seen with septic arthritis prior to fusion.

RHEUMATOID ARTHRITIS

The disease is first seen in the feet rather than the hands, most commonly at the fifth metatarsophalangeal joint, least commonly at the first metatarsophalangeal joint. The metatarsal heads are involved before the adjacent phalanges.

Table 4.4 Causes of widespread changes in epiphyseal shape.

Osteoarthritis
Rheumatoid arthritis, juvenile chronic arthritis, psoriatic arthritis
Hypothyroidism
Haemophilia
Following avascular necrosis
Acromegaly
Rickets
Dysplasias of bone:
  Achondroplasia
  Pseudoachondroplasia
  Dysplasia epiphysealis multiplex (Fairbank)
  Dysplasia epiphysealis hemimelica (Trevor)
  Spondyloepiphyseal dysplasia
  Mucopolysaccharidoses
  Enchondromatosis

Table 4.5 Generalized changes at epiphyses—diseases of joints.

Seropositive arthritides
  Rheumatoid arthritis
  Juvenile chronic arthritis
Seronegative arthritides
  Psoriasis
  Reiter's syndrome
  Ankylosing spondylitis
  Enteropathic spondylarthritides
Osteoarthritis
Septic arthritis
Gout
Haemophilia
Synovial tumours

Table 4.6 Erosive changes around joints.

Commonly occur in these main disease groups:
• Seropositive arthritides
• Seronegative arthritides
• Osteoarthritis
• Infections
• Synovial tumours:
    benign—pigmented villonodular synovitis, synovial osteochondromatosis
    malignant—malignant synovioma (synovial sarcoma)
• Gout
• Haemophilia

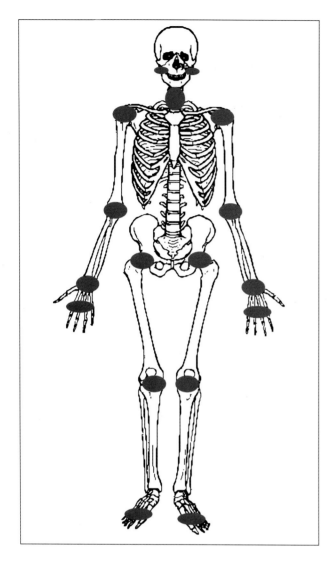

Figure 4.14 *Distribution of rheumatoid disease (shaded areas).*

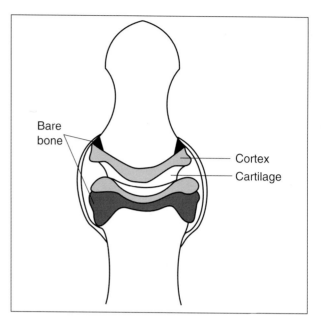

Figure 4.15 *Diagrammatic representation of a distal interphalangeal joint in the hand. The reciprocity of cartilage thickness is demonstrated. The black shaded areas are bare bone and are uncovered by either cartilage or synovium. Erosions arise first at these sites. (Reproduced from Martel W, Stuck KJ, Dworin AM et al, Erosive osteoarthritis and psoriatic arthritis: a radiologic comparison in the hand, wrist and foot, Am J Roentgenol (1980)* **134**:*125–35, with permission.)*

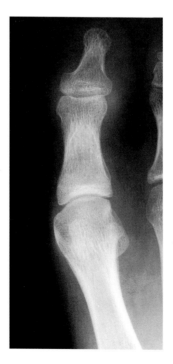

Figure 4.16 *In this patient with rheumatoid arthritis, there is soft tissue swelling around the great toe metatarso-phalangeal joint. Fine lamellar periosteal reactions can be seen along the metatarsal and phalangeal shafts. The metatarsophalangeal joint is narrower than the interphalangeal joint. There is demineralization.*

Abnormal joints are symmetrically affected and show local soft tissue swelling and osteoporosis. Erosions are the definitive change in rheumatoid arthritis. The distribution of erosions is illustrated in Figure 4.14. They occur initially in the para-articular regions, at the cartilage/synovium interface (Figure 4.15). Cartilage destruction results in joint space narrowing (Figure 4.16), followed by erosion of articular surfaces (Figure 4.17). Migration of pannus below the articular cortex results in subchondral erosions and collapse of articular cortex. Erosive changes around joints occur in other disease groups (Table 4.6).

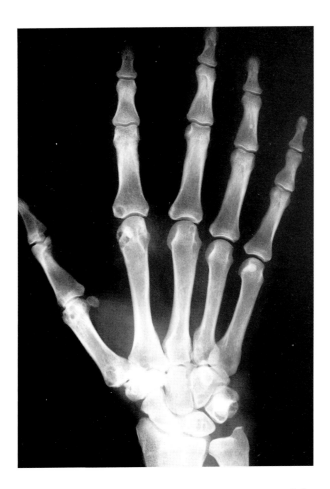

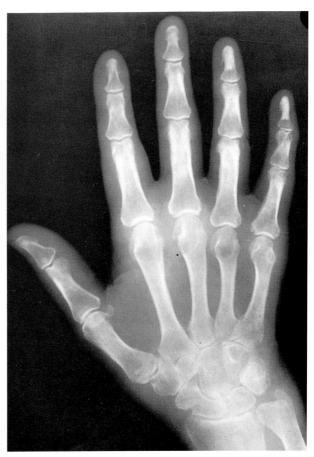

Figure 4.17 *Rheumatoid arthritis. Narrowing of the thumb and index metacarpophalangeal joints is associated with local erosive change. Further erosions are seen in the carpal bones.*

Figure 4.18 *In this patient with rheumatoid arthritis there is soft tissue swelling, particularly over the index and middle finger metacarpophalangeal joints and proximal phalanges. Bone density is reduced overall. The distal phalanges, however, show terminal phalangeal sclerosis, which is associated with, and often pre-dates, the onset of an erosive arthritis. Erosive change is also present at the fourth and fifth metacarpophalangeal joints.*

Reactive sclerosis can occur but overall bone density is diminished (Figure 4.18). New bone proliferation is not a prominent feature of rheumatoid arthritis, and erosions do not fill in. Secondary osteoarthritis occurs. Malalignment at joint surfaces is the result of bone destruction and local soft tissue changes, ligamentous laxity and tendinous attrition (Figure 4.19). Neurotrophic or 'cup and pencil' deformities are also seen. Where two normally separate bone surfaces approximate, usually due to alteration of the adjacent soft tissues, pressure erosions arise where one bone moves on the other.

This occurs, for instance, in rheumatoid arthritis with chronic rotator cuff tears. The humeral head migrates upward through the tear and its movements erode or scallop the undersurface of the acromion. The elevated humeral neck is subsequently eroded by the adjacent inferior lip of the glenoid (Figure 4.20). In scleroderma and Jaccoud's arthritis, subluxed phalangeal bases erode adjacent metacarpal necks (Figure 4.21). The upper surfaces of the third to sixth ribs are eroded in rheumatoid arthritis (Figure 4.20) and in any condition associated with muscle wasting—polio, old age, scleroderma.

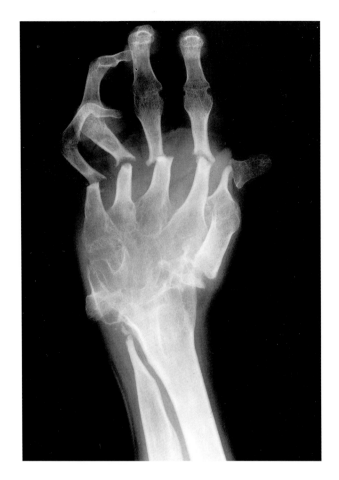

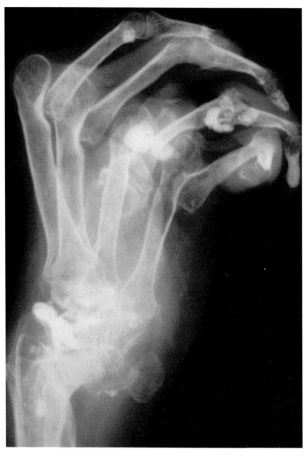

Figure 4.19 *End-stage rheumatoid arthritis with radiocarpal fusion. Cup and pencil deformities with bone resorption are present at the metacarpophalangeal joints, while the interphalangeal joints are fused. There is overall demineralization and soft tissue wasting.*

Figure 4.21 *Scleroderma. There is terminal phalangeal sclerosis and soft tissue calcification. In addition, there is subluxation at the metacarpophalangeal joints. Proximal subluxation of the phalangeal bases results in pressure erosion of the metacarpal necks; these erosions are well corticated and smooth.*

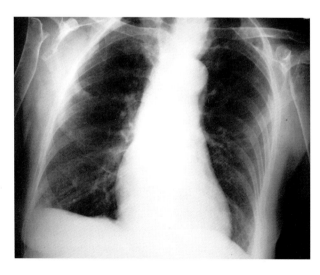

Figure 4.20 *The resorption of bone around the glenohumeral joints is almost neuropathic. The bone surfaces are no longer in alignment, and are smooth and sclerotic. Also, there is erosion of the upper surfaces of the third, fourth and fifth ribs. This phenomenon is probably related to muscle wasting and scapular attrition.*

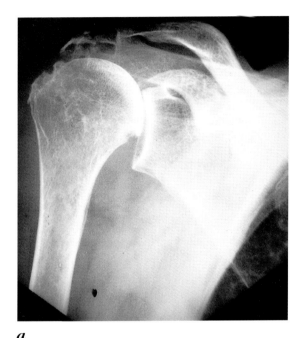
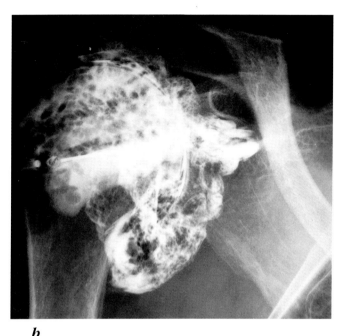

a   *b*

Figure 4.22 *Arthrography in rheumatoid arthritis.* **(a)** *The plain film shows generalized demineralization with substantial soft tissue swelling in the subaxillary region. Fat displacement indicates capsular distension. There are marginal erosions. Upward subluxation of the humeral head is shown together with obliteration of the gleno-humeral joint.* **(b)** *At arthrography the soft tissue swelling shown on the plain film is seen to correspond with a distended joint capsule. This is filled with numerous defects, some loose. There is synovial proliferation; debris and fibrin bodies lie within the joint. The rotator cuff is torn, as shown by filling of the subacromial bursa.*

Arthrography in rheumatoid arthritis demonstrates the distended joint and shows synovial proliferation (Figure 4.22). Debris is shown in the joint space and large geodes, or subarticular cysts, fill with contrast.

Baker's cyst is an enlarged gastrocnemius-semimembranosus bursa seen on a plain film as a mass posterior to the knee joint which fills with contrast at arthrography. Loose bodies may be seen within; if more than four loose bodies are present, synovial osteochondromatosis may be inferred (Figure 4.23). Rupture of the cyst causes a very painful leak of synovial fluid into the muscles of the calf, mimicking the symptoms of a deep vein thrombosis (Figure 4.24). This leak can be shown on arthrography, as well as ultrasound (Figures 4.25 and 4.26) or MRI (Figure 4.27). Ultrasound excludes a deep vein thrombosis, as does venography.

Baker's cysts are associated with meniscal tears (see below) and other forms of internal derangement because of increased fluid pressure in the joint. MRI shows a 5% incidence of popliteal cysts

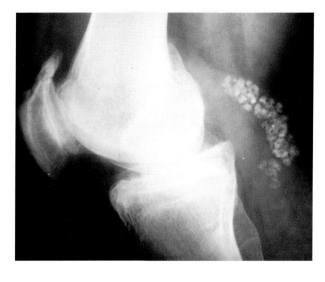

Figure 4.23 *Baker's cyst. A Baker's cyst is demonstrated posterior to the knee joint. It contains numerous loose bodies, compatible with a diagnosis of synovial osteochondromatosis.*

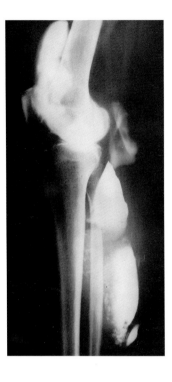

Figure 4.24 *Baker's cyst at arthrography. The cyst has ruptured and contrast medium passes into the calf and thigh. This lesion is chronic, as shown by the smooth wall of the contained leak.*

in patients with internal derangement of the knee joint and a 13% incidence in patients with a ruptured anterior cruciate ligament, but arthrography, which distends the joint, shows a higher incidence of these cysts.

Hyperaemia in the pre-erosive state and subsequent erosive change are demonstrated with great sensitivity using isotope scans. The distribution of the disease can be analysed and a distinction made between seronegative and seropositive arthropathies (Figure 4.28).

CT scanning demonstrates joint space narrowing and erosions (Figure 4.29).

Erosions are seen earlier and better at MRI than on plain films. Subchondral cysts (Figure 3.71), effusions and extra-articular collections of fluid are all clearly imaged, as are tendons and tendon sheaths. Small part coils demonstrate the joints of the hand and foot and surrounding structures with great detail (see Chapter 10, page 459). Intravenous paramagnetic contrast media give further enhancement of vascular (but not

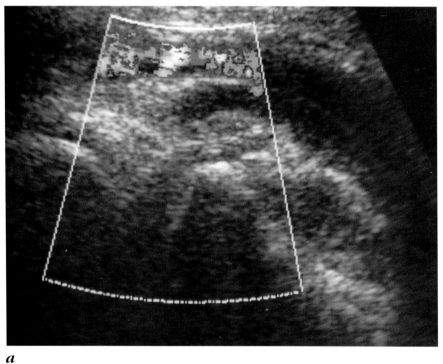

a

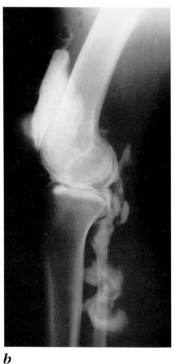

b

Figure 4.25 *Ruptured Baker's cyst. The patient presented with chronic pain in the calf. A deep vein thrombosis was suspected and a Doppler ultrasound scan was performed. (a) This scan shows a patent but compressed popliteal vein. This is the posterior of the two hypoechoic structures in the calf. The more anterior represents the fluid in the leak from the Baker's cyst, which is compressing the adjacent vein (patient examined prone). (b) An arthrogram was then performed, confirming the presence of a ruptured Baker's cyst. The suprapatellar pouch is also ruptured.*

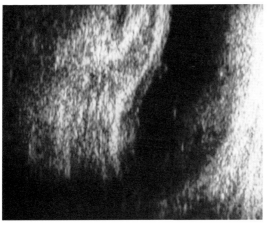

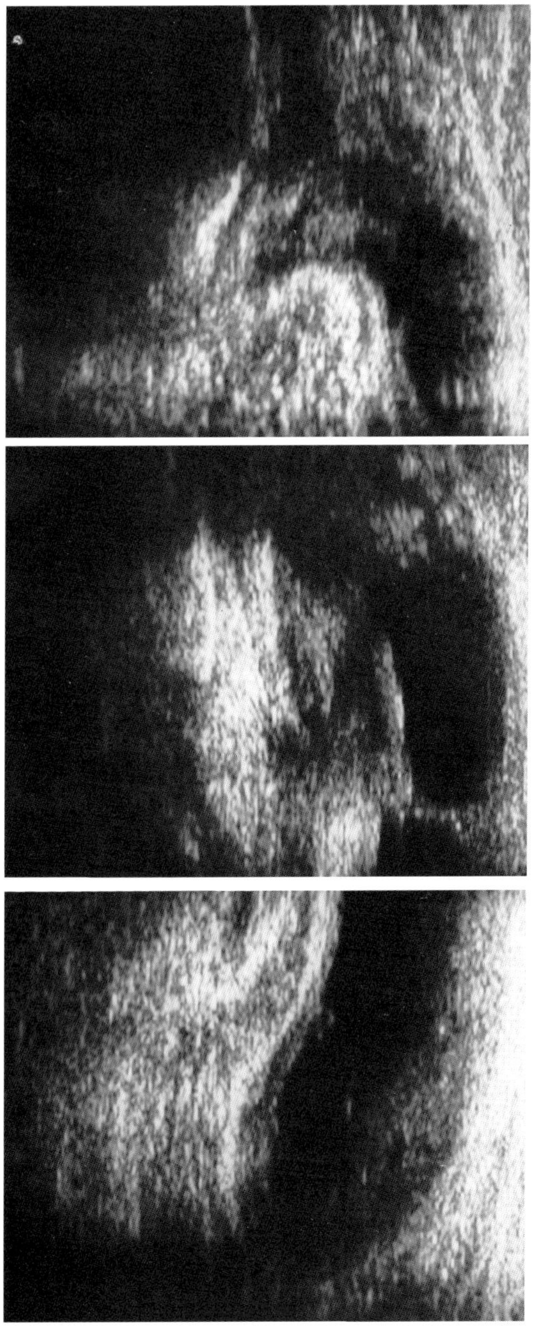

Figure 4.26 *Baker's cyst. Three serial images passing inferiorly behind the knee showing a Baker's cyst which has ruptured. There is a smooth and well defined hypoechoic collection of fluid extending down into the calf. Compare with Figure 4.24.*

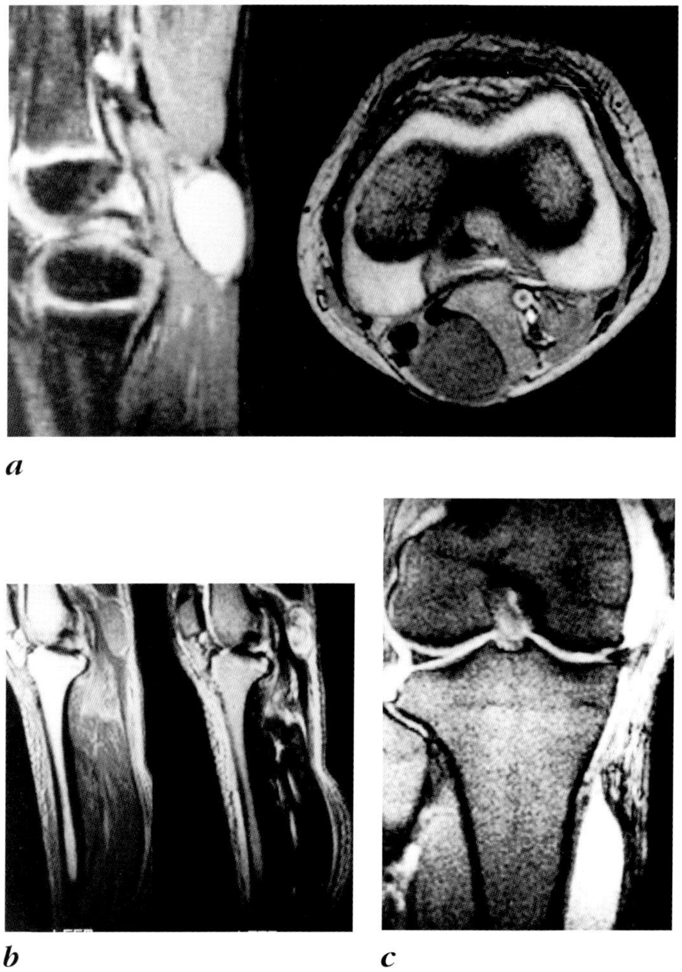

a

b   *c*

Figure 4.27 *Baker's cyst. (**a**) Sagittal fat suppression (left) and axial T$_1$-weighted gradient echo (right) MR sequences. The sagittal image demonstrates a well defined and intact Baker's cyst posterior to the knee joint in this child. The axial image shows the medial situation of the Baker's cyst and demonstrates its origin between the tendons of the medial gastrocnemius head and distal semimembranosus muscles. (**b**) T$_1$- and T$_2$-weighted images showing a posteriorly situated cyst, seen to contain debris. The leak disrupts the adjacent musculature. (**c**) Ruptured cyst (coronal T$_2$-weighted gradient echo MR sequence). Degenerative change is demonstrated at the medial compartment of the knee joint. There is marginal osteophytosis. A large effusion displaces the medial collateral ligament. The rather blunted hypoplastic meniscus is displaced together with the collateral ligament which itself is substantially disrupted. There is a leak of synovial fluid in and around the disrupted structures of the medial collateral ligament and a better loculated collection extending for a substantial distance into the calf.*

Anterior   Posterior

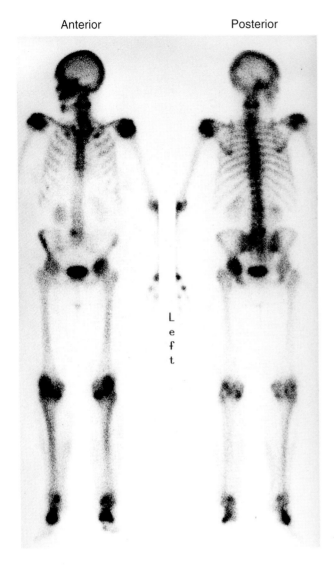

L
e
f
t

Figure 4.28 *Rheumatoid arthritis—radionuclide bone scanning. Increase in uptake is shown at major joints, sparing the right hip. (By courtesy of Dr A Hilson, Royal Free Hospital.)*

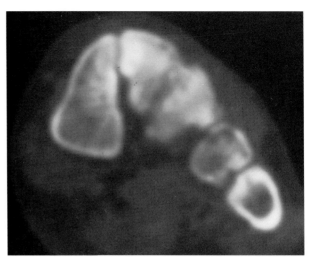

Figure 4.29 *Rheumatoid erosions in the foot, shown at CT scanning. Cortical changes are well demonstrated, as expected, on CT scans.*

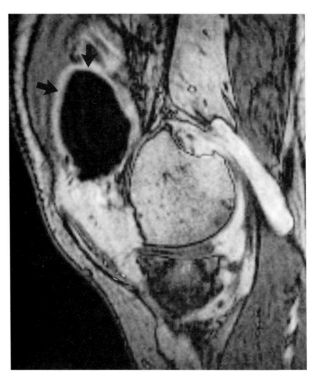

Figure 4.30 *Gadolinium-enhanced synovium in rheumatoid arthritis (modified sagittal T_1-weighted MR sequence following intravenous gadolinium). The effusion exhibits a low signal, while the surrounding area of bright signal (arrows) represents hypertrophic vascular synovium. (By courtesy of Dr G Clunie, UCL Hospitals.)*

fibrous) pannus (Figure 4.30). Cartilage loss too is best shown at MR scanning (Figure 4.31), so that rheumatoid arthritis and osteoarthritis are better shown on MR imaging than on plain films.

MRI is certainly the investigation of choice in the investigation of rheumatoid arthritis at the C1/2 region. Pannus is clearly shown, as is bone (see Chapter 8, page 375). The images are superior to those obtained with CT myelography, especially in the sagittal plane.

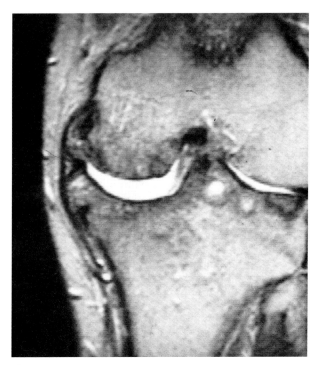

a

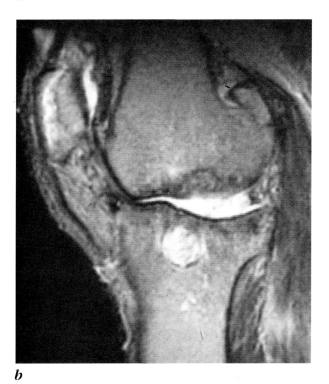

b

Figure 4.31 *(a, b) Rheumatoid arthritis at MR (coronal and sagittal T₂-weighted sequences). There is loss of meniscal and articular cartilage, irregularity of articular surfaces and subchondral cysts filled with fluid. There is also debris within the joint.*

PSORIATIC ARTHRITIS

Between 5 and 20% of psoriatics have an associated arthritis. The distribution of lesions in this disease is shown in Figure 4.32. Typical psoriatic arthritis is found in only 30% of patients with both psoriasis and arthritis; the remaining 70% have either rheumatoid-like changes or a mixed pattern.

Soft tissue swelling is seen. Density at affected joints is usually preserved, but this is not inevitable. Increase in the density of affected digits occurs in the presence of marked periostitis ('sausage' digit) (Figures 4.33 and 4.34).

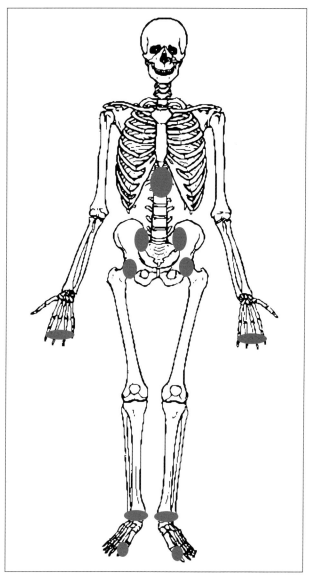

Figure 4.32 *Distribution of lesions in psoriasis (shaded areas).*

Erosions at affected joints, particularly the great toe and distal phalanges, occur on the articular surfaces rather than at joint margins, and are associated with marked local new bone formation. At distal phalangeal bases a 'gull's wing' appearance results (Figure 4.35);

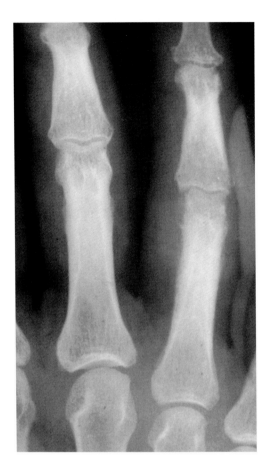

Figure 4.33 *In this psoriatic patient, swelling of the ring finger is associated with a periostitis of the proximal and middle phalanges and an increase in bony density.*

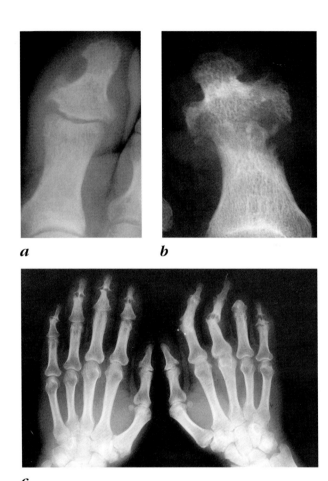

a   *b*

c

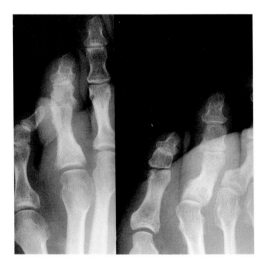

Figure 4.34 *Psoriasis. The proximal phalanx of the fourth toe shows expansion with sclerosis and overlying soft tissue swelling.*

Figure 4.35 *Psoriasis. (**a**) Soft tissue swelling is seen over the great toe and the erosions at the bases of the distal phalanges are on the articular, rather than the periarticular surface, producing a gull's wing appearance (**b**). (**c**) The distal interphalangeal joints are involved in this condition. Bone density is often preserved. Erosions proceed along the bases of the distal phalanges and there is splaying of bone locally. Despite the erosive change, the joints may be increased in width or, alternatively, fused. These changes are totally unlike those seen in rheumatoid arthritis both in appearance and distribution. There is also a neurotrophic change at the distal and middle phalanges, with longitudinal and concentric bone resorption, producing a 'licked candy stick' appearance.*

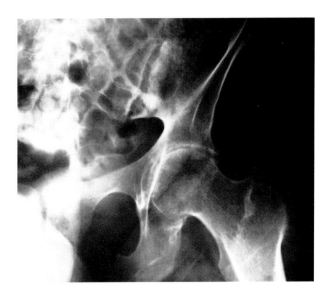

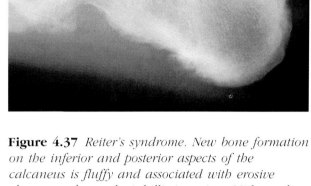

Figure 4.36 *Psoriasis. The left sacroiliac joint is eroded laterally with underlying reactive sclerosis. The left hip joint is narrowed, particularly superomedially, and the articular surfaces are irregular. There is no reactive new bone formation. Erosions are seen at the musculotendinous insertions on the ischium.*

Figure 4.37 *Reiter's syndrome. New bone formation on the inferior and posterior aspects of the calcaneus is fluffy and associated with erosive change at the tendo-Achillis insertion. Mid-tarsal new bone formation is also present on the plantar aspect.*

this may be associated with articular ankylosis. Bony proliferation at erosions is a feature of psoriatic arthritis, and occurs at joints and also at musculotendinous and ligamentous insertions into bone, known as the entheses. Changes at major joints are similar to those seen in rheumatoid disease (Figure 4.36).

REITER'S SYNDROME

This disease involves soft tissue swelling around affected joints but the changes are asymmetrical, unlike those seen in rheumatoid arthritis. Metatarsophalangeal joints are involved, and the feet are more often involved than the hands. New bone formation is prominent (Figure 4.37).

ANKYLOSING SPONDYLITIS AND ENTEROPATHIC SPONDYLARTHRITIS

Peripheral joint disease is not prominent but may precede the spinal changes, particularly in children. Erosive change can be followed by fusion of affected joints.

OSTEOARTHRITIS

The distribution of lesions in osteoarthritis is shown in Figure 4.38. Primary osteoarthritis has no obvious underlying aetiology whereas secondary disease usually follows articular malalignment, for example, after congenital anomalies or acquired, traumatic or infective lesions. Soft tissue swelling around the affected joints reflects underlying new bone proliferation, particularly at the distal interphalangeal joints (Figure 4.39). Bone density is unaffected by this condition, which is not associated with significant hyperaemia. Joint narrowing due to cartilage loss occurs primarily at areas of maximal stress, for example, the weight-bearing areas, and is followed by loss of articular bone (Figure 4.40). New bone is laid down in the non-weight-bearing areas of joints. Subarticular cysts collapse (Figure 4.41). Marginal osteophytes are characteristic features. Osteoarthritis is rare in the gleno-humeral joint as it is not weight-bearing, but unusual stresses here do cause osteoarthritis (Figures 4.42 and 4.43).

Change in osteoarthritis affects cortical bone and so is well seen at CT scanning, where axial images

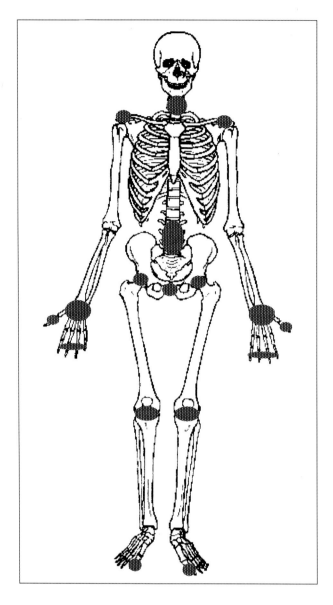

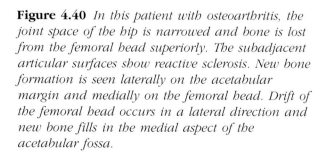

Figure 4.38 *Distribution of osteoarthritis (shaded areas).*

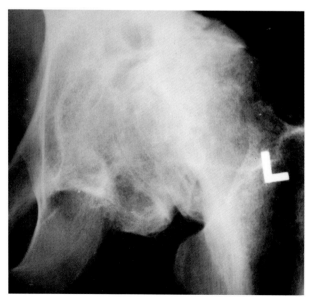

Figure 4.39 *Osteoarthritis. Involvement of the proximal and distal interphalangeal joints is shown with joint space narrowing and sclerosis of the articular surfaces. At the distal interphalangeal joints particularly there is proliferation of new bone around the joints.*

Figure 4.40 *In this patient with osteoarthritis, the joint space of the hip is narrowed and bone is lost from the femoral head superiorly. The subadjacent articular surfaces show reactive sclerosis. New bone formation is seen laterally on the acetabular margin and medially on the femoral head. Drift of the femoral head occurs in a lateral direction and new bone fills in the medial aspect of the acetabular fossa.*

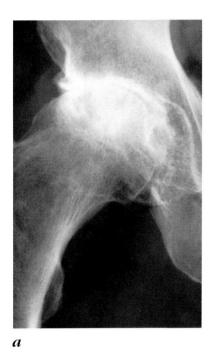 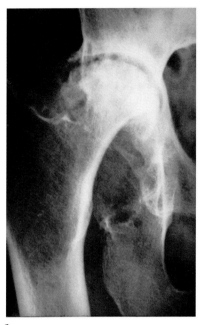

a *b*

Figure 4.41 *Progression of osteoarthritis. (a) The initial radiograph shows severe degenerative change with loss of the superior joint space, and subarticular cyst formation. (b) The subarticular cysts have collapsed with deepening of the acetabulum and loss of the superior part of the femoral head. The articular surfaces remain congruous but show eburnation.*

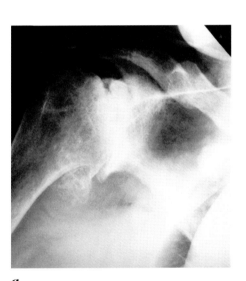 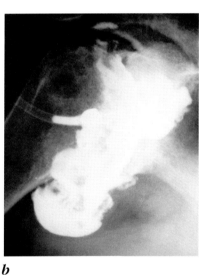

a *b*

Figure 4.42 *Osteoarthritis of the right shoulder. (a) Degenerative change is unusual at the gleno-humeral joint but usually follows excessive use of this joint in weight bearing, i.e. in paralysed patients who use artificial walking aids. The joint space is obliterated and there is resorption of subarticular bone with eburnation and marginal osteophytosis. (b) The arthrogram shows a very distended, irregular capsule. Numerous loose fragments are seen within the joint.*

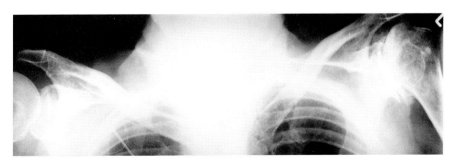

Figure 4.43 *Osteoarthritis of the left shoulder. The patient had been a famous English cricketer, who bowled with his left arm. The chest X-ray, taken in old age, shows severe degenerative change at the left shoulder joint with a normal right shoulder.*

and coronal and sagittal reconstructions show osteo-phytes, subarticular cysts and calcified loose bodies (Figure 4.44).

MRI has the benefit of demonstrating effusions, cysts (Figure 3.73) and non-mineralized loose bodies. Osteophytes are particularly well shown at articular margins, as are subarticular cysts and bone oedema. Cartilage loss is shown better than by any other imaging modality (Figures 4.31 and 4.45). It is the modality of choice.

Isotope scanning demonstrates the distribution of change in osteoarthritis (Fig 4.46).

GOUT

Eccentric soft tissue swelling around joints, which may calcify, is associated with deep erosions which undercut the cortex, often some distance from the joint margin (Figure 4.47). Large, curved bony spurs are seen at the margins of erosions. Distribution may be random but gout classically affects the metatar-sophalangeal joint of the big toe. Bone density is preserved, and chondrocalcinosis is common. (For a list of causes of chondrocalcinosis, see Table 9.2, page 437.)

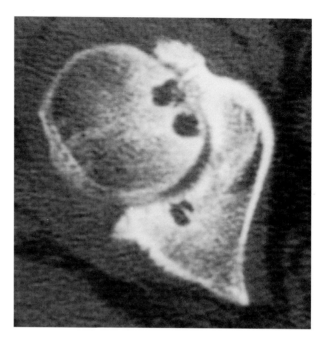

Figure 4.44 *Osteoarthritis at CT scanning. Joint space narrowing, subarticular cyst formation, eburnation and osteophyte formation are demonstrated.*

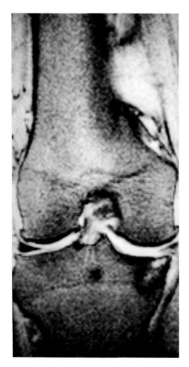
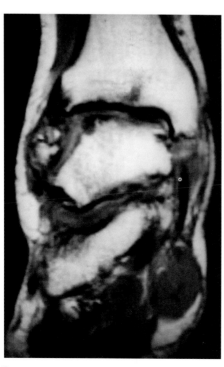

a   *b*

Figure 4.45 *Osteoarthritis at MR imaging (see also page 150). (**a**) On this coronal T$_2$-weighted MR sequence marginal osteophytes are demonstrated, together with a subarticular cyst in the medial tibial plateau. This is surrounded by a zone of low signal intensity compatible with sclerosis of bone on a plain film. A substantial effusion is present. The medial meniscus is torn. (**b**) A coronal T$_1$-weighted MR image demonstrates severe degeneration at the ankle and subtalar joints, with marked irregularity of the articular surfaces, joint space narrowing and new bone formation at the articular margins. There is subchondral low signal intensity compatible with bone sclerosis.*

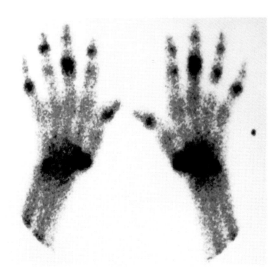

Figure 4.46 *Osteoarthritis. Radioisotope bone scan of the hands. Extensive increase in uptake is shown in the wrist, especially at the first carpometacarpal joints.*

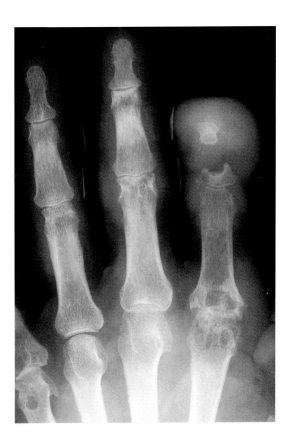

Figure 4.47 *Gout. There is massive soft tissue swelling around the affected digits. Large, punched-out cystic defects are shown. On occasion, the gouty tophi calcify.*

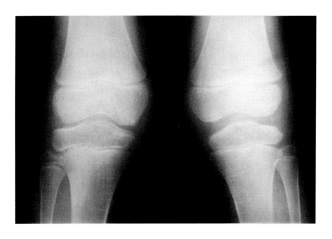

Figure 4.48 *Juvenile chronic arthritis. The right knee shows overgrowth of its epiphyses with a resultant apparent narrowing of the joint space. The overgrowth is not smooth and is associated with angularity rather than roundness of articular margins. This feature follows synovial hyperplasia and hyperaemia in this disease. Growth arrest lines are also seen superimposed on osteoporosis.*

JUVENILE CHRONIC ARTHRITIS

In juvenile chronic arthritis, 90% of patients are seronegative. The remaining seropositive patients have an erosive pattern of disease similar to adult rheumatoid arthritis. Usually the erosions are not prominent, which may be because the ossific nuclei of the epiphyses are protected by a thicker cover of cartilage. Soft tissue swelling and osteoporosis are seen and bone growth is accelerated because of local hyperaemia (Figure 4.48). Epiphyses become enlarged and abnormal in shape, often angular and squared rather than round and smooth. Overgrowth results in joint space narrowing, and premature fusion at growth plates results in small stature, which is often compounded by corticosteroid administration (Figure 4.49).

Because the bony changes in juvenile chronic arthritis are due to synovial disease, they are similar to those seen with two other diseases, tuberculosis (Figure 4.50) and haemophilia (Figure 4.51), in which identical epiphyseal modelling abnormalities are seen. In haemophilia (see below), a deepened intercondylar notch occurs, said to be due to bleeding into the cruciate ligament origins (Figure 4.51); this deepening, however, may be a reflection of condylar overgrowth. In both haemophilia and tuberculosis, cartilage and bone destruction can occur because of synovial proliferation.

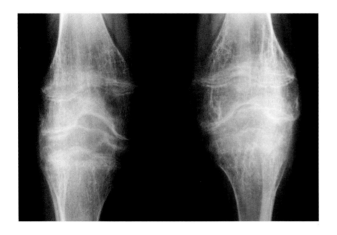

Figure 4.49 *In this extreme case of juvenile chronic arthritis, both knees are affected after 5 years of illness. There is osteoporosis, which is compounded by steroid administration, and marked muscle wasting. Overgrowth of epiphyses results in bulbous and angular articular surfaces. The only remaining trabeculae are along the lines of stress.*

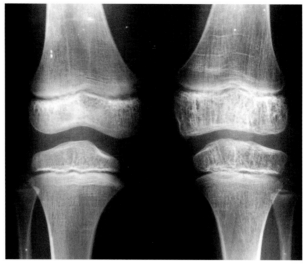

Figure 4.50 *Synovial tuberculosis. The left knee is affected and the appearances are basically identical to those seen with juvenile chronic arthritis. There is overgrowth of epiphyses, which are squared. Stress trabeculae and growth arrest lines are prominent.*

Table 4.7 shows that spinal changes and sacroiliitis are features of seronegative arthritides (see also Chapter 8, page 376). Rheumatoid arthritis only occasionally causes sacroiliitis, which is often unilateral. Spinal changes below the upper cervical spine are infrequent in rheumatoid arthritis but they may result in fusion there. Psoriasis is associated with joint disease to a greater extent than Reiter's syndrome, although both have a form of spinal ankylosis which may differ slightly in appearance from the classical

Table 4.7 Distribution of changes in arthritis.

Condition	SI Joints	Spine	Hands	Feet	Hips	Knees	Shoulders
Osteoarthritis	Unilateral or bilateral	C + L	DIP CMC	Hallux MTP	++	++	—
Rheumatoid arthritis	—	C	MCP Carpus	MTP Tarsus	+	++	+
Reiter's syndrome	Unilateral	T + L	Occasional	Hallux MTP + IP	Occasional	Occasional	Occasional
Psoriatic arthritis	Unilateral	T + L	DIP	DIP	Occasional	Occasional	Occasional
Ankylosing spondylitis	Bilateral	C + T + L	Occasional	Occasional	Occasional	Occasional	Occasional
Enteropathic spondylarthritis	Bilateral	C + T + L	Occasional	Occasional	Occasional	Occasional	Occasional
Juvenile chronic arthritis	Occasional	C	All over	All over	+	+	+

C	=	Cervical	
CMC	=	Carpometacarpal	
DIP	=	Distal interphalangeal	
IP	=	Interphalangeal	
L	=	Lumbar	
MCP	=	Metacarpophalangeal	
MTP	=	Metatarsophalangeal	
SI	=	Sacroiliac	
T	=	Thoracic	

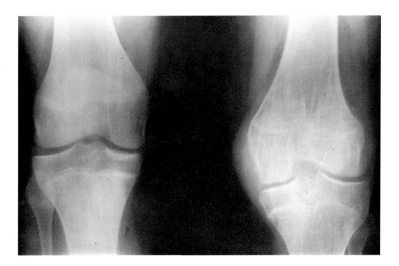

Figure 4.51 *Haemophilia. The affected limb shows soft tissue swelling around the joint and quadriceps wasting when compared with the normal side. There is an effusion or blood in the joint. The bones are demineralized and increased in length and the joint space is narrowed, which is partly due to overgrowth of epiphyses. The intercondylar notch appears deepened and stress trabecular lines are prominent (see also Figure 4.49).*

'bamboo spine' of ankylosing spondylitis, and a sacroiliitis which may be unilateral. An enthesopathy is prominent in the seronegative spondylarthropathies, but is less common in rheumatoid arthritis. In ankylosing spondylitis, spinal and sacroiliac changes predominate over joint changes. Erosions are prominent at the entheses in all the seronegative disorders.

HAEMOPHILIA

Lesions occur in joints of the lower limbs as these tend to be more easily traumatized. Bleeding occurs into soft tissues, resulting in haematomas (Figure 4.52), and into joints. Acute bleeding in the joint results in capsular distension, especially in the knee—a 'lax' joint. Hyperaemia results in epiphyseal overgrowth. At the knee, condylar overgrowth results

in a deepened intercondylar notch, joint narrowing and epiphyseal squaring (Figure 4.51). The appearances resemble juvenile chronic arthritis. A tibio-talar slant is seen at the ankle (see page 241). Osteoporosis occurs as a result of hyperaemia and immobilization.

Increased density of periarticular tissue, shown on plain films (Figure 4.53) and, on CT scanning, is the result of long-term haemosiderin deposition in the synovium. Synovial proliferation occurs and marked irregularity results. Erosions occur.

Synovial proliferation and pigment deposition are especially well seen at MRI. Haemosiderin gives signal void in the irregular synovium. Articular cartilage and the menisci are eroded. Subarticular cysts are seen, as in degenerative disease (Figure 4.54). Intramuscular bleeds result in pseudotumours (Figure 4.55).

Avascular necrosis occurs, presumably as a result of intra-articular bleeding or tamponade (Figure 4.56).

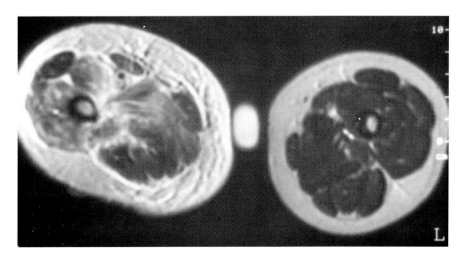

Figure 4.52 *Haemophilia (axial T_2-weighted MR sequence). Chronic bleeding into the thigh muscles is associated with muscle atrophy and a diffuse increase in signal in the affected muscles.*

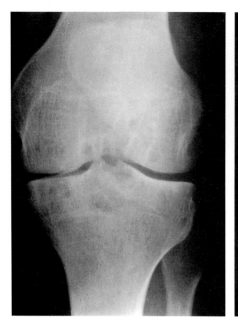
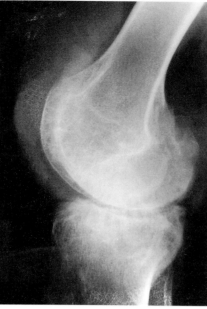

Figure 4.53 *Haemophilia. The AP view is unremarkable, showing changes similar to those seen in degeneration, with joint space narrowing and subarticular cyst formation. The lateral radiograph shows extreme density of the synovium in the suprapatellar pouch due to haemosiderin deposition.*

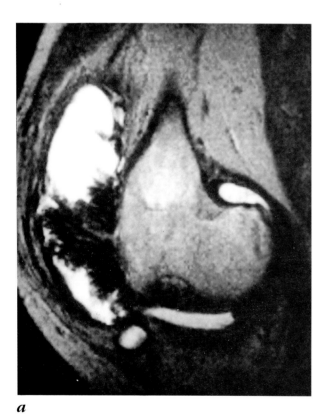

a

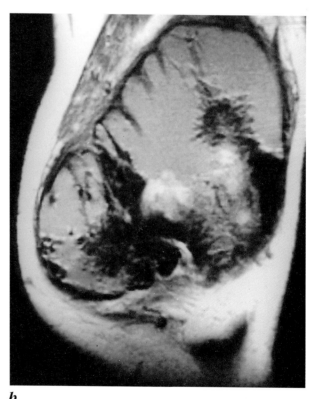

b

Figure 4.54 *Haemophilia at MR imaging. (**a**) There is marked distension of the suprapatellar pouch; the synovium is grossly hypertrophied and shows decrease in signal due to haemosiderin deposits. The menisci and articular cartilages are destroyed and a subarticular cyst is seen on the sagittal T$_2$-weighted MR sequence. (**b**) A coronal T$_1$-weighted MR image through the anterior aspect of the suprapatellar pouch shows its distension and the florid hypertrophy of synovium containing haemosiderin.*

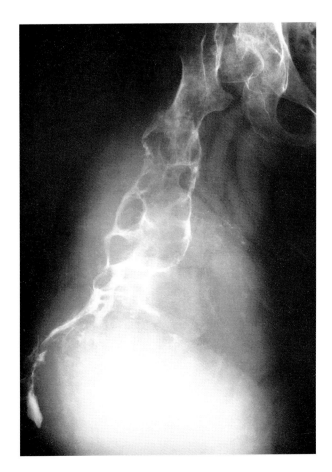

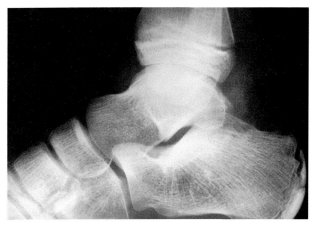

a

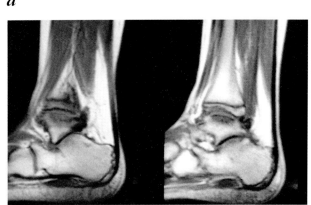

b

Figure 4.55 *Haemophilia in the femoral shaft causing pseudotumour formation. The change is extensive and associated with a soft tissue haematoma. These appearances are similar to hydatid disease.*

Figure 4.56 *Haemophilia. (a) The plain film shows a distended capsule with some increase in synovial density. There is sclerosis of the dome of the talus. (b) The sagittal T_1-weighted MR images show a subarticular zone of low signal compatible with avascular necrosis in the talar dome. The proliferating synovium also exhibits diminished signal.*

SEPTIC ARTHRITIS

When the epiphyseal plate is open between the ages of 1 to 16, it acts as a barrier to the direct spread of infection from the metaphysis into the epiphysis and joint (Figure 4.57). If the metaphysis is intracapsular, the focus of infection originating there may enter the joint through the metaphyseal cortex. Joint effusions and osteoporosis are followed by bone and cartilage destruction and joint narrowing (Figure 4.58), and the epiphyses overgrow in children.

Osteoporosis in subarticular regions may initially allow the thinned cortex to appear prominent, but the cortex then becomes destroyed.

Radiological change may not be apparent for 10–14 days, but is seen early in the disease, even within hours, at radionuclide bone scanning using Tc-99m. Only occasionally, especially in infants, pus causes tamponade of blood vessels to the affected area so that the isotope does not reach the area of infection. Under these circumstances, gallium or indium labelling of white cells may be positive. Gallium scans are also positive with soft tissue infections, so that good quality scans are needed to discriminate between bone and soft tissue infection.

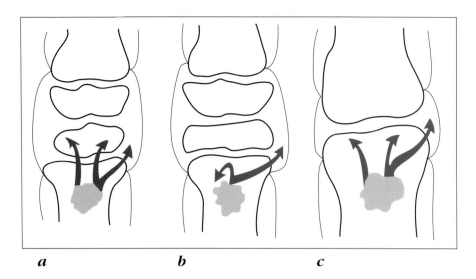

a   *b*   *c*

Figure 4.57 *The shaded area in the metaphysis represents a focus of osteomyelitis. From 1 to 16 years of age the epiphyseal plate acts as a barrier to infection but, if the metaphysis is intracapsular, the joint can still be affected. (a = 0–1 years; b = 1–16 years; c = 16 years onwards)*

With conventional Tc-99m scanning, uptake is increased in all phases—the initial angiographic, the subsequent blood pool and the delayed scan obtained after 3 hours; cellulitis alone does not result in increased uptake in the local bone or joint.

Ultrasound confirms the presence of excess fluid in a distended capsule (Figure 4.59) and allows

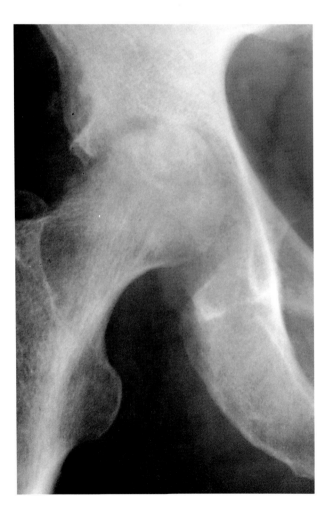

Figure 4.58 *Septic arthritis. The hip joint shows bone and cartilage destruction. The articular cortices are no longer visible and the joint is narrowed, particularly superiorly.*

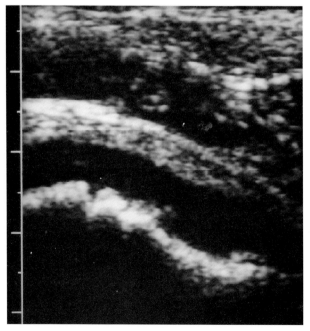

Figure 4.59 *On ultrasound a large effusion lifts the capsule over the femoral head and neck (normal bone–capsule distance is less than 2 mm over the femoral neck). The closing physis is shown.*

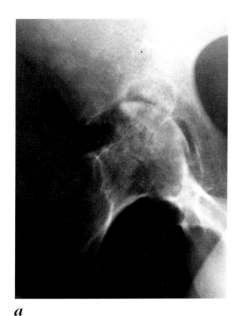

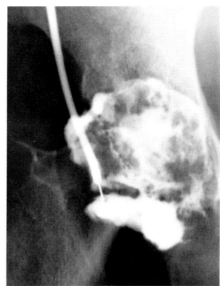

a   *b*

Figure 4.60 *Tuberculosis of the hip. (**a**) The joint space is narrow and irregular, and destruction of bone is seen on both sides of the joint. (**b**) Arthrography. Following aspiration of pus, contrast is injected into the joint. The synovium is irregular, erodes the underlying bone and the capsule is contracted.*

immediate aspiration of joint contents for culture. Contrast medium can be installed into the joint after fluoroscopic aspiration. Arthrography demonstrates abnormal synovium and irregular bone (Figure 4.60), but the rise in intra-articular pressure may give rise to septic emboli and septicaemia.

MRI is as sensitive as isotope scanning in the diagnosis of bone or joint infection, but also specific. Anatomical detail is shown. Effusions, cartilage destruction and cortical erosion are demonstrated. Marrow infiltration by fluid in the active phase of infection is seen as an area of increased signal on T_2-weighted or fat suppression images, and decreased signal on T_1-weighted sequences. Central areas of necrosis enhance only at the periphery with intravenous gadolinium, but inflamed synovium enhances after intravenous gadolinium.

Changes in bone are superimposed on marrow which may be fatty, red or both. The demonstration of inflammation at MRI thus varies according to the type of marrow involved. Marrow oedema also may be difficult to distinguish from infection in subarticular bone.

Joint effusions are bright on T_2-weighted and fat suppression sequences, as is infected fluid in the joint. Similarly, oedema surrounding the infected area may be difficult to distinguish from infection. Intravenous gadolinium distinguishes vascular from necrotic or fibrous tissue; hyperaemic synovium enhances in septic arthritis.

SYNOVIAL TUMOURS

These are uncommon and may be benign or malignant. They erode bone on both sides of the joint but, unlike rheumatoid disease, infection or haemophilia, do not necessarily destroy articular cartilage or subcartilaginous bone. The erosions are often para-articular only (Figure 4.61). Their margins are well defined if the tumour is benign, for example, in pigmented villonodular synovitis or synovial osteochondromatosis.

Pigmented villonodular synovitis

This benign lesion is the result of hypertrophy of synovium which becomes progressively darker due to haemosiderin deposition. The arthrographic appearance is of frond-like synovial hypertrophy (Figure 4.61), usually at the hip or knee. At MRI, the haemosiderin deposits result in low signal in proliferating synovium on T_1- and T_2-weighted sequences (Figure 4.62). Similar change occurs in haemophilia.

In pigmented villonodular synovitis, smooth bone erosion is seen in 'tight' joints—the hip rather than the knee—while in haemophilia substantial osteoarticular abnormality is seen. Large erosions of bone are well shown at CT scanning (Figure 4.63).

Pigmented villonodular synovitis also occurs in tendon sheaths in the hand, causing erosion of the underlying mid-shafts of the phalanges (Figure 4.64).

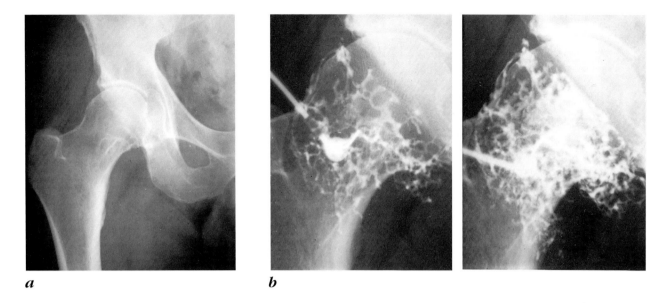

a   *b*

Figure 4.61 *Pigmented villonodular synovitis. (**a**) Well demarcated erosions are seen on the medial aspect of the femoral neck and in the medial wall of the acetabulum. Superiorly the joint space is intact. (**b**) After injection, contrast medium is shown around the proliferating synovium. The cartilage-covered areas are spared.*

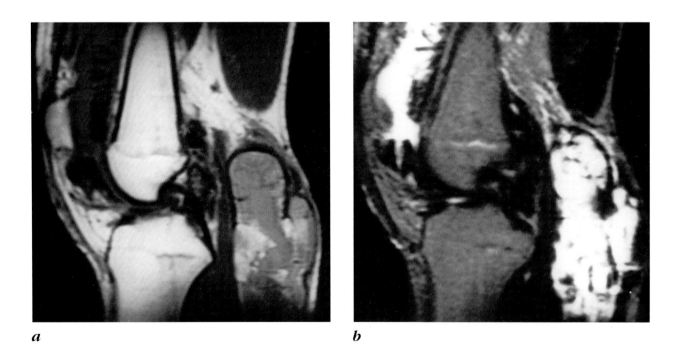

a   *b*

Figure 4.62 *(**a**, **b**) Pigmented villonodular synovitis at MRI (sagittal T$_1$-weighted and fat suppression sequences). The changes resemble those seen in haemophilia but without the osteoarticular abnormalities. There is distension of the capsule and frond-like hypertrophy of synovium, which is low in signal due to haemosiderin deposition.*

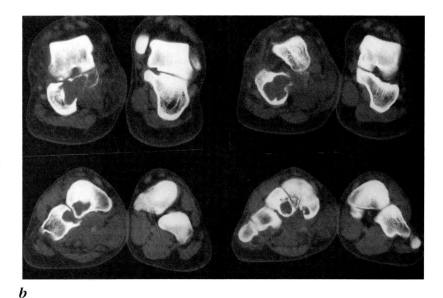

a   *b*

Figure 4.63 *Pigmented villonodular synovitis. (**a**) A plain radiograph of the hindfoot indicates a widespread abnormality of synovium, with well defined multiple erosions of adjacent bones. (**b**) The CT scan confirms the presence of widespread destruction of bone by a non-mineralizing synovium-based soft tissue tumour which erodes adjacent articular surfaces.*

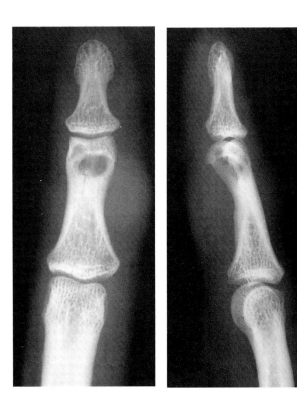

Figure 4.64 *Pigmented villonodular synovitis of the tendon sheath causing smooth scalloping of the underlying phalanx.*

Synovial osteochondromatosis

More than four apparently loose bodies in a joint are a feature of synovial osteochondromatosis (Figure 4.65). These are seen in major joints (Figure 4.66) and also in Baker's cysts (Figs. 4.23 and 4.67). They result from cartilaginous metaplasia in hypertrophied synovium. The cartilaginous masses may remain in synovium or may become truly loose. Ossification may be rather irregular or total, giving an appearance resembling pearls. Filling defects are seen at arthrography (Figure 4.68).

The ossified masses may show fatty marrow signal on T_1-weighted sequences but dense mineralization is seen as low signal change (Figure 4.67).

Smooth bone scalloping occurs in this lesion.

Synovial sarcoma

Synovial sarcoma is a rare lesion, usually affecting the knee, but any synovial surface may be involved (Figures 4.69 and 4.70). The underlying bone is not scalloped but is invaded, so that the cortical irregularities are ill defined. The tumour shows an irregular ossification in one-third of cases.

Tumours appearing in the epiphyseal region are listed in Table 3.5.

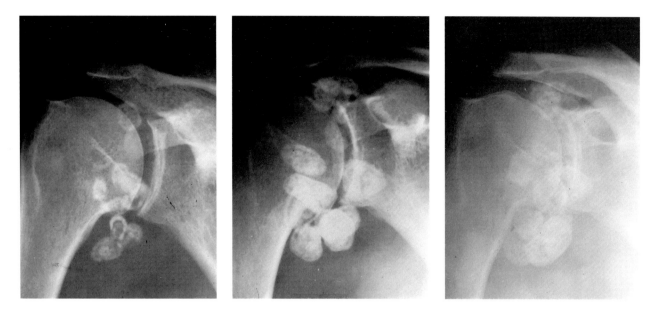

Figure 4.65 *Synovial osteochondromatosis. Multiple, mineralized loose bodies are seen to grow in this patient over 5 years.*

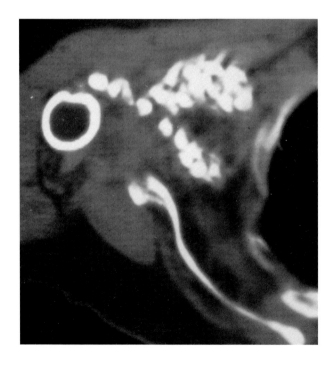

Figure 4.66 *Synovial osteochondromatosis. Multiple densities are demonstrated in the shoulder joint. (By courtesy of Professor I McCall, Oswestry.)*

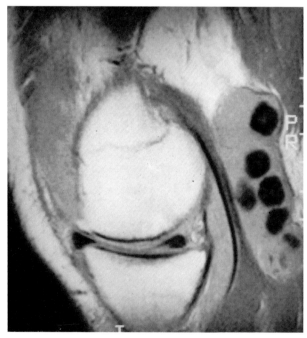

Figure 4.67 *Synovial osteochondromatosis in a Baker's cyst is shown on a sagittal T_1-weighted MR image. Note a meniscal tear.*

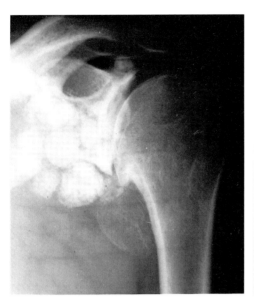
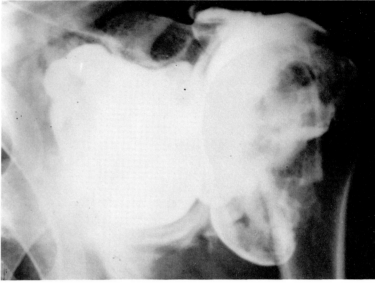

Figure 4.68 *Synovial osteochondromatosis. (**a**) The plain film shows numerous loose bodies in the shoulder joint. (**b**) A single-contrast arthrogram shows the filling defects due to loose bodies in the joint.*

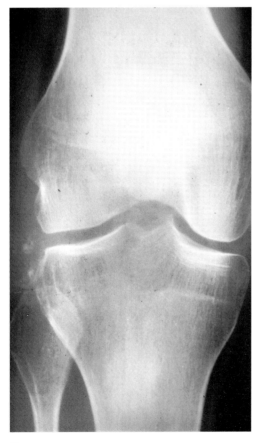
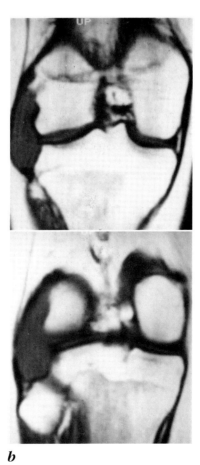

Figure 4.69 *Synovial sarcoma. (**a**) The plain film shows a mineralized soft tissue mass eroding the lateral tibial plateau. (**b**) On the coronal T$_1$-weighted MR sequences a soft tissue mass erodes the underlying bone and displaces the lateral collateral ligament.*

a   *b*

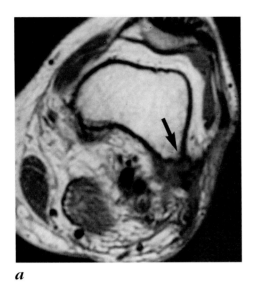

a

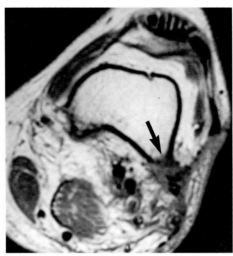

b

Figure 4.70 *Synovial sarcoma. (**a**) Pre-gadolinium and (**b**) post-gadolinium axial T₁-weighted MR sequences showing an enhancing soft tissue tumour eroding the posterior aspect of the lateral femur (arrow).*

ABNORMAL EPIPHYSEAL CONTOURS IN CHILDREN

PERTHES' DISEASE

Perthes' disease is the commonest cause of flattening and irregularity of the femoral head in children. In the early phase, hip pain is associated with widening of the joint space (Figure 4.71); an ultrasound scan may show an effusion in the joint, while an isotope bone scan may show diminished or no uptake in the femoral head (Figure 4.72). When the disease becomes established, there is fissuring beneath the articular cortex and loss of its normal contour, often best seen with a 'frog' lateral view, which demonstrates the anterosuperior aspect of the head (Figure 4.73). This part is often the first and more severely affected, but as the disease becomes established the ossific nucleus becomes flattened, fragmented and fissured to varying degrees. Cystic changes also occur in the metaphysis. Arthrography reveals that the cartilaginous portion of the head is only slightly altered (Figure 4.73c) by being mildly flattened. MRI shows loss of signal and later flattening of the femoral head (Figure 4.74). Although

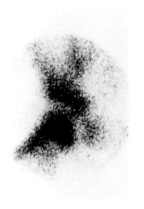
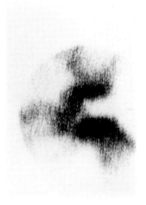

Figure 4.72 *Radioisotope bone scan in Perthes' disease showing absence of uptake in the left femoral head.*

Figure 4.71 *Irritable hip syndrome. (**a**) An effusion in the right hip joint is shown on the plain film by widening of the joint space. (**b**) The subsequent film shows reversion to the normal width.*

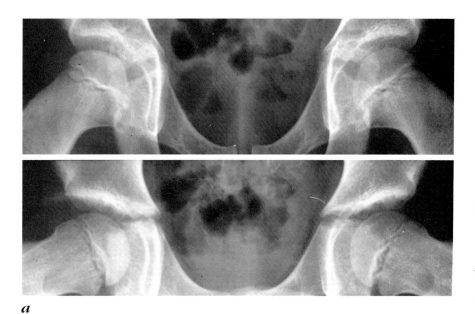

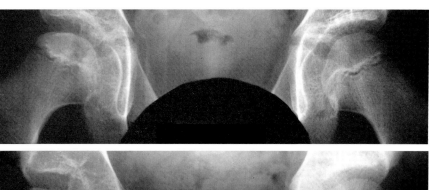

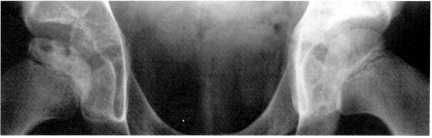

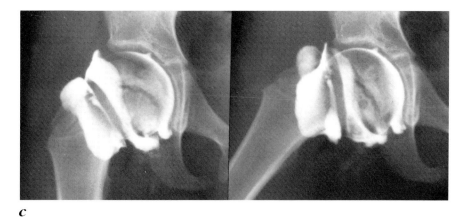

Figure 4.73 *Perthes' disease. (**a**) In the right hip, a crescentic rim of radiolucency is seen beneath the anterosuperior aspect of the femoral head on both the anteroposterior (top) and frog lateral (bottom) views. The disease develops from here. (**b**) Eight months later there is progressive flattening and condensation of the femoral head. (**c**) The cartilaginous dome, containing the flattened ossific nucleus, has a more normal appearance at arthrography. Pooling of contrast is somewhat greater medially in the film taken in abduction. This indicates that joint incongruity is maximal in this position.*

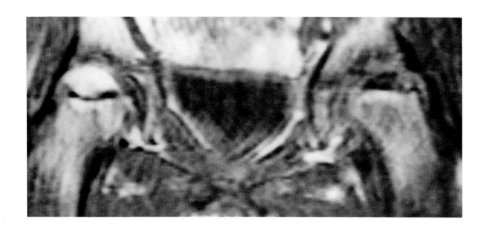

Figure 4.74 *Perthes' disease of the left hip. The coronal T$_1$-weighted MR sequence shows late flattening and loss of signal in the medial part of the left femoral head.*

in 50% of cases the change is bilateral, it is only very rarely symmetrical. No other joints will be affected. The flattened ossific nucleus reforms with resorption of osteonecrotic fragments, but residual deformity remains, which depends on the initial extent of the avascular process (Figure 4.75). The flattened head extends beyond the acetabulum laterally and reaches the medial acetabular wall.

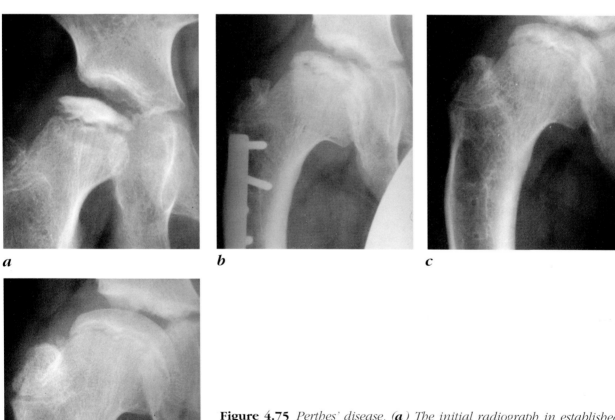

a *b* *c*

d

Figure 4.75 *Perthes' disease. (**a**) The initial radiograph in established Perthes' disease shows a flattened sclerotic femoral head which is uncovered laterally. (**b**) Subsequently a proximal femoral osteotomy was performed to attain maximal congruity. (**c**) The avascular ossific nucleus resorbs to be replaced by vital but deformed bone. (**d**) The reformed head is flat, smooth and uncovered laterally.*

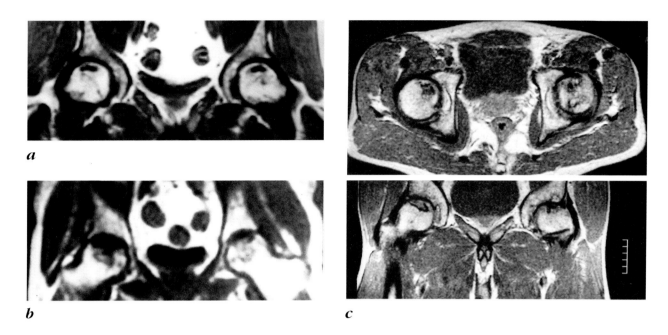

Figure 4.76 *Avascular necrosis of the femoral heads secondary to steroids. (**a**) A broad band of subcortical infarction is demonstrated bilaterally on this coronal T₁-weighted MR study. (**b**) Further change has resulted in structural failure in another patient (coronal T₁-weighted MR sequence). (**c**) Bilateral avascular necrosis (axial and coronal T₁-weighted MR images). The coronal T₁-weighted MR image (bottom) shows structural failure on the left with an acetabular cyst. On the right, a serpiginous zone of low signal is shown, together with an adjacent bright zone within which there is loss of the normal marrow signal, compatible with local infarction and fibrosis.*

MRI scanning detects early change in Perthes' disease and other forms of avascular necrosis of the femoral head, as well as at other joints. Pathologically, red marrow cells die in the first day, then osteoblasts and osteoclasts and finally, at 48 hours, the fat cells. Oedema in the avascular area and hyperaemia around it both cause characteristic MR changes.

If oedema replaces fat, signal is lowered on T_1-weighted and raised on T_2-weighted sequences. Hyperaemia around the avascular area may result in peripheral increase in signal, just as the radionuclide bone scan shows reactive increase in uptake around the infarcted region. Necrosing or fibrotic change in the avascular region causes further lowering of signal in affected areas. Avascular areas do not enhance with intravenous gadolinium.

The characteristic finding at MR in established avascular necrosis is the 'double line' sign. A low signal serpiginous band is shown, and adjacent to this on T_2-weighted images is a bright zone. This phenomenon represents an artefact related to chemical shift but is very specific for avascular necrosis.

Fibrosis, necrosis or even vacuum phenomena may be demonstrated by subcortical low signal bands. Cortical failure, seen on plain films, also occurs.

Change at MR imaging represents the variety and complexity of radiological change in the bone, but the 'double line' sign is the most useful (Figures 4.76 and 4.77).

Flattened, or fragmented and irregular femoral capital ossific nuclei are also found in cretinism and dysplasia epiphysealis multiplex (Figure 4.78).

DYSPLASIA EPIPHYSEALIS MULTIPLEX (MULTIPLE EPIPHYSEAL DYSPLASIA; FAIRBANK'S DISEASE)

This produces flattened epiphyses at the hip which persist through adolescence and adult life. Changes, ranging from minor to severe, vary from patient to patient, and are associated with premature degeneration (Figures 4.79 and 4.80). The abnormalities are symmetrical, unlike those seen in Perthes' disease, and also affect other major joints. At the shoulder, humerus varus and epiphyseal hypoplasia are similar in appearance to

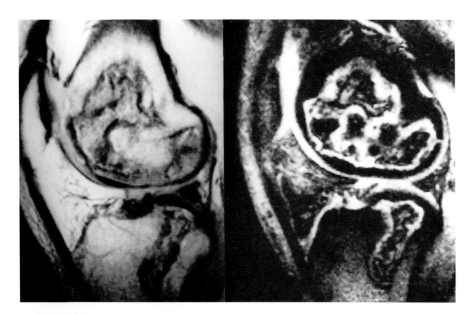

Figure 4.77 *Avascular necrosis in a patient on steroids (same patient as in Figure 4.76a); sagittal T_1-weighted (left) and fat suppression (right) MR sequences. Infarcts are distributed around the knee joint. Fluid is demonstrated within the infarcted area together with necrotic bone of low signal.*

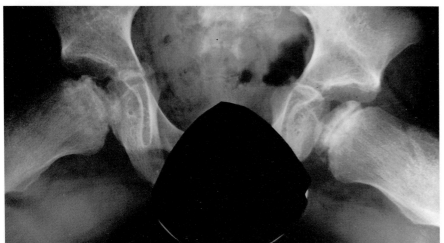

Figure 4.78 *Dysplasia epiphysealis multiplex. Bilateral and symmetrical Perthes-like changes are seen in the femoral heads.*

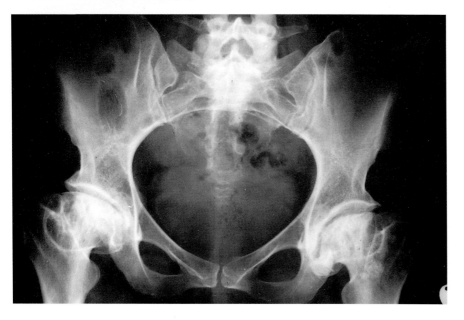

Figure 4.79 *Dysplasia epiphysealis multiplex. In adults, flattening of the femoral head results in secondary degeneration. Secondary acetabular dysplasia is seen.*

a telephone receiver (Figure 4.81). At the knees, the femoral condyles may be hypoplastic or even absent (Figure 4.82), and changes are also seen in the spine which resemble widespread Scheuermann's disease with end-plate irregularity (Figure 4.83) and minor platyspondyly. At the ankle, a characteristic tibio-talar slant is seen. The plafond of the ankle joint, which is the distal tibial articular surface, is no longer parallel to the weight-bearing plane but slopes, with hypoplasia of part of the distal tibial epiphysis and overgrowth of the adjacent talus (Figure 4.84; Table 4.8). Changes are also present in the hands and feet (Figure 4.85).

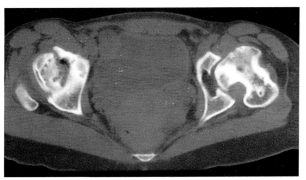

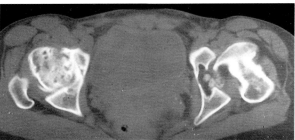

Figure 4.80 *Dysplasia epiphysealis multiplex. CT scanning shows anteverted and degenerate hip joints with loose bodies.*

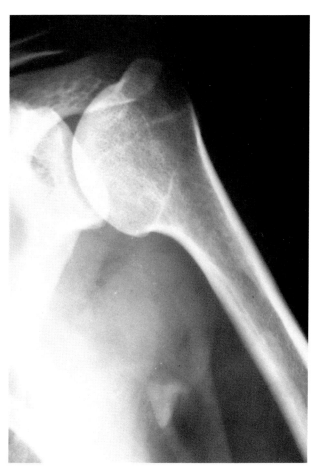

Figure 4.81 *Dysplasia epiphysealis multiplex. Hypoplasia of the humeral head results in a varus deformity which has been likened in appearance to a telephone receiver. Similar changes are seen in cretinism (see Figure 1.49c).*

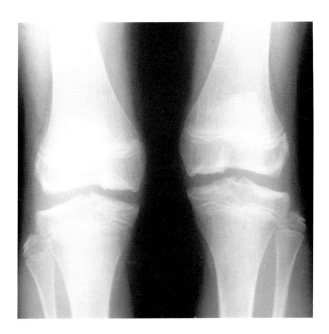

Figure 4.82 *Dysplasia epiphysealis multiplex. Hypoplasia of the femoral condyles is a variable but prominent feature of this disease. There is also irregularity of the proximal tibial and fibular epiphyses in this patient.*

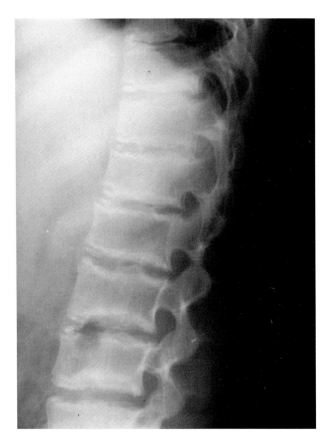

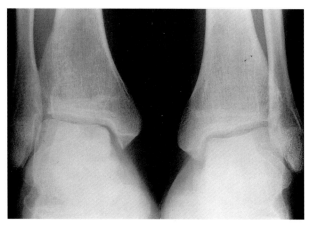

Table 4.8 Causes of tibio-talar slant.

Dysplasia epiphysealis multiplex
Haemophilia
Mucopolysaccharidoses
Dysplasia epiphysealis hemimelica
Asymmetrical epiphyseal plate fusion eg. following
   infection or trauma in childhood and in sickle-cell
   disease

Figure 4.83 *Dysplasia epiphysealis multiplex. Changes in the spine include platyspondyly and end-plate irregularity resembling Scheuermann's disease.*

Figure 4.84 *Dysplasia epiphysealis multiplex. There is a bilateral tibio-talar slant. The upper surface of the talus is no longer parallel to the weight-bearing plane.*

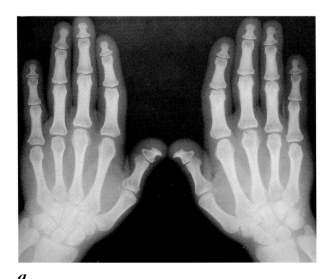

a

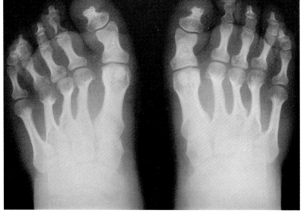

b

Figure 4.85 *Dysplasia epiphysealis multiplex. (**a**) Dysplastic changes are demonstrated at the distal phalanges in the hands. (**b**) The metatarsals are short and broad. The distal phalanges of the great toes are similarly affected.*

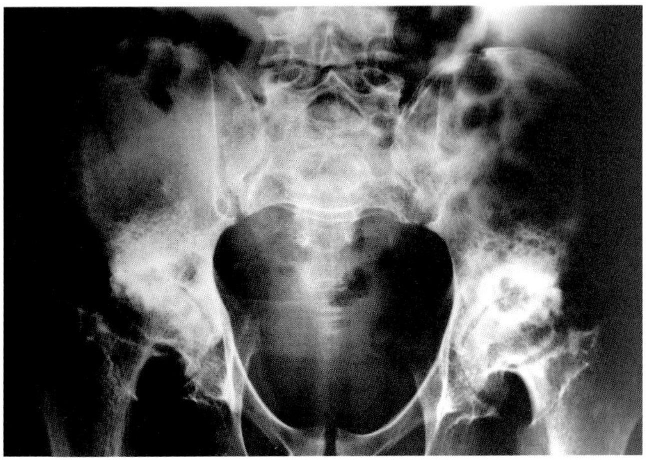

Figure 4.86 *Spondyloepiphyseal dysplasia tarda. Minor incongruity at the hip joints results in gross secondary degenerative changes at the hips. The diagnosis is made on inspection of the lumbar vertebral bodies which show a central hump on the anterior view.*

CRETINISM

Cretinism presents with symmetrically flattened and fragmented femoral heads in the presence of delayed skeletal maturity (Figure 4.3). With growth and treatment, epiphyseal fusion takes place, but the femoral head may remain fragmented. Again, changes may be seen in the other major joints, and humerus varus is present (Figure 1.49c). The vertebral bodies may be hypoplastic.

None of these three conditions is seen in the neonate. Radiologically, Perthes' disease occurs at about 6 to 8 years of age. Cretinism will be evident earlier, while dysplasia epiphysealis multiplex may not present clinically until adult life, often with joint pain. Earlier presentation is associated with dwarfism in severe cases.

SPONDYLOEPIPHYSEAL DYSPLASIA TARDA

This is a rare condition with a minor incongruity of the hips due to a femoral head dysplasia which can result in premature osteoarthritis (Figure 4.86). There are spinal changes particularly in the tarda form, which distinguish these lesions. The spinal abnormality consists of a heaping up of bone primarily posteriorly on the end-plates, which is associated with severe discal degeneration (Figure 4.87).

CHONDRODYSTROPHIA CALCIFICANS CONGENITA (CHONDRODYSPLASIA PUNCTATA; STIPPLED EPIPHYSES)

This occurs in mild and severe forms. Both show punctate calcification of cartilages at birth, particularly

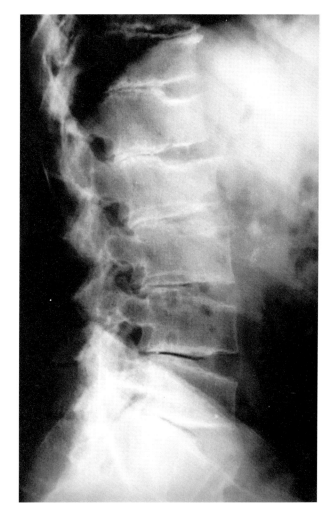

Figure 4.87 *Anterior defects in the lumbar vertebral bodies with a characteristic posterior hump are seen in this patient with spondyloepiphyseal dysplasia tarda.*

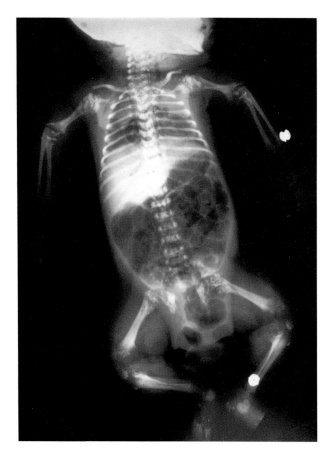

Figure 4.88 *This child with chondrodystrophia calcificans congenita survived for a short time after birth. Inguinal hernias are visible as well as gas in the pericardial sac. The lung fields are almost totally opaque. There is gross short-limbed dwarfism and the epiphyses are fragmented and stippled. Similar changes are seen in the tracheal cartilages. There is platyspondyly and vertebral defects.*

at the epiphyses, but also in the trachea (Figure 4.88). The mild form may develop into a dysplasia similar or identical to dysplasia epiphysealis multiplex. Cleft vertebrae are seen in the severe form in association with a gross form of short-limbed dwarfism which is markedly rhizomelic.

DYSPLASIA EPIPHYSEALIS HEMIMELICA (TREVOR'S DISEASE)

First recognized in the French literature, it was later described in England by Trevor as a disease localized to the ankle (tarso-epiphyseal aclasia). Fairbank showed that the other major joints were also involved. Changes are unilateral and maximal on one side of the epiphysis. The most prominent feature is a cartilage-capped exostosis arising on one half of the epiphysis. An epiphyseal lesion never occurs in diaphyseal aclasia. At the talus, a lateral osteochondroma causes a lateral defect at the plafond of the tibia, so that a form of tibio-talar slant is produced (Figure 4.89). Other local growth anomalies may be present, with overgrowth of other epiphyses (distal fibular) and fusion between the local long bones. Similar epiphyseal osteochondromas are seen at all the major joints.

MUCOPOLYSACCHARIDOSES

These are a complex group of heterogeneous conditions.

In MPS I-H (Hurler's syndrome) changes are progressive during infancy and eventually the entire skeleton is affected. The ring epiphyses in the carpus and tarsus become progressively irregular and

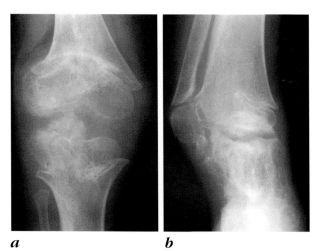

a   *b*

Figure 4.89 *Dysplasia epiphysealis hemimelica. (**a**) In this patient a chevron sign is seen at the distal femur and proximal tibia, with a large osteochondromatous excrescence on the lateral tibial plateau. (**b**) Premature fusion at one part of the epiphyseal plate at the ankle results in a tibio-talar slant. Articular irregularity due to osteochondromatous lesions is prominent. The fibular epiphysis is overgrown and has fused with the distal tibia.*

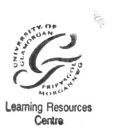

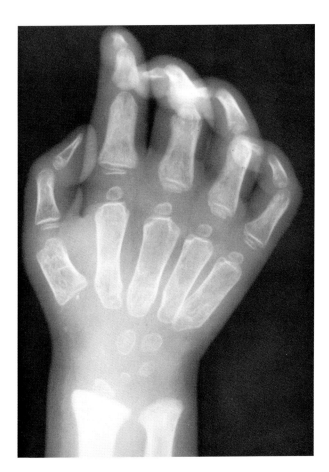

Figure 4.90 *MPS I-H (Hurler's syndrome). There is overall demineralization and thin cortices are apparent. The distal radius and ulna slope towards each other, and the proximal aspects of the metacarpals are pointed. Overall, the bones are broadened, and the phalanges resemble bullets.*

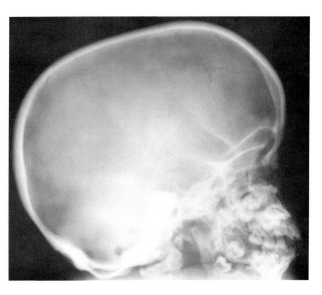

Figure 4.91 *The skull in MPS I-H. Enlargement of the pituitary fossa is seen. It is described as J-shaped. The condyle of the mandible is hypoplastic, and the odontoid peg is similarly underdeveloped.*

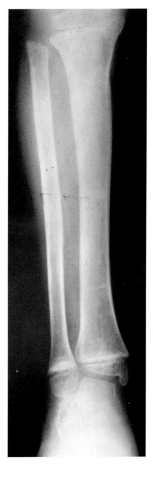

Figure 4.92 *In this patient with MPS I-H, a tibio-talar slant is visible at the ankle and the paired long bones show undertubulation. The proximal metaphyses show an abnormal slant.*

fragmented, the proximal metacarpals taper (Figure 4.90), and the phalanges become bullet-shaped. The skull shows enlargement with a J-shaped sella. The mandibular condyles become irregular and hypoplastic with an upward concavity (Figure 4.91). It is probable that this condylar defect is specific for mucopolysaccharidoses. The ankle also shows a tibio-talar slant, but with overgrown, hyperplastic epiphyses (Figure 4.92) and the metaphyses and diaphyses are also broad. A similar V deformity is also seen at the distal radius and ulna.

The ribs become paddle-shaped with a posterior constriction (Figure 4.93) and the spine has a thoracolumbar hook associated with a kyphos, probably due to local postural instability

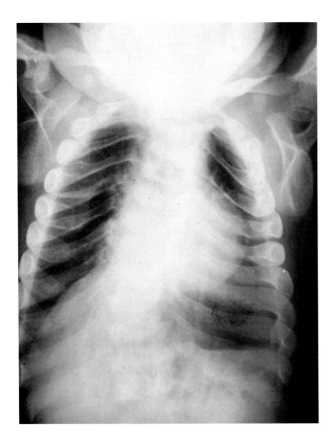

Figure 4.93 *This chest X-ray in an MPS I-H patient shows that the ribs are constricted posteriorly and broadened anteriorly. A scoliosis is shown.*

MPS IV (Morquio–Brailsford syndrome) is perhaps the next best known, but is extremely rare (see Chapter 7, page 342).

FRAGMENTATION OF EPIPHYSES AND APOPHYSES

Fragmentation of epiphyses or apophyses may be generalized or unifocal, and occurs in many different diseases, although often the end appearances are identical. The femoral heads in Perthes' disease, cretinism and multiple epiphyseal dysplasia may all be similar in appearance. The causes of epiphyseal fragmentation vary. Perthes' disease may be due to a rise in intracapsular pressure causing vascular occlusion in the ligamentum teres, while fragmentation at the second metatarsal head and tibial tuberosity are due to trauma (Tables 4.9 and 4.10).

Table 4.9 Causes of widespread epiphyseal fragmentation.

Cretinism
Cushing's syndrome
Steroid excess
Alcoholism
Renal failure, dialysis
Systemic lupus erythematosus
Gaucher's disease
Sickle-cell disease
Pancreatic disease
Caisson disease
Hodgkin's disease
Dysplasia epiphysealis multiplex
Dysplasia epiphysealis hemimelica
Chondrodystrophia calcificans congenita
Haemophilia

Table 4.10 Local causes of epiphyseal fragmentation in the hip.

Perthes' disease
Following treatment for congenital dislocation of the hip and slipped epiphysis
Following dislocations, fractures and surgery
Following local irradiation
Following infection
All the causes of generalized fragmentation

CAUSES OF WIDESPREAD EPIPHYSEAL FRAGMENTATION

CRETINISM

There is multiple joint involvement with flattening and fragmentation, and skeletal growth and maturity is retarded. Beaking at the thoraco-lumbar junction of the spine is due to diminished tone. Bone density is normal or increased.

CUSHING'S SYNDROME AND STEROID EXCESS

Generalized osteoporosis is present in these conditions. Spinal collapse is associated with callus. Resorption of bone in subarticular regions of joints results in a local crescentic rim of radiolucency beneath the articular cortex. Structural failure with collapse of joint surfaces then follows (Figure 4.94).

Patients with systemic lupus erythematosus show similar changes, but they are often receiving steroids. Patients with rheumatoid arthritis can also show articular collapse, and these changes are compounded in steroid therapy by the concomitant euphoria and diminution of pain induced by the drug (Figure 4.95). Following collapse of the cortex and subarticular area, there may be a local increase in bone density due to trabecular compression, as well as dystrophic calcification in necrotic tissue.

RENAL DISEASE, PANCREATITIS AND ALCOHOLISM

Similar changes are also seen at the hips and, particularly, the shoulders in patients with renal disease who are often receiving steroids or dialysis.

Infarcts and avascular necrosis in pancreatitis may be due to fat emboli, and alcoholism may cause avascular necrosis by inducing pancreatitis, hepatic failure and elevated steroid levels (see Chapter 1, page 16).

CAISSON DISEASE

Avascular necrosis and infarction in caisson disease result from nitrogen emboli. Cortical infarcts can occur, but a ring of serpiginous sclerosis in the subarticular bone—the zone of creeping substitution—is more typical and represents the edge of revascularization around the infarcted area of bone (Figure 3.66). These changes can occur beneath all major joints, and may also be seen following chemotherapy and radiotherapy, for example, in Hodgkin's disease. The avascular areas also suffer structural failure, leading to collapse of articular surfaces.

GAUCHER'S DISEASE AND SICKLE-CELL ANAEMIA

Changes of avascular necrosis also occur in Gaucher's disease and sickle-cell disease. Avascular necrosis at the hips in an Afro-Caribbean child is usually due to sickle-cell disease rather than Perthes' disease (Figure 4.96). Cortical infarcts occur in both disorders, but Erlenmeyer flask changes are more usual in Gaucher's disease, and generalized osteosclerosis is more common in sickle-cell anaemia. The joint space does not narrow until secondary osteoarthritis supervenes.

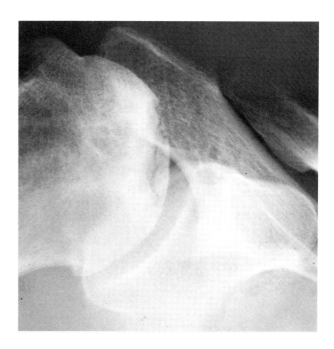

Figure 4.94 *Avascular necrosis following steroid therapy. A crescentic rim of lucency is seen beneath the fragmented articular cortex. Overall, the humeral head shows sclerosis and structural failure.*

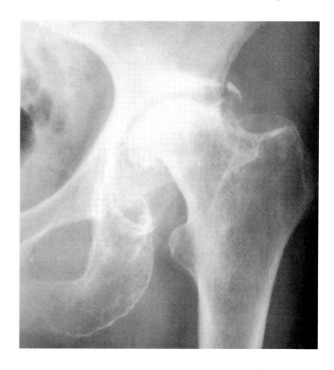

Figure 4.95 *Iatrogenic arthropathy. There is total resorption of the femoral head and deepening of the acetabulum. Loose bone fragments are demonstrated in the joint. The patient had been on indomethacin for 5 years.*

CAUSES OF A MUSHROOM-SHAPED FEMORAL HEAD (Table 4.11)

Avascular necrosis of the femoral head in children follows vigorous treatment for congenital dislocation of the hip (Figure 4.97), pinning of the head for slipped epiphysis, sickle-cell anaemia and Gaucher's disease. It may also follow trauma or surgery to the femoral head and neck in adults. Infection in childhood may destroy the femoral head either partially or totally (Figure 4.98). The ossific nucleus may disappear permanently or a deformed flattened head may result. Premature fusion of the growth plate results in local shortening.

PERTHES' DISEASE

In Perthes' disease, the femoral head ends up flattened in a mildly dysplastic acetabulum. The joint

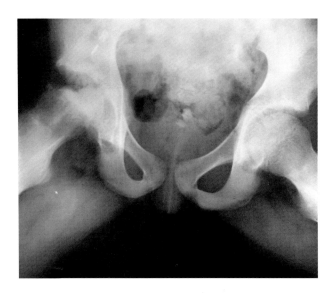

Figure 4.96 *There is a generalized increase in density and avascular necrosis of the right femoral head in this patient with sickle-cell disease.*

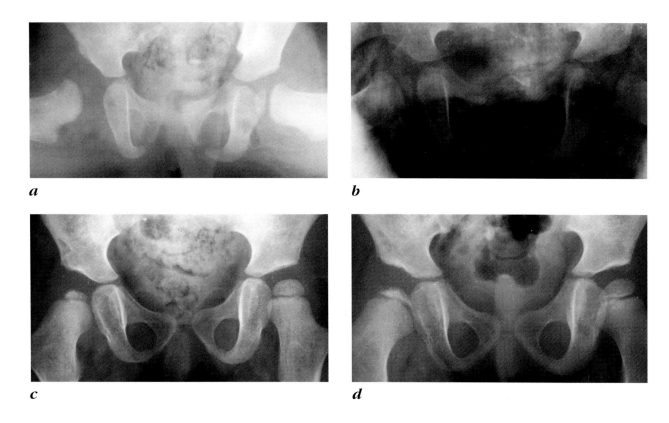

a

b

c

d

Figure 4.97 *Congenital dislocation of the hip and Perthes' disease. (**a**) The initial radiograph shows a dysplastic right acetabulum and, in abduction, the femoral head is well placed. (**b**) The hips are kept in abduction in splints. (**c**, **d**) Subsequently the patient develops Perthes' disease.*

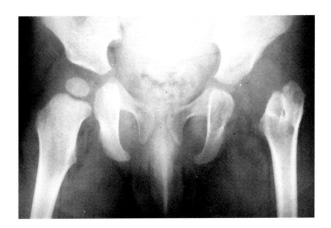

Figure 4.98 *Infantile septic arthritis. The left femoral head has failed to appear and healed metaphyseal defects are seen in this patient following septic arthritis in early childhood.*

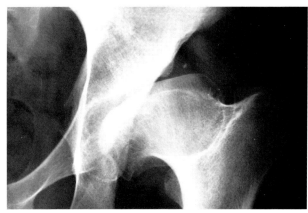

Figure 4.99 *Old Perthes' disease.*

Table 4.11 Causes of a mushroom-shaped femoral head.

Perthes' disease and other causes of avascular necrosis in childhood
Congenital dislocation of the hip complicated by avascular necrosis
Slipped capital femoral epiphysis
Osteomyelitis
Avascular necrosis in adult life
Secondary osteoarthritis

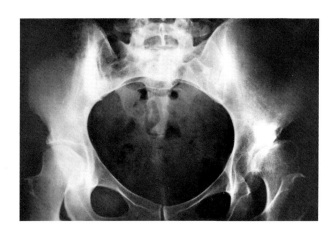

Figure 4.100 *Congenital dislocation of the hip. The right hip is normal, but the left acetabulum is dysplastic and shows internal new bone formation. The femoral head is uncovered laterally, where it is slightly bulbous, but flattened where it bears weight. Secondary osteoarthritic changes have supervened. The sacro-iliac joints show stress sclerosis.*

space is preserved for many years. The head is slightly uncovered laterally and the medial aspect of the acetabulum is essentially normal (Figure 4.99).

CONGENITAL DISLOCATION OF THE HIP

Lateral uncovering of the head is more marked than in Perthes' disease and the medial wall of the acetabulum is much thicker, due to the absence of the stimulus of a normal head against it (Figure 4.100). Again, the joint space narrows when secondary osteoarthritis supervenes. Avascular necrosis superimposed on congenital dislocation of the hip as a result of treatment can cause gross flattening of the femoral head (Figure 4.97).

SLIPPED CAPITAL FEMORAL EPIPHYSIS

In slipped epiphysis, the femoral head usually slips inferomedially, and the contour seems deficient superolaterally (Figure 4.101). The femoral neck is displaced laterally by the head and now no longer has its medial portion overlapped by the posterior acetabular wall. Normally, a line drawn centrally up

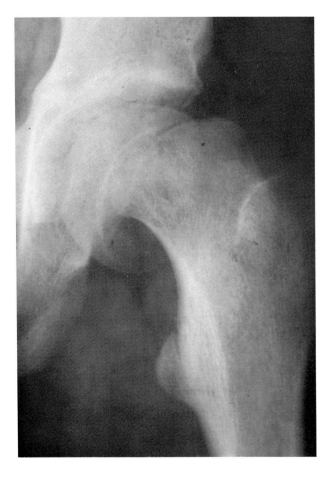

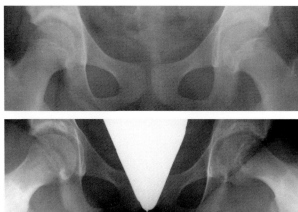

Figure 4.102 *Slipped capital femoral epiphysis. The anteroposterior radiographs (top) do not show obvious slip but there is asymmetry of the epiphyseal plates. On the right, a normal appearance is seen but, on the left, the margins of the plate are poorly defined. The left femoral head has also lost height, indicating a posterior slip. The lateral view (bottom) demonstrates the left-sided slip.*

Figure 4.101 *Slipped capital femoral epiphysis. The slip is both medial and posterior.*

the femoral neck, along its long axis, bisects the head; with medial slip it no longer does so.

In 15% of patients the femoral head is displaced purely posteriorly and medial slip is not in evidence, but the growth plate is abnormal in appearance and

the height of the head lessened (Figure 4.102). The displacement can however be seen on frog views. The medial acetabulum is normally formed. Secondary osteoarthritis supervenes (Figure 4.103).

INFECTION

With infection, the joint space may be narrowed or widened, but bone is destroyed on either side of the joint. Again, secondary osteoarthritis supervenes.

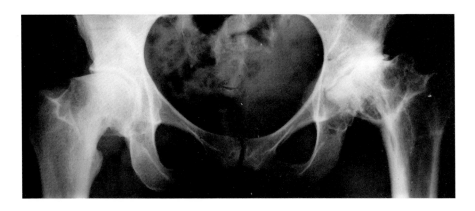

Figure 4.103 *Slipped capital femoral epiphysis. This patient has bilateral slipped epiphyses with quite marked degeneration of the left hip.*

CLASSICAL OSTEOARTHRITIS

In osteoarthritis of the hip, loss of cartilage and bone occurs, particularly at the dome of the femoral head on the anteroposterior view. The acetabulum also becomes dysplastic and secondary cystic change is often followed by articular collapse (Figure 4.41). This causes the head to migrate laterally. New bone is laid down internally on the medial acetabulum, and laterally as retaining osteophytes on the acetabulum and femoral head (Figure 4.40).

COMMON SITES OF OSTEOCHONDRITIS (Table 4.12)

THE TIBIAL TUBERCLE

Here, the disorder occurs in adolescents, often those with a history of sporting activity. Traction causes fragmentation of the tibial tubercle. Pain and soft tissue swelling are essential features of the diagnosis (Figure 4.104). Ultrasound also demonstrates the soft tissue changes and CT and MRI in particular, even if a little superfluous, are of value in demonstrating both bone and soft tissue changes.

THE METATARSAL HEAD

The second metatarsal head is usually involved in adolescent girls. The epiphysis flattens and fragments

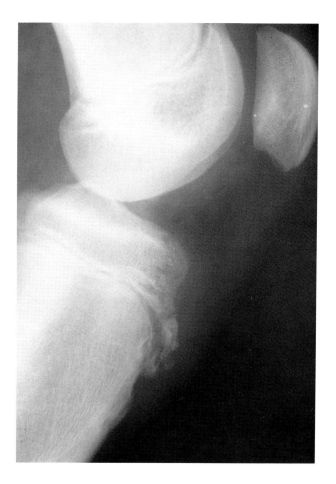

Figure 4.104 *Osgood–Schlatter's disease. Fragmentation of the tibial tubercle is associated with overlying soft tissue swelling in this painful lesion.*

Table 4.12 Common sites of osteochondritis.

Disease	Cause	Site
Perthes	Primary aseptic necrosis	Femoral head
Köhler	? Primary aseptic necrosis	Tarsal navicular
	? Necrosis following fracture	
Freiberg	? Primary aseptic necrosis	Metatarsal head
	? Necrosis following fracture	
Kienböck	? Primary aseptic necrosis	Lunate
	? Necrosis following fracture	
Osgood–Schlatter	Necrosis following partial avulsion of patellar tendon	Tibial tubercle
Sinding–Larsen	Necrosis following partial avulsion of patellar tendon	Lower pole of patella
Sever	Necrosis following partial avulsion of tendo-Achillis	Calcaneal apophysis
Calvé	Eosinophilic granuloma	Vertebral body
Scheuermann	Disc herniation through defective end-plate	Ring-like epiphysis of vertebra

Adapted from Catto M, *Aseptic Necrosis of Bone*, (Excerpta Medica: Amsterdam 1976) with kind permission.

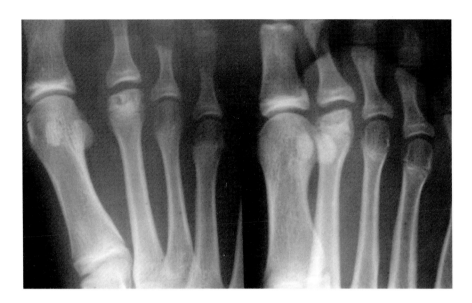

Figure 4.105
Osteochondritis of the second metatarsal head (Freiberg's disease). Collapse and sclerosis of the epiphysis is shown. The adjacent phalangeal base soon remodels to correspond to the altered appearance of the metatarsal head.

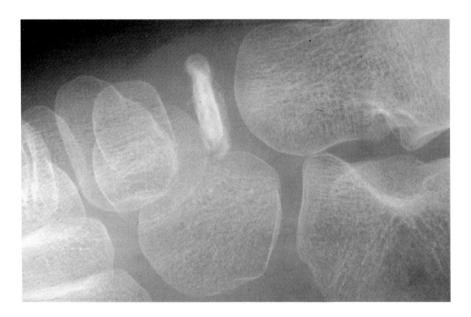

Figure 4.106
Osteochondritis of the tarsal navicular (Köhler's disease). Flattening and fragmentation with sclerosis are features of this disorder, which is self-limiting. There is disuse osteoporosis.

and, after epiphyseal fusion and healing, a flat, broad head results, often accompanied by local degeneration (Figure 4.105).

THE TARSAL NAVICULAR

The affected bone becomes flattened, sclerotic and fissured, but the adjacent joint spaces are not narrowed. The lesion is painful, but the bone usually reverts to normal (Figure 4.106).

THE CARPAL LUNATE

This bone flattens, fissures and scleroses (Figure 4.107).

THE SESAMOID FOR THE FIRST METATARSAL HEAD

Weight-bearing stress traumatizes this small ossicle, which fragments. Changes are symptomatic and the radionuclide bone scan is abnormal (Figure 4.108).

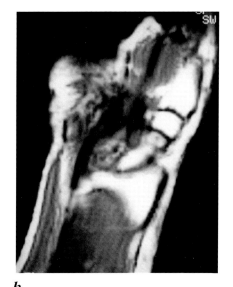

a

b

Figure 4.107
*Osteochondritis of the lunate (Kienböck's disease). (**a**) This bone is flattened, sclerotic and fragmented. (**b**) The coronal T₁-weighted MR sequence shows loss of signal and irregularity of the lunate.*

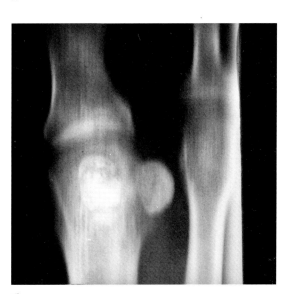

a

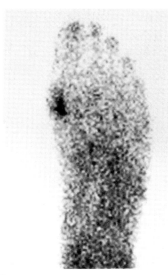

b

Figure 4.108
*Osteochondritis of the sesamoid of the great toe metatarsal. (**a**) The medial sesamoid is usually affected, and it fragments. (**b**) Increased uptake on the radionuclide bone scan.*

OSTEOCHONDRITIS DISSECANS (Table 4.13)

At the knee, changes of osteochondritis dissecans may be bilateral (Figures 4.109 and 4.110) and a familial history is often found. The dissecting fragment is usually (85%) on the internal aspect of the medial femoral condyle, on the convexity (Figure 4.111). It is seen on tunnel views. Some 15% occur on the lateral femoral condyle. The lesion is also likely to be related to local trauma.

The bed of the cleft smoothes off with time and gradually becomes less visible. A loose body may remain within the joint. Premature degeneration can result.

Table 4.13 Sites of osteochondritis dissecans.

Knee
Talus
Capitellum
Humeral head

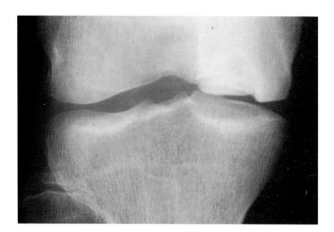

Figure 4.109 *Osteochondritis dissecans. A defect of the medial femoral condyle is present on its internal aspect. A well defined fragment is seen within the bed. There is articular incongruity. The underlying bone looks normal. The lesion is becoming well defined.*

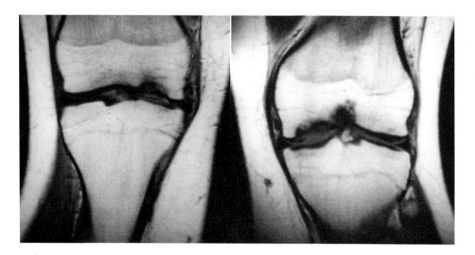

Figure 4.110 *Bilateral symmetrical osteochondritis dissecans of the medial femoral condyles—coronal T₁-weighted MR image. The left side shows the larger defect with significant irregularity of the articular cortex. Reactive changes are seen in the underlying bone.*

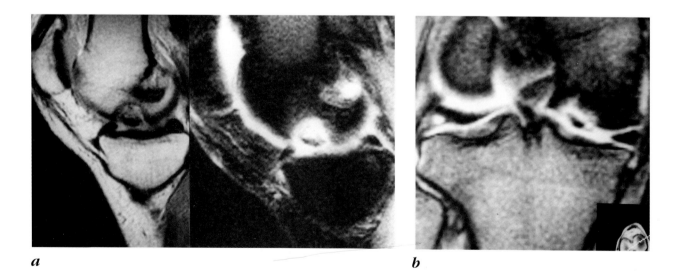

a *b*

Figure 4.111 *Osteochondritis dissecans—(**a**) sagittal T₁-weighted (left) and fat suppression (right) MR images, (**b**) radial gradient echo MR sequence. A well defined defect of the medial femoral condyle is demonstrated. Fluid separates the dissected loose fragment from underlying bone. An effusion is present.*

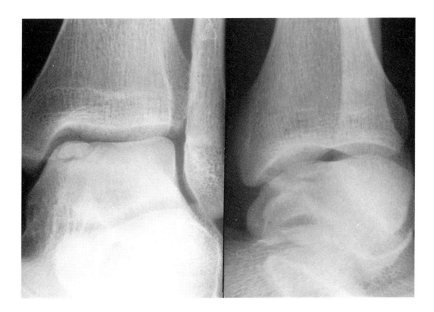

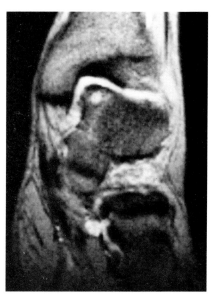

Figure 4.112 *Osteochondritis dissecans. A well defined defect is seen on the convexity of the medial aspect of the dome of the talus. This is a common site for such a lesion. The dissected fragment appears vital. It has the same density as the underlying bone.*

Figure 4.113 *Post-traumatic subcortical cyst of the medial dome of the talus. A common appearance in the same situation as osteochondritis dissecans (see Figure 4.112) The cystic nature of the lesion is demonstrated on the coronal T₂-weighted MR image, together with irregularity of the overlying articular cortex.*

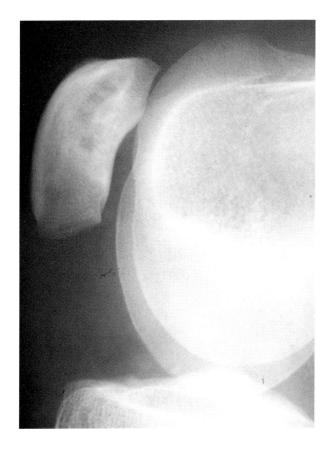

Figure 4.114 *Dorsal defect of patella.*

Trauma to the talar dome results in a cartilaginous or an osteochondral shear lesion. Changes are seen both medially and laterally and, on the convexity of the dome, a flake of cartilage alone, or cartilage with underlying bone, may be avulsed. A plane of cleavage is seen in the presence of a bony lesion (Figure 4.112). Sometimes the overlying cartilage is intact but the underlying bone fractured. The bed of underlying bone is vascular, unlike the situation in avascular necrosis, where the bed beneath a loose flake is also avascular. If a layer of fluid—seen as bright signal on T₂-weighted MR images (Figure 4.111)—lies between the bed and the dissected segment, the latter is likely to be loose and may require pinning. CT will also demonstrate the plane of cleavage, especially if combined with arthrography.

Often a well corticated cyst is seen on AP or oblique views of the talus, just below the convexity of the dome. The defect is also seen at CT scanning and is shown to contain fluid at MRI. Presumably there is a local post-traumatic cortical defect which allows the cyst to form (Figure 4.113).

DORSAL DEFECT OF THE PATELLA

A well defined lytic lesion on the posterior surface of the patella is seen on plain films and at tomography (Figure 4.114). Arthrography and MR imaging reveal the cartilage over the lesion to be intact in this normal variant.

IMAGING OF JOINTS

THE SHOULDER JOINT

Plain films: acromioclavicular joint degeneration is shown by joint space narrowing and local osteophyte formation. Soft tissue swelling accompanies this change. The glenoid parallels the humeral head. Mahoney's line is smooth and continuous.

Ninety-five per cent of rotator cuff tears result from subacromial impingement (Neer, 1983).

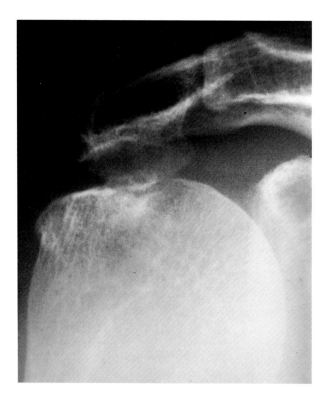

Figure 4.115 *A large subacromial osteophyte is demonstrated. There is irregularity of the subadjacent humeral head with loss of cortex. Cyst formation is evident but is best demonstrated at MRI.*

Osteophytic change is seen on the undersurface of the acromion and this compresses the subjacent supraspinatus tendon (Figure 4.115). Hypertrophy of the acromioclavicular joint impinges upon the supraspinatus muscle proximal to the tendon. The humeral head and greater tuberosity may show cystic or osteophytic change at the rotator cuff insertion (Figure 4.115).

Axial images show the acromioclavicular joint and gleno-humeral relationships. The Stryker's view demonstrates hatchet or Hill–Sachs defects. These mainly follow the more common form of dislocation, which is anterior, so that the defect is on the posterior aspect of the humeral head. An anterior defect is seen after the less common posterior dislocation. Here, the posterior glenoid impinges upon the anterior humerus.

On the AP radiograph, an apparently cystic lesion of the humeral head may be shown laterally but the defect is better seen on a film obtained in internal rotation (Figure 4.116a). An axial (Figure 4.116b), or better still, a Stryker's view, shows the defect (Figure 4.116c,d), which fills with contrast medium at arthrography (Figure 4.117). Subsequent CT scans show the defect and also show post-traumatic abnormality of the anterior glenoid and stripping of the capsule from its attachment to the neck of the scapula (Figure 4.118). Identical change is seen at MRI (Figure 4.119).

Cystic change at the greater tuberosity of the humerus may also be due to rheumatoid arthritis (Figure 4.120) or tuberculosis (Figures 4.121 and 4.122).

A bicipital groove view shows local osteophytosis, or a shallow groove. CT and MRI show the groove optimally.

Upward subluxation of the humeral head indicates the presence of a rotator cuff tear. Calcific tendinitis may be present, usually at the supraspinatus insertion (see Chapter 9, page 434).

Arthrography: single- or double-contrast studies are used to show:

(1) the presence of a partial or total rotator cuff tear. Filling of the subacromial bursa indicates a complete rotator cuff tear (Figure 4.123). A partial tear is seen as contrast staining of the inferior surface of the tendon (Figure 4.124);
(2) the long head of biceps tendon is seen on the AP (Figure 4.125) and bicipital groove views. The tendon may be thickened or ruptured, in which case it retracts and is no longer seen in the groove (Figure 4.118);

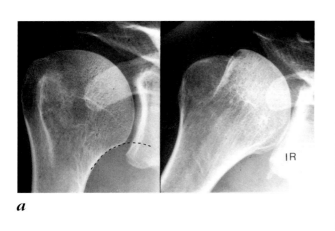

a

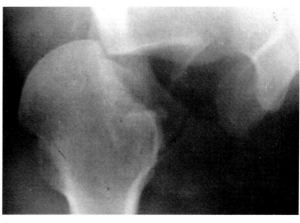

b

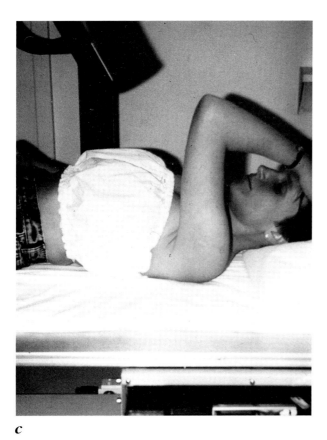

c

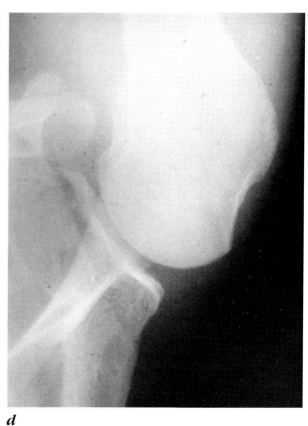

d

Figure 4.116 *Hatchet (Hill–Sachs) defect. (**a**) A hatchet defect is well demonstrated on the radiograph on the right taken in internal rotation. Note the almost total normality of the conventional radiograph (left), but the humeral head is upwardly subluxed and Mahoney's line discontinuous. (**b**) An axial image showing a posteriorly dislocated humeral head with an anterior hatchet defect. (**c**) Positioning of the patient to obtain a Stryker's view. (**d**) The X-ray obtained shows the hatchet defect.*

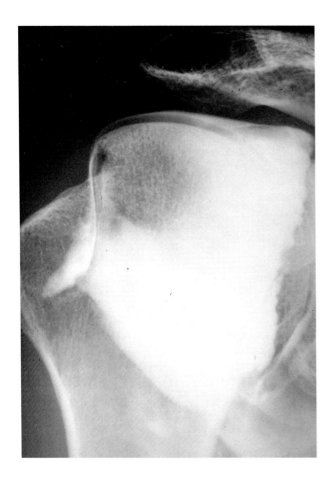

Figure 4.117 *Hatchet defect. At arthrography the defect fills with contrast but there is no rotator cuff tear.*

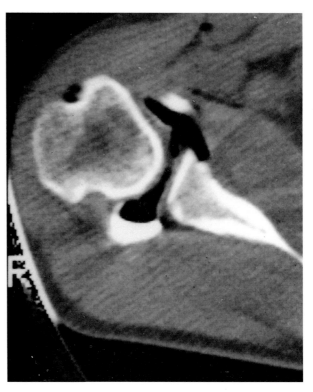

Figure 4.118 *Hatchet defect—CT arthrogram. The anterior lip of the labrum glenoidale is defective. The long head of biceps tendon is no longer seen in the air-filled sheath. The capsule is stripped back from the neck of the glenoid anteriorly and distended posteriorly. There is a large posterior defect of the humeral head.*

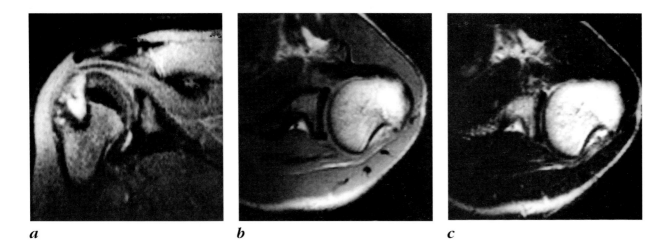

a   *b*   *c*

Figure 4.119 *Hatchet defect. (**a**) The coronal fat suppression MR sequence shows upward subluxation of the humeral head in association with a large defect in the humeral head. The axial T$_1$- (**b**) and T$_2$-weighted (**c**) MR images demonstrate a large posterior defect which shows increased signal intensity on T$_2$-weighting.*

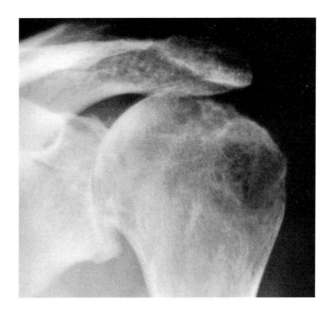

Figure 4.120 *Rheumatoid arthritis. A lytic lesion is present in the greater tuberosity on the anteroposterior view. This change may be found in rheumatoid arthritis, tuberculosis or may even follow repeated anterior dislocation (hatchet defect). In this patient there is also upward subluxation of the humeral head with para-articular erosions and eburnation of the articular surface. The joint space is narrow.*

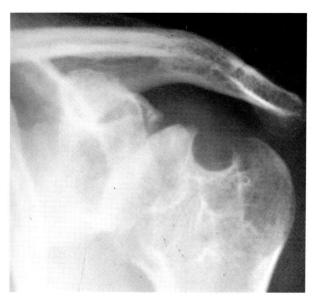

Figure 4.121 *Caries sicca (tuberculosis) in the region of the greater tuberosity. The shoulder joint space is also obliterated.*

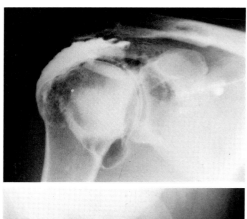

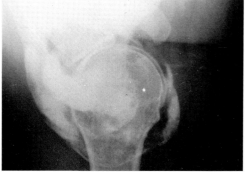

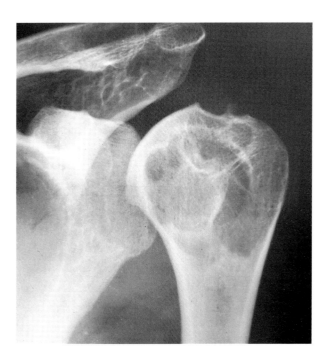

Figure 4.122 *Cystic tuberculosis. In another patient a much more extreme example of erosion at the proximal humerus is demonstrated.*

Figure 4.123 *Rotator cuff tear. The glenohumeral articulation is normal in this double-contrast study. The large pool of contrast medium beneath the acromion is in the subacromial bursa and indicates a communication between the two structures, that is, a rotator cuff tear must be present.*

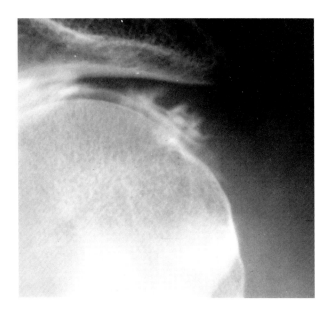

Figure 4.124 *Partial tear of the rotator cuff. There is irregularity of the undersurface of the rotator cuff tendon at arthrography and contrast medium stains much of the tendon locally, but does not fill the subacromial bursa.*

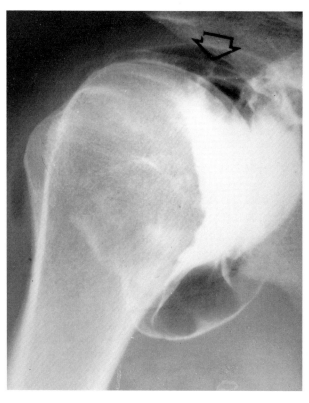

Figure 4.125 *The normal double-contrast arthrogram shows the tendon coated with contrast medium and surrounded by air in the distended capsule (arrow).*

(3) frozen shoulder, or restrictive capsulitis, presents with similar symptoms to a rotator cuff tear. Here, the volume of the joint is severely restricted, often admitting only 5–6 ml of gas and contrast medium (n = 20–30 ml). The margins of the joint capsule are constricted and irregular. Contrast medium is forced into the tendon sheath, which may rupture (Figure 4.126).

Ultrasound: unlike the knee, the intra-articular structures of the shoulder joint are of little relevance to function, while the tendons, muscles and ligaments around the shoulder are more superficially situated, can be cleared from overlying bone and are more amenable to examination by ultrasound (Figure 4.127).

The normal rotator cuff is seen as a hyper-reflective band tapering to the greater tuberosity. Calcification is seen earlier than on plain films, and is shown on or in the tendon as a hyper-reflective area with acoustic shadowing. The subacromial bursa is a reflective line beneath the deltoid.

Rotator cuff tears are shown by failure to demonstrate the tendon, i.e. it is retracted, or by a bare area filled with fluid or granulation tissue. Thinning of the cuff can be assessed. Excess fluid in the subacromial bursa is rarely seen in rotator cuff tears.

Tendinitis and partial thickness tears are difficult or impossible to assess by ultrasonography.

CT scanning in the axial plane is used following arthrography to demonstrate structures coated by contrast medium. The labrum and associated bone are seen (Figure 4.128), as is the long head of biceps in its sheath. The hatchet defect is shown (Figure 4.118). Loose bodies can be demonstrated. The rotator cuff tear will have been seen on the preceding arthrogram.

MR imaging: this technique is said to have 100% sensitivity in the diagnosis of complete rotator cuff tears, and differentiates tendinitis with impingement from tears.

Changes at the acromioclavicular joint are seen on coronal scans. T_2-weighted images show both hypertrophy and oedema in and around the joint. The subjacent supraspinatus may be compressed, oedematous or even torn (Figure 4.129).

The acromion is the site of a spur seen on T_1-weighted and fat suppression sequences. The subjacent

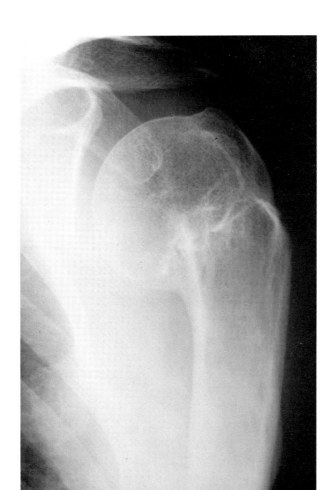

Figure 4.126 *Frozen shoulder. (**a**) The patient initially sustained a fracture of the neck of the humerus which had healed with varus deformity, but still complained of pain in the shoulder and limitation of movement. (**b**) The arthrogram shows the typical features of restrictive capsulitis. There is a narrow and constricted synovium, which is irregular. (**c**) In a different patient, contrast medium is forced down into the bicipital tendon sheath, which is itself irregular. This is a high pressure system. (**d**) In this high pressure joint space, the bicipital tendon sheath ruptures.*

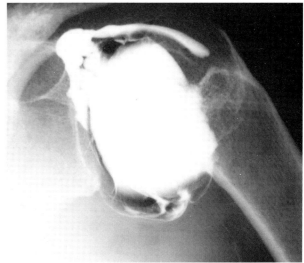

a

b

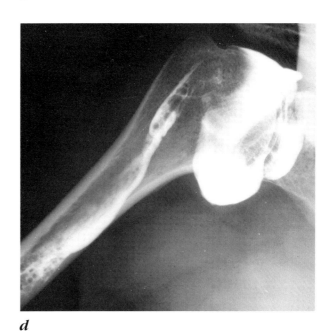

c

d

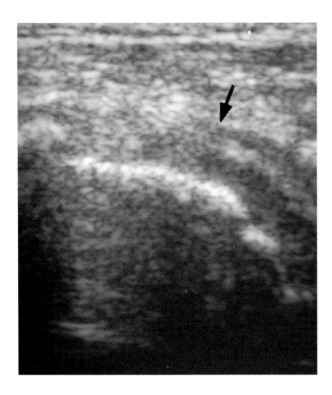

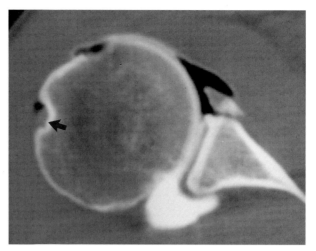

Figure 4.128 *CT arthrography. Recurrent anterior dislocation has resulted in avulsion of the anterior lip of the glenoid labrum and the underlying bone. The changes are well demonstrated by this technique. The long head of the biceps tendon is shown in the bicipital groove (arrow).*

Figure 4.127 *Rotator cuff tear at ultrasonography. The supraspinatus tendon is retracted and the free end can be identified (arrow). A bare area is seen over the humeral head.*

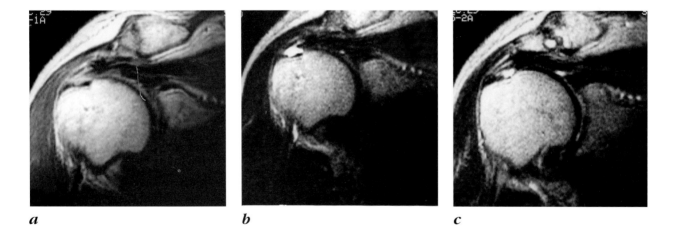

a   *b*   *c*

Figure 4.129 *Hypertrophy of the acromioclavicular joint. (**a**) This is bony and seen in both a superior and inferior direction on this coronal proton density weighted MR sequence. Inferiorly, there is compression of the subjacent supraspinatus tendon. A distal rotator cuff tear is demonstrated. (**b**) A coronal T₂-weighted MR sequence at the same level demonstrates a rotator cuff tear with retraction. (**c**) The acromioclavicular joint is better shown on an adjacent T₂-weighted slice. Fluid is demonstrated within the joint. The subjacent supraspinatus is compressed and slightly oedematous. Here, the tendon is not retracted and a horizontal cleft is demonstrated within it, which contains fluid.*

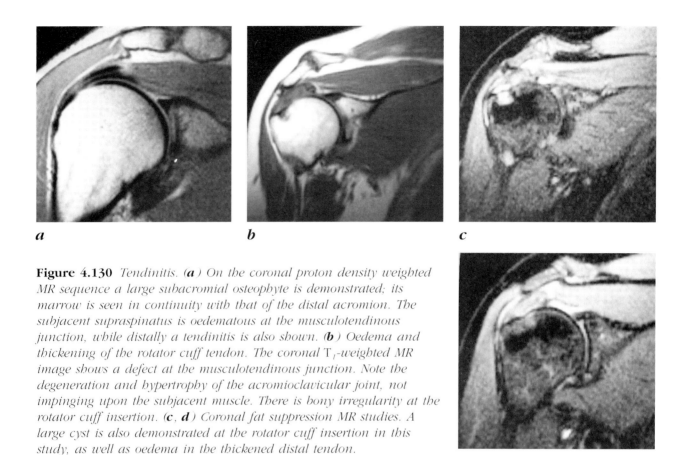

a   *b*   *c*

d

Figure 4.130 *Tendinitis. (**a**) On the coronal proton density weighted MR sequence a large subacromial osteophyte is demonstrated; its marrow is seen in continuity with that of the distal acromion. The subjacent supraspinatus is oedematous at the musculotendinous junction, while distally a tendinitis is also shown. (**b**) Oedema and thickening of the rotator cuff tendon. The coronal T₁-weighted MR image shows a defect at the musculotendinous junction. Note the degeneration and hypertrophy of the acromioclavicular joint, not impinging upon the subjacent muscle. There is bony irregularity at the rotator cuff insertion. (**c**, **d**) Coronal fat suppression MR studies. A large cyst is also demonstrated at the rotator cuff insertion in this study, as well as oedema in the thickened distal tendon.*

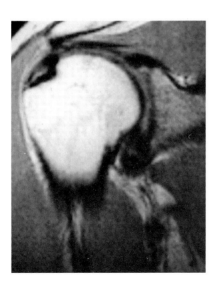

Figure 4.131 *Subacromial impingement by a spur is shown on a coronal* T₁*-weighted MR image. The subjacent tendon is thinned and deficient beneath the spur. Distally there is a tear of the tendon just proximal to its insertion.*

tendon may be oedematous on T_2-weighted and fat suppression images (Figure 4.130a), and thickened (Figure 4.130b–d), thinned (Figure 4.131), torn (Figure 4.132) or retracted (Figures 4.129b, 4.133 and 4.134). A band of fluid, seen as an increase in signal, may be aligned along the long axis of the tendon as well as vertically (Figures 4.129c and 4.135). Cystic change may be present in the greater tuberosity (Figure 4.135b). The subacromial bursa is seen on T_1-weighted images as a bright band beneath the acromion due to fat around it. Fluid distends it in disease, seen on T_2-weighted and fat suppression sequences. Fluid is also seen in the gleno-humeral joint. The deltoid may be atrophied.

Axial scans in the T_2-weighted mode demonstrate the long head of biceps tendon in the groove. The tendon sheath may be distended. The labrum is shown. It should be of low signal intensity and be pointed, but may be normally rounded. Articular cartilage of brighter signal may lie between it and the bony lip of the glenoid simulating a labral detachment. Labral detachment may be seen with avulsion

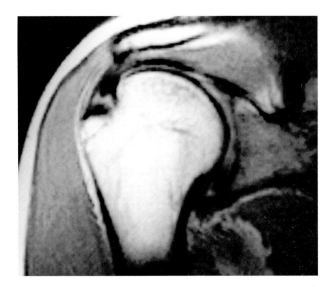

Figure 4.132 *Distal rotator cuff tear in the presence of a subacromial spur with subjacent tendinitis (coronal T₁-weighted MR sequence).*

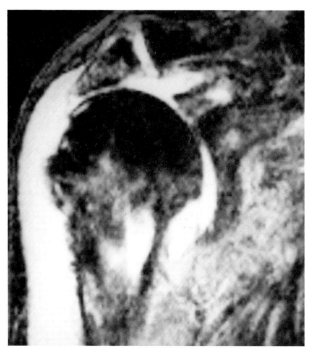

Figure 4.133 *Coronal fat suppression MR sequence showing obliteration of the subacromial space due to upward subluxation of the head of humerus through a totally retracted tendon. Note the cystic changes in the region of the rotator cuff insertion and also the fluid in the acromioclavicular joint.*

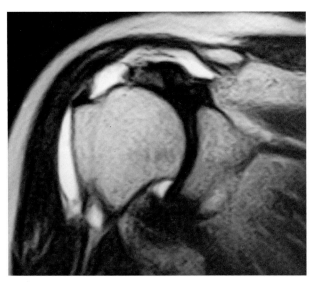

a

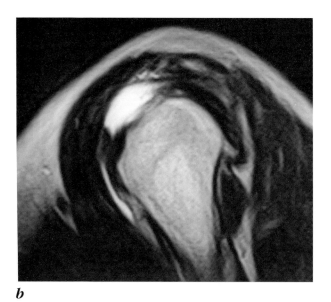

b

Figure 4.134 *Rupture of the rotator cuff. (**a**) Coronal and (**b**) sagittal T₂-weighted MR sequences showing total rupture of the rotator cuff with retraction of the muscle belly, seen in both the coronal and sagittal planes. There is a large subacromial/subdeltoid bursa.*

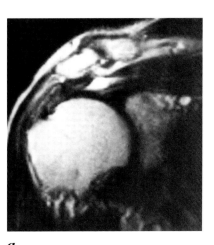
a

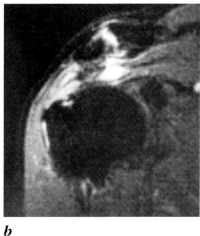
b

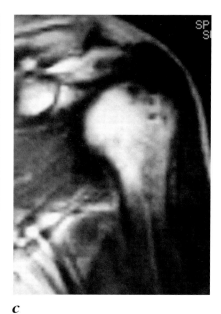
c

Figure 4.135 *Cystic degeneration of the rotator cuff—(**a**) coronal T₂-weighted and (**b**) fat suppression MR images. There is substantial degeneration at the acromioclavicular joint and this contains much fluid. Hypertrophy is present, both superiorly and inferiorly. The supraspinatus muscle belly is compressed beneath the hypertrophied distal clavicle and acromioclavicular joint. A large, transversely inclined cyst is demonstrated at the musculotendinous rotator cuff junction. The distal tendon is thinned, irregular and oedematous. Fluid is seen in the subacromial and subdeltoid bursae and cystic change is demonstrated in the greater tuberosity.*
*(**c**) Irregularity of the greater tuberosity and mixed signal is demonstrated on this coronal T₁-weighted MR image. These changes are often associated with rotator cuff abnormality. (**d**) Double-contrast shoulder arthrogram demonstrating a rotator cuff tear with filling of the subacromial bursa. There is communication with the acromioclavicular joint, the irregular and hypertrophied synovial cavity of which fills with contrast medium.*

d

of the underlying bone (Figure 4.136). Hatchet defects are shown (Figure 4.119).

THE KNEE JOINT

Plain films: these are of great value. Experience shows that the changes on the plain film, certainly in

severe osteoarthritis, relate closely to the changes subsequently seen at MRI.

Joint symmetry is normally present. With a *discoid*, or non-involuted meniscus, usually the lateral, retaining its fetal form, the joint space is widened and the tibial plateau dished (Figure 4.137). Joint space *narrowing* must imply loss of articular or meniscal cartilage, or both, in full or in part. Marginal

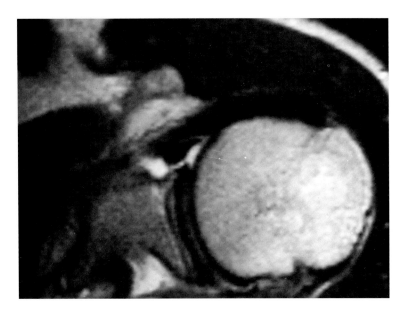

Figure 4.136 *Axial T$_2$-weighted MR sequence showing detachment of the anterior labrum. The long head of the biceps tendon is seen passing over the anterior aspect of the head of the humerus and entering the bicipital groove. Compare with Figure 4.128.*

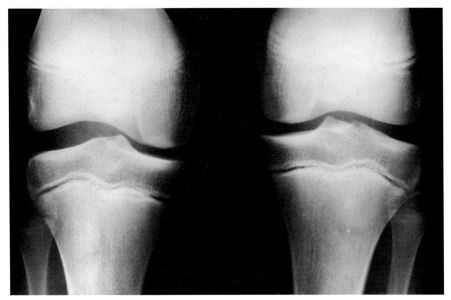

a

Figure 4.137 *Discoid meniscus. (a) The plain film shows widening of the lateral compartment on the right. (b) An arthrogram in a different patient shows a thickened meniscus which, instead of being pointed internally, has a rather bulbous aspect. (c) The coronal (left) and sagittal T$_2$-weighted gradient echo (right) MR sequences shows the thickened lateral meniscus, which is often degenerate or torn.*

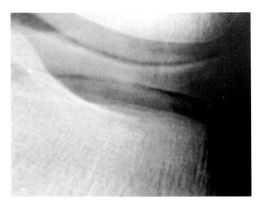

b

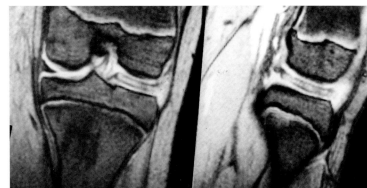

c

osteophytes and subarticular cysts may be seen in arthritis (Figure 4.138). The subcutaneous soft tissues are normally thicker medially; there is more fat there. Poor definition of the fat–capsule interface may indicate a tear of the medial collateral ligament (Figure 4.139). Subsequent ossification of a local haematoma at the site of ligamentous avulsion is the *Pellegrini–Stieda lesion* (Figure 4.140).

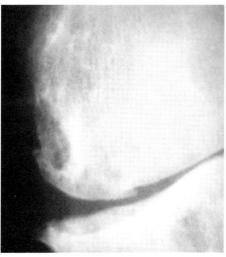

Figure 4.138 *Degenerative changes at the medial compartment of the knee. There is joint space narrowing and marginal osteophytosis extending over the articular surface, together with subarticular sclerosis and early cyst formation.*

Figure 4.139 *Poor definition of thickened medial soft tissues of the right knee may indicate a tear of the medial collateral ligament (arrow).*

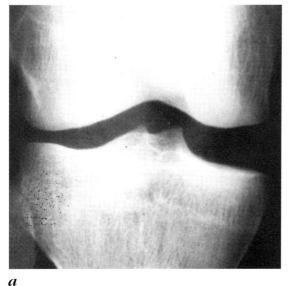

a

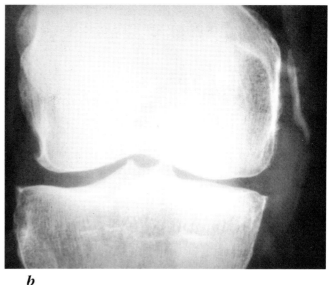

b

Figure 4.140 *Pellegrini–Stieda lesion. (a) The initial radiograph shows a severe valgus strain on the joint with widening of the medial compartment. (b) Subsequent imaging 14 months later shows the spur of new bone lying proximally along the line of the avulsed ligament.*

On a lateral view of the knee, the soft tissues should be assessed first. Effusions are seen in the suprapatellar pouch (Figure 4.141) and behind the joint in the popliteal fossa (see Chapter 9, page 423). On an anteroposterior view of the knee, the fat planes are displaced from the region of the distal femoral metaphysis and bow convexly outwards in the presence of a suprapatellar effusion. The displacement is confirmed

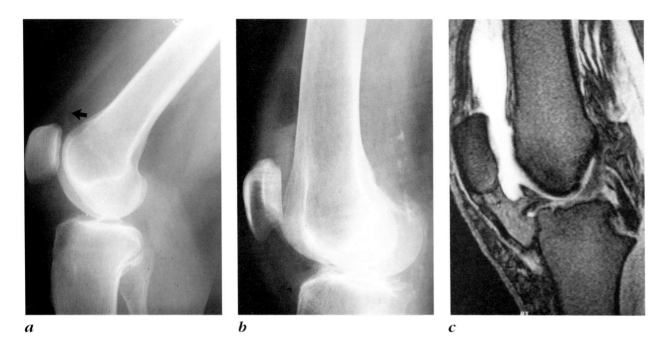

a   *b*   *c*

Figure 4.141 *Lateral radiograph of the knee (**a**) showing the normal suprapatellar pouch, seen as a soft tissue stripe arising from the superior patello-femoral joint space, surrounded by fat anteriorly and posteriorly (arrow). (**b**) Effusion in the suprapatellar pouch. Note the fat–fluid level in the erect position. The suprapatellar effusion has a lenticulate appearance. (**c**) Sagittal fat suppression MR image showing the lenticulate-shaped effusion, separating the patella from the femur.*

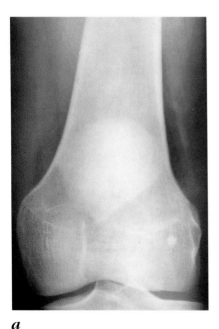
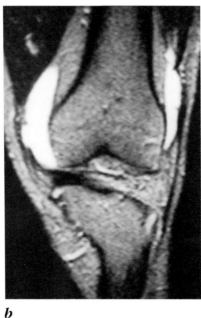

a   *b*

Figure 4.142 *(**a**) Displaced fat lines on the anteroposterior radiograph indicate the presence of an underlying effusion. (**b**) The coronal T_1-weighted MR image demonstrates soft tissue displacement by a knee joint effusion.*

at MR imaging (Figure 4.142). Contained densities or synovial calcinosis may be seen (see Chapter 9, page 437). The quadriceps insertion and retropatellar joint space should be assessed. A posterior patellar bony defect is described, filled with cartilage or fibrous tissue (Figure 4.114). The ligamentum patellae may be thick-

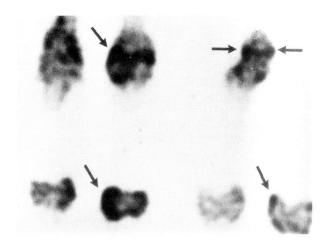

Figure 4.143 *Anterior, lateral and axial SPECT scans of the knee show increased activity related to adjacent meniscal abnormality (arrowed). (Reproduced with permission from Ryan PJ, SPECT bone scanning in the 1990s.* Appl Radiol *(1994)* **23***: 30–46.)*

ened, especially inferiorly, in the presence of Osgood–Schlatter's disease, where the soft tissues over the tibial tubercle are thickened (Figure 4.104).

Radionuclide bone scanning: increase in uptake is to be expected in degenerative disease of the knee. Bone sclerosis and osteophytosis at areas of stress will be seen as foci of increase in uptake. SPECT scanning of the knee in the axial plane is sensitive in detecting adjacent meniscal abnormality (Figure 4.143).

Ultrasound: because the menisci and cruciate ligaments lie deep within the joint, they are essentially inaccessible to the ultrasound beam but superficial structures are shown. Tendons and ligaments, especially the patellar, are demonstrated (Figure 4.144). Baker's cysts are seen, as is leak of synovial fluid from them (see Figures 4.25 and 4.26). Superficial meniscal cysts can also be imaged (Figure 4.144b). Peripheral meniscal parts are seen as hyperechoic triangular structures.

Arthrography demonstrates the internal structures of the joint, coated by contrast medium. Demonstration of meniscal abnormalities, especially partial (Figure 4.145a) or total tears, is as accurately shown as at arthroscopy. Tears may be bucket-handle (Figure 4.145b), total or partial, or horizontal. Contrast medium and air enter the tear. Cystic change within the meniscus can only infrequently be shown at arthrography, unlike at MR imaging.

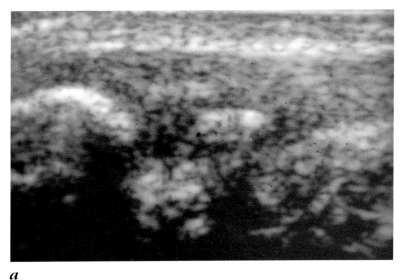
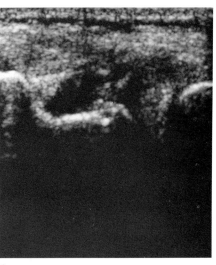

a   *b*

Figure 4.144 *Ultrasonography of the knee. (**a**) Severe patellar tendinitis in a chauffeur. Thickening and oedema of the tendon are shown with a large focus of calcification. (**b**) A fluid collection communicates with a cleft in the lateral meniscus. This is a lateral meniscal cyst associated with a torn meniscus.*

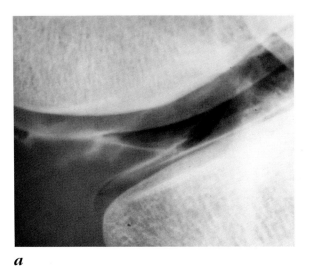 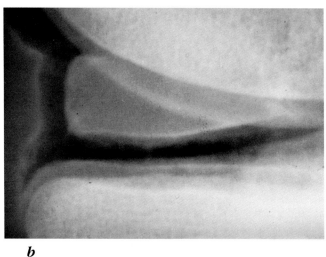

a　　　　　　　　　　　　*b*

Figure 4.145 *Double-contrast arthrography of the knee. (**a**) A partial tear of the medial meniscus is demonstrated towards the posterior horn. Note the partial overlap of the femoral condyles. Contrast medium leaks into the upper portion of the meniscus. (**b**) Total peripheral detachment.*

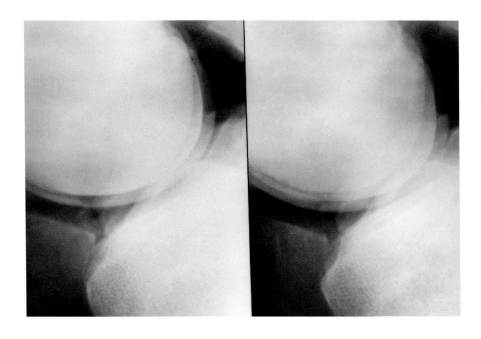

Figure 4.146 *The cruciate ligaments are fairly well defined. The anterior cruciate ligament in particular looks kinked and was judged to be torn. This was confirmed at surgery.*

Arthrography does not demonstrate the cruciate ligaments well, even when adrenaline is added to the contrast medium and tomography is used (Figure 4.146). Failure to visualize the cruciate ligaments may be due to an effusion and cannot be taken as conclusive evidence of cruciate abnormality.

Articular cartilage loss and osteochondritis dissecans (Figure 4.147) may be shown at arthrography. Extra-articular structures are not demonstrated.

CT scanning: chondromalacia patellae is shown at CT arthrography. Irregularity of retropatellar cartilage and absorption of contrast medium occur. The patellar tendon is well demonstrated on CT scanning.

MR imaging demonstrates not only superficial meniscal lesions but also changes *within* the meniscus to which contrast medium would not have access at arthrography. Fluid or myxoid degeneration within the meniscus are shown as areas of bright signal,

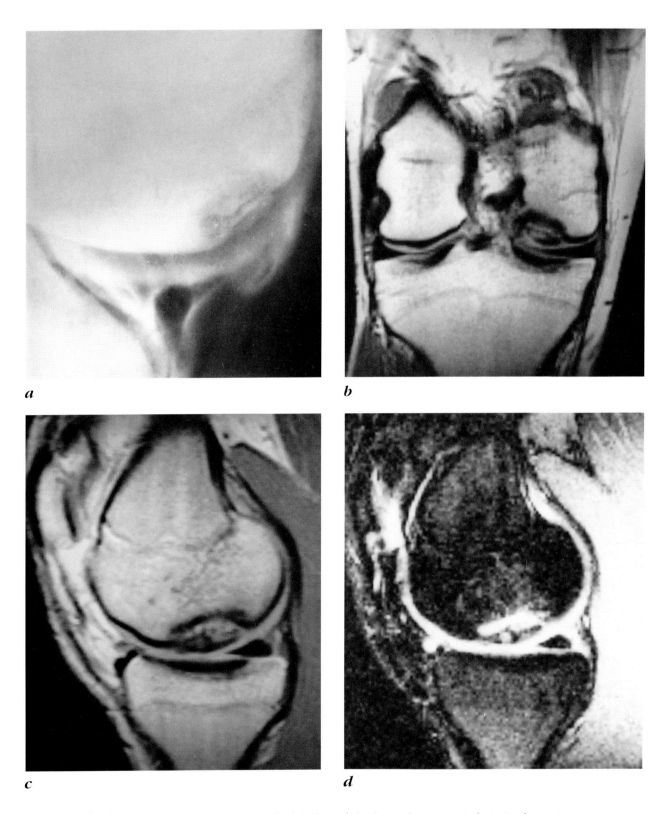

Figure 4.147 *(a) Post-traumatic osteochondral defect of the knee demonstrated at single-contrast arthrography. (b–d) Osteochondritis dissecans. Coronal (b) and sagittal (c) T₁-weighted MR sequences show a dissected fragment lying within a well-corticated bed of bone. (d) The sagittal fat suppression MR image shows fluid separating the underlying bone from the dissected fragment.*

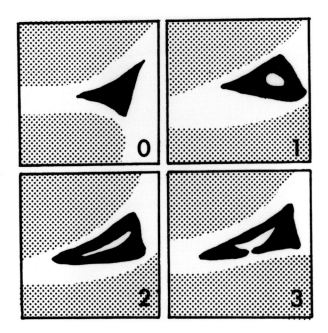

Figure 4.148 *Classification of meniscal lesions at MR imaging (after Stoller et al, 1987). Grade 0—normal. There is no increase in signal in the meniscus. Grade 1—a circular focus of increased signal. Grade 2—a linear focus of increased signal that does not extend to an articular surface and is not likely to be seen at arthroscopy as a tear. Grade 3—increased signal reaching an articular surface. A tear is present.*

especially on T_2-weighted and fat suppression images. The change has been graded (Figures 4.148 and 4.149). If the bright signal extends to the superficial meniscal surface, a tear is diagnosed (Figures 4.150 and 4.151). If the change is not shown unequivocally to reach the surface, a tear should not be diagnosed. Progression from grade 2 to grade 3 usually only occurs with severe stress, for example, in professional footballers.

The meniscus is also assessed after surgery. Substantial meniscal remnants may be present despite a 'meniscectomy' (Figure 4.152) and the remnant may be torn with recurrence of symptoms.

Cysts lying within the meniscus or at the menisco–capsular junction can be seen by this technique, but usually not at arthrography (Figure 4.149c). The cyst may communicate with a meniscal tear internally (Figures 4.149c and 4.153) and enlarge peripherally to come to lie beneath the skin (Figures 4.153 and 4.154). Baker's cysts are shown (Figure 4.27), as is leak.

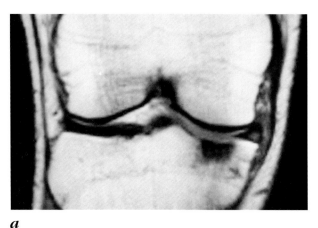

a

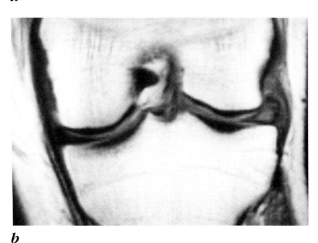

b

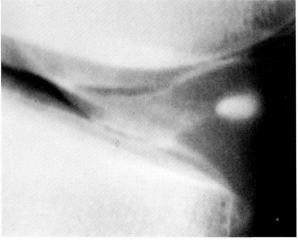

b

Figure 4.149 *(**a**) Type 1 medial meniscal lesion according to the classification of Stoller et al, 1987. (**b**) More extensive cyst formation within the lateral meniscus (coronal T_1-weighted MR images). (**c**) An unusual demonstration at arthrography of a cyst in a meniscus communicating with a tear.*

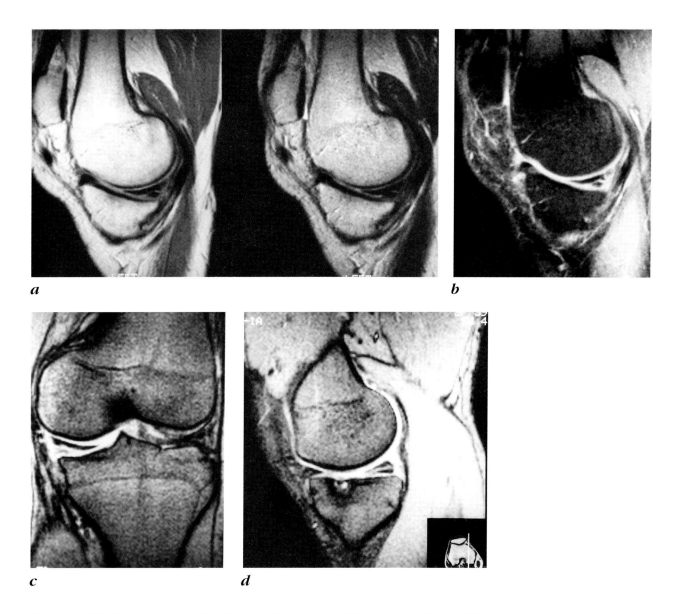

Figure 4.150 *Meniscal tears. (a) Sagittal T₁- (left) and T₂-weighted (right) MR images showing the tear extending to the inferior surface of the posterior third of the medial meniscus. (b) The same patient showing the tear on a fat suppression study and (c) on a radial T₂-weighted gradient echo MR image. (d) Fat suppression MR sequence in another patient showing a horizontal tear of the posterior horn of the medial meniscus in association with a degenerative cyst of the adjacent medial tibial plateau.*

Cruciate ligaments are better demonstrated than at arthroscopy; diagnostic accuracy approaches 100%. The normal anterior cruciate ligament is thinner and is less well seen than the posterior cruciate ligament, which is always well visualized. The anterior cruciate ligament is also more obliquely oriented.

Tears in the acute stage may be partial or total. The anterior cruciate ligament is straight in extension. If damaged, it may be concave anteriorly. Anterior laxity may be associated with kinking of the ligamentum patellae, which is normally straight. Fluid may be seen in the torn anterior cruciate ligament on T_2-weighted and fat suppression sequences (Figure 4.155). Total rupture and fragmentation may be present.

The posterior cruciate ligament may be torn. Increase in signal indicates local oedema or haemorrhage (Figure 4.156). Avulsion of the tibial cortex at

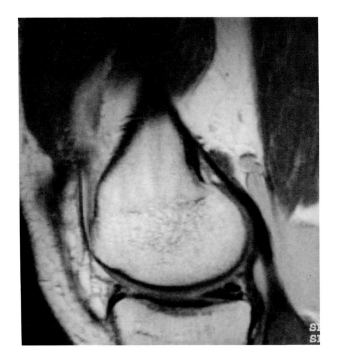

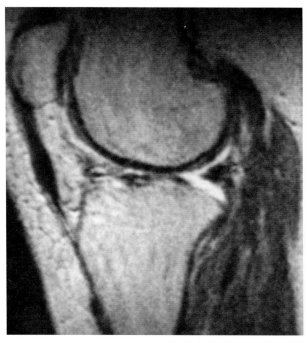

Figure 4.151 *A tear of the medial meniscus is shown in association with a Baker's cyst on this sagittal T₁-weighted MR sequence.*

Figure 4.152 *Post-meniscectomy. A remnant of the meniscal rim is demonstrated on this T₂-weighted MR sequence. It is irregular.*

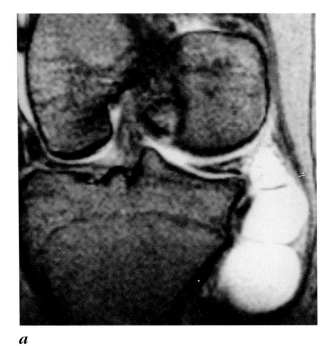

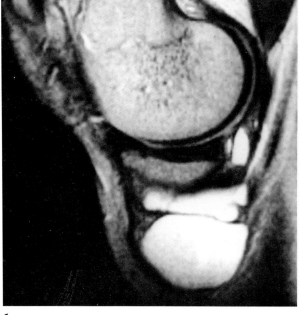

a

b

Figure 4.153 *Tear of the meniscus and superficial cyst. (a) The medial meniscus on this radial T₂-weighted gradient echo MR image is shown to have a central linear band of increased signal extending to the superior surface of the meniscus as a tear. At the meniscal periphery there is communication with a very large cyst, which is multilocular. (b) Sagittal T₂-weighted MR sequence.*

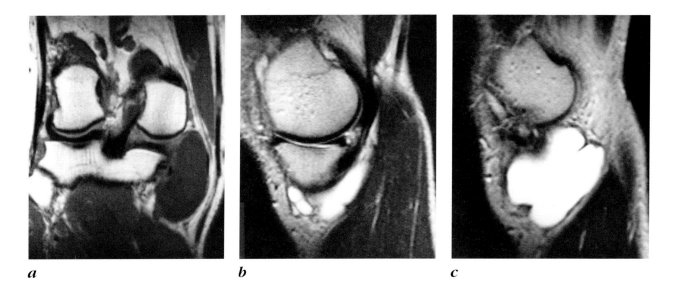

a   *b*   *c*

Figure 4.154 *Another case of a tear of the posterior horn of the medial meniscus associated with a cyst extending into the subcutaneous soft tissues. (**a**) coronal T$_1$-weighted and (**b**, **c**) sagittal T$_2$-weighted MR sequences.*

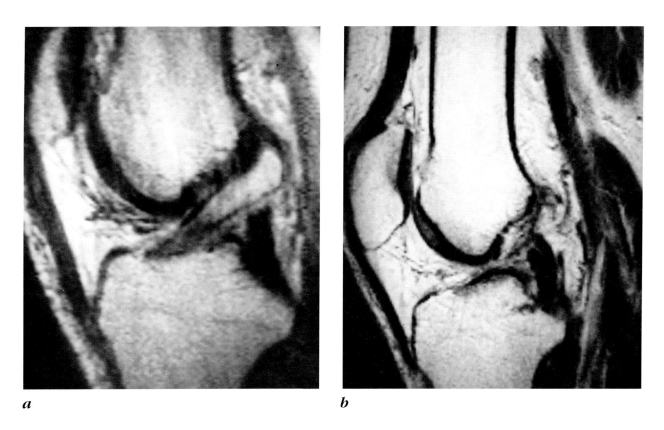

a   *b*

Figure 4.155 *(**a**) Haemorrhage into the anterior cruciate ligament is shown as increase in signal on the sagittal T$_1$-weighted MR study. (**b**) A disrupted anterior cruciate ligament is demonstrated; it is thinned, irregular and bowed. The posterior cruciate ligament is not shown in its entirety. The superior portion would be seen on the next slice, but the structure is otherwise normal.*

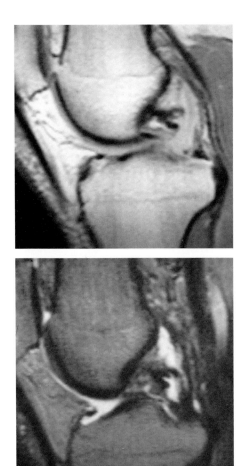

Figure 4.156 *Sagittal T₁-weighted (top) and fat suppression (bottom) MR images showing a tear of the posterior cruciate ligament.*

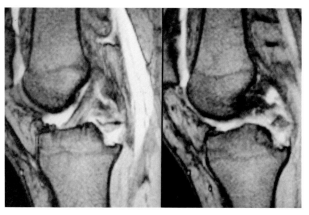

a

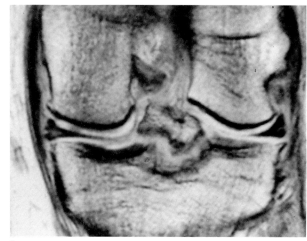

b

Figure 4.157 *Rupture of the posterior cruciate ligament with avulsion of its insertion. (a) Sagittal fat suppression MR images show the cortical plate lifted superiorly by a torn and irregular posterior cruciate ligament. (b) Note oedema of the anterior cruciate ligament on the coronal gradient echo MR image. Note too the marginal osteophytosis and the thickening of the medial collateral ligament.*

the insertion of the posterior cruciate ligament may occur; a cortical plate of bone is avulsed and the defect fills with fluid (Figure 4.157). Healing of the cruciate ligaments results in fibrosis and abnormal contours, but fluid need no longer be present in the structure (Figure 4.158).

Articular cartilage is demonstrated at MRI. Its loss can be assessed. Osteochondral defects are shown; fluid is seen in the defects (Figure 4.147).

Chondromalacia patellae is shown as an alteration of local signal in cartilage (Figure 4.159).

The collateral structures are well defined on coronal and axial MR imaging. Disruption of the medial collateral ligament is seen on T_1-weighted coronal sequences and on T_2-weighted and fat suppression studies, where haemorrhage or oedema around the torn ligament are shown (Figure 4.160). The plain film may also show

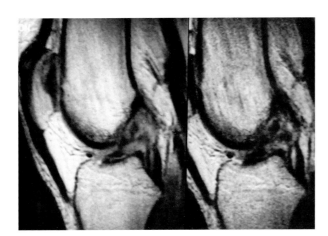

Figure 4.158 *Sagittal T$_1$- and T$_2$-weighted MR images showing a chronic tear of the anterior cruciate ligament which has healed by fibrosis. The contour is now step-like.*

oedema and irregularity of the medial soft tissues beneath the subcutaneous fat (Figure 4.139). The valgus strain which disrupts the medial collateral ligament may simultaneously result in impaction of the lateral femoral condyle on the lateral tibial plateau. A fracture may then be seen on the plain film, perhaps with a fat–fluid level in the joint. The fat suppression MR sequence shows tibial bone oedema following impaction (see Figure 1.19). Oedema or haemorrhage after trauma may be extensively distributed around the joint (Figure 4.161). Subsequently a Pellegrini–Stieda lesion may arise (Figure 4.140).

The anterior fat pad may be disrupted and contain fluid, and prepatellar oedema is a common finding.

Direct anterior trauma to the knee results in a firm prepatellar bursitis, best seen on T$_2$-weighted and fat suppression images (Figure 4.162).

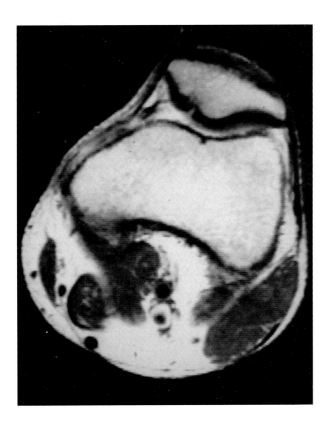

Figure 4.159 *Chondromalacia patellae. On an axial T$_1$-weighted MR image a defect is seen in the articular cortex and overlying cartilage of the medial facet.*

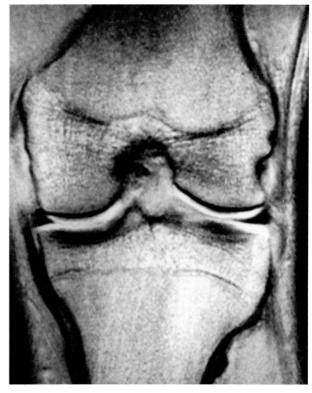

Figure 4.160 *Disruption of the medial collateral ligament with fluid in the local soft tissues.*

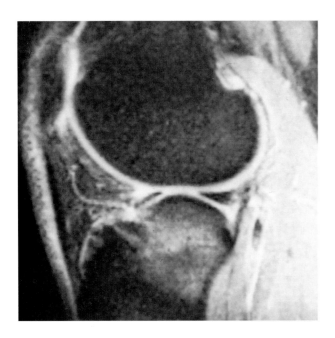

Figure 4.161 *Bone bruising. Sagittal fat suppression MR image showing bone bruising in the lateral tibial plateau.*

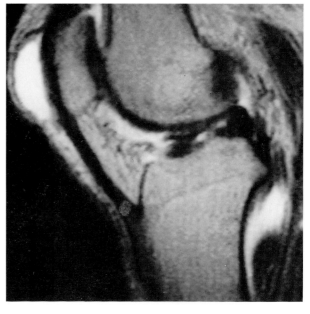

Figure 4.162 *Prepatellar bursitis. On the sagittal T₂-weighted MR image, a large, well defined, fluid-containing bursa sits upon the anterior patella following trauma.*

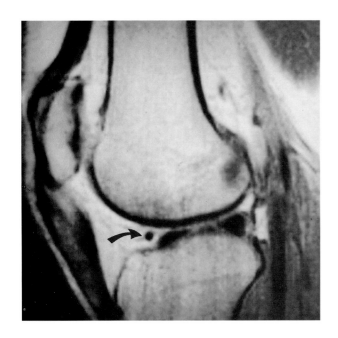

Figure 4.163 *Patellar tendinitis (sagittal T₁-weighted MR sequence). There is extensive thickening and cystic degeneration of the ligamentum patellae in its mid-portion. Note the transverse ligament (arrowed). This is not to be confused with an abnormality of the anterior horn of the adjacent meniscus.*

The ligamentum patellae may also be the site of thickening and cystic degeneration (Figure 4.163), also well seen on CT scanning. Osgood–Schlatter's disease (see page 250) shows local fragmentation of the tibial tubercle and soft tissue oedema in and around the distal patellar tendon. A bursa is occasionally seen between the tendon and tibial tubercle in a situation analogous to the retrocalcaneal bursa.

With degenerative disease, articular cartilage thins and cysts form beneath cortical defects; these are better seen at MRI than on plain films (Figure 3.71). Marginal osteophytes are seen on plain films, CT and especially well at MRI (Figure 4.164). Menisci beneath such osteophytes may be degenerate or torn and associated with overlying cysts and oedema in bone. Large marginal osteophytes displace the collateral ligaments and attached menisci (Figures 4.164 and 4.165).

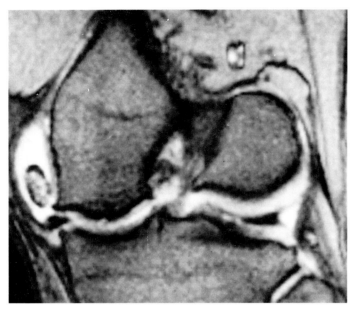
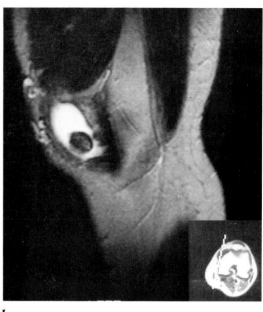

a   *b*

Figure 4.164 *Degenerative joint disease. (**a**) On the radial* T$_2$-*weighted gradient echo MR image there is an effusion, marginal osteophytosis and a loose body situated beneath the medial collateral ligament. The displacement of this ligament removes the degenerate attached meniscus from its normal intra-articular situation. (**b**) The sagittal* T$_2$-*weighted MR sequence shows the loose body in the distended joint capsule.*

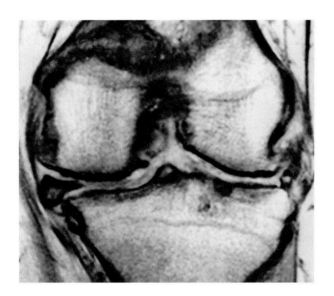

Figure 4.165 *Degenerative joint disease. The coronal* T$_1$-*weighted MR image shows extensive cystic degeneration of the medial meniscus, which is displaced because of its attachment to the adjacent collateral ligament. The osteophyte on the medial femoral condyle is the cause of the ligamentous displacement. Only a remnant of the lateral meniscus remains.*

THE ANKLE JOINT

Effusions are seen on plain films (Figure 4.166a) and at MRI (Figure 4.166b).

Tenosynovitis

Tendons around the ankle involved in pathology are:

1 tendo-Achillis;
2 the peroneal tendons behind the lateral malleolus, brevis anterior to longus;
3 tibialis posterior and flexor digitorum longus posterior to it behind the medial malleolus;
4 tibialis anterior over the dorsum of the foot;
5 flexor hallucis longus behind the tibia.

Tendons 2–5 are surrounded by synovial tendon sheaths. Tendons may be thickened, degenerate or torn. The sheaths may be distended with fluid or constricted and irregular with tenosynovitis.

Swelling of the tendo-Achillis and its margins by oedema are seen on soft tissue radiographs because this structure is surrounded by fat, but the other tendons are not seen on plain radiographs (Figures 4.167 and 4.168).

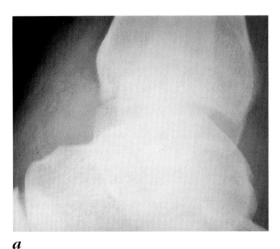

a

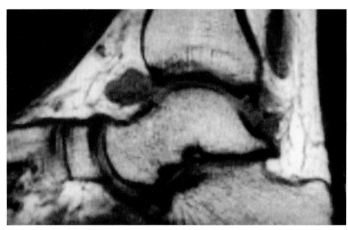

b

Figure 4.166 *(a) Ankle joint effusion demonstrated on a soft tissue lateral radiograph. There is a soft tissue density anterior to the ankle joint which displaces the overlying fat plane. (b) Sagittal T$_1$-weighted MR image demonstrates the synovial distension against the overlying fat.*

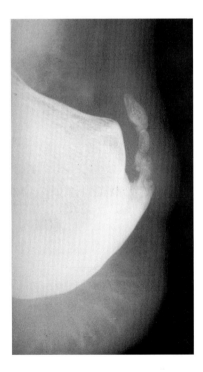

Figure 4.167 *Degeneration of the tendo-Achillis. The distal tendon is substantially thickened and ossified.*

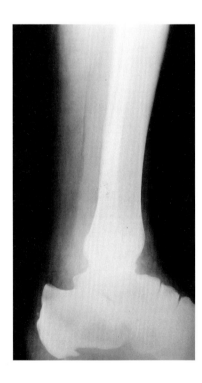

Figure 4.168 *Acute tear of tendo-Achillis. The tendo-Achillis is thickened and its anterior aspect poorly defined. Kager's fatty triangle, which normally lies anterior to the tendo-Achillis, is no longer seen because of local oedema and soft tissue swelling.*

Tenosynography: injection of a tendon sheath demonstrates the thickness of the tendon, or its absence following a tear and retraction, and the state of the sheath itself (Figure 4.169). The examination is supplemented by CT scanning which, on its own, demonstrates the size of the tendons around the ankle.

Arthrography has been used at the ankle to demonstrate capsular tears after injury. *Ultrasound* shows tendinous change around the ankle, including rupture, oedema, distension of the tendon sheaths, and tendon rupture and retraction (Figure 4.170). Ligamentous injuries are also shown.

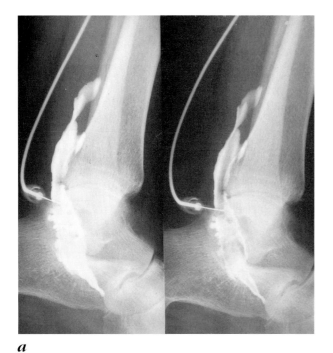

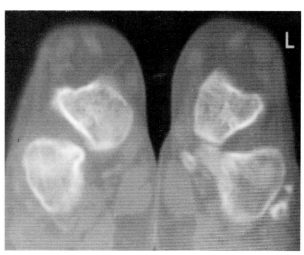

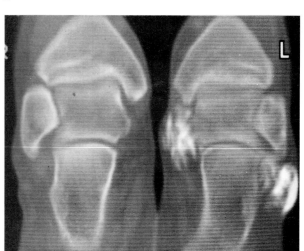

Figure 4.169 *Tenosynovitis. (**a**) Injection of the peroneal tendon sheath shows it to be irregular with diverticulum formation. The contained tendon is thickened. (**b**, **c**) CT tenosynogram following injection of the posterior tendon sheaths. This shows relative normality superiorly (**b**), though some distension of the peroneus longus sheath is demonstrated. More distally (**c**), thickening of the tendon and distension of the sheath is shown at the tip of the lateral malleolus.*

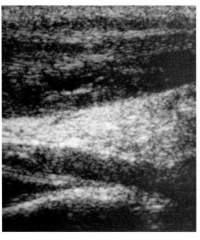

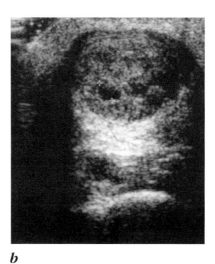

Figure 4.170 *Ultrasonography shows severe Achilles tendinitis with gross thickening and multiple degenerative cysts. The paratenon is normal; (**a**) longitudinal; (**b**) transverse.*

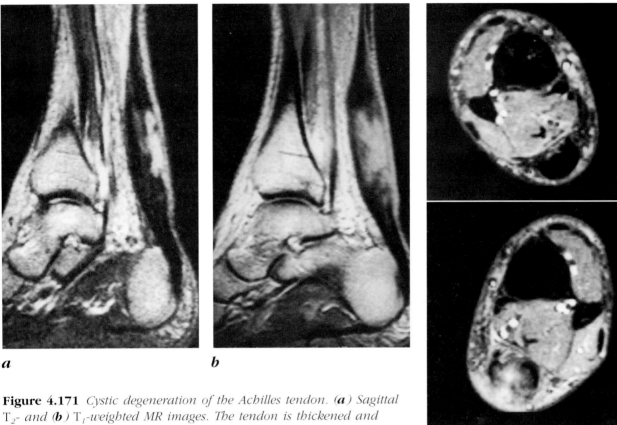

a

b

c

Figure 4.171 *Cystic degeneration of the Achilles tendon. (**a**) Sagittal T$_2$- and (**b**) T$_1$-weighted MR images. The tendon is thickened and shows extensive degeneration. (**c**) The axial fat suppression study compares the abnormal (bottom) with the normal side (top). The tendo-Achillis is normally bean-shaped, concave anteriorly.*

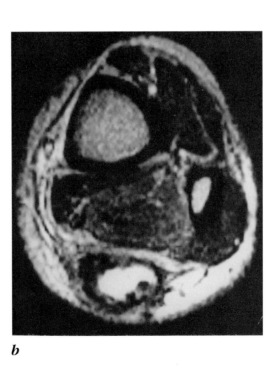

a

b

Figure 4.172 *Total rupture of the tendo-Achillis. (**a**) On the sagittal T$_2$-weighted MR sequence fluid lies between the separated, thickened parts. (**b**) On the axial image a pseudocapsule is seen around the fluid at the site of the rupture.*

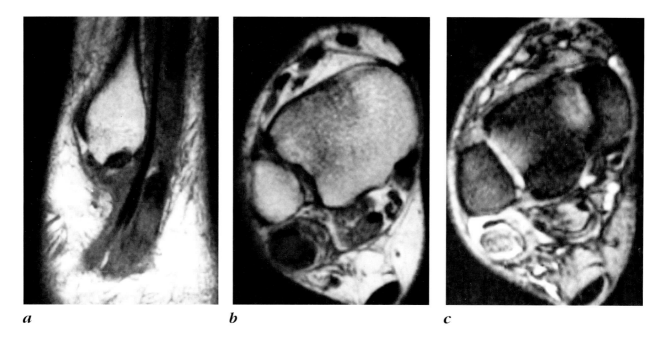

a   *b*   *c*

Figure 4.173 *Tendinitis of peroneus longus. (**a**) Sagittal* T*₁-weighted, (**b**) axial* T*₁-weighted and (**c**) axial fat suppression MR sequences. The tendon is grossly thickened, oedematous and the tendon sheath is distended with fluid.*

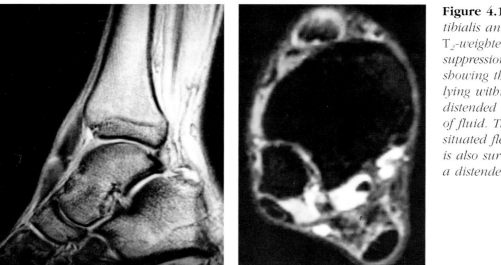

a   *b*

Figure 4.174 *Tendinitis of tibialis anterior. (**a**) Sagittal* T*₂-weighted and (**b**) axial fat suppression MR images showing the swollen tendon lying within a much distended tendon sheath full of fluid. The posteriorly situated flexor hallucis longus is also surrounded by fluid in a distended tendon sheath.*

MRI demonstrates degenerative change within tendons, seen as thickening and local increase in signal. These changes are especially well seen in the Achilles tendon (Figures 4.171 and 4.172). MRI also shows fluid in and around the thickened tendon, which may subsequently rupture and retract. T_2-weighted and fat suppression sequences are essential. Axial images often show an intact low signal capsule surrounding fluid lying between the retracted parts. There is often much surrounding oedema (Figures 4.172, 4.173 and 4.174).

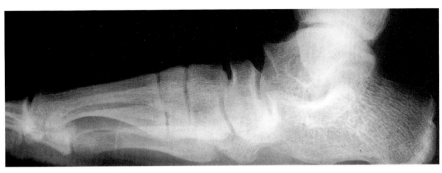

a

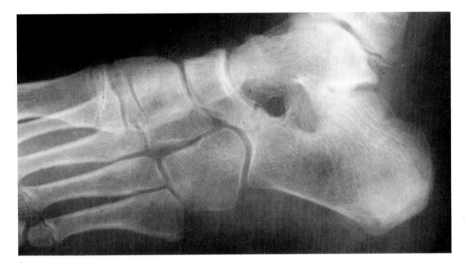

b

Figure 4.175 *Peroneal spastic flat foot due to tarsal coalition.* (*a*) *The lateral view, taken weight bearing, demonstrates typical features. These are loss of visualization of the subtalar joint together with apparent beaking of the anterior talus in a patient with flattening of the longitudinal arch.* (*b*) *The oblique view of the foot demonstrates the nature of the coalition. It is an almost total calcaneonavicular fusion with enlargement of the navicular towards the calcaneus. A talar beak may be also be demonstrated on the oblique view.*

Subtalar and talonavicular coalition

Hindfoot coalition is associated with flattening of the longitudinal arch. This causes stretching of the peroneal muscles, resulting in pain and spasm—the peroneal spastic flat foot. As bony coalition between tarsal bones occurs in infancy or adolescence during ossification of cartilaginous masses, symptoms occur then as hindfoot mobility is limited.

A lateral weight-bearing radiograph shows a flat foot (Figure 4.175a). Oblique views show total or partial calcaneonavicular synostosis (Figure 4.175b). An axial view (Figure 4.176a) shows subtalar fusion, usually at the middle facet; this is confirmed at axial CT (Figure 4.176b) and MR scanning (Figure 4.176c). The radionuclide bone scan shows increase in uptake around the remaining patent but stressed joints (Figure 4.177).

Abnormal movement of the navicular on the talus elevates the talonavicular ligament, resulting in a talar beak or spur. Other causes of excess local stress, e.g. in professional footballers, also cause a local talar beak to form (Figure 4.178).

THE ELBOW JOINT

Plain films show irregularity, thickening and ossification in musculotendinous insertions around the joint, on the olecranon and on the medial and lateral epicondyles (Figure 4.179). Anterior and posterior fat pad elevation follows trauma and is also seen in rheumatoid arthritis and infection.

Bursae enlarge over the triceps insertion at the olecranon (Figure 4.180). Loose bodies are occasionally seen on plain films, but are difficult to identify at arthrography, often being hidden by dense contrast medium or confused with bubbles at a double-contrast study. Loose bodies may be seen at CT and MRI (Figure 4.181). MRI also shows inflammatory changes in the flexor and extensor origins (Figure 4.182). Ultrasound is also of value in showing soft tissue change (Figure 4.183).

THE WRIST JOINT

Plain films: fat planes around the wrist are described in Chapter 9, page 421.

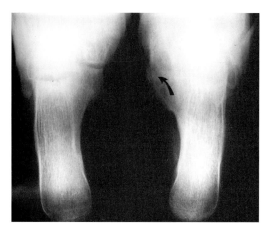

a

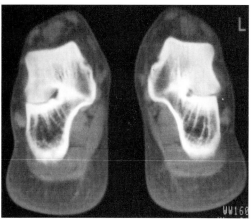

b

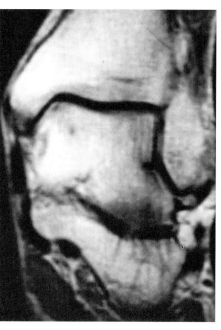

c

Figure 4.176 *Tarsal coalition. (**a**) The axial, or Korvin–Harris, view. On the left the middle and posterior facets are well demonstrated, while on the right there is congenital total fusion of the middle facet (arrow). (**b**) CT scans in another patient showing bilateral subtalar fusion. There is cortical thickening and joint narrowing at the patent part of the joint. (**c**) Coronal T$_1$-weighted MR sequence showing fusion at the subtalar joint, together with cortical thickening and loss of signal in the adjacent bone.*

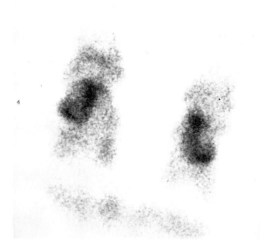

Figure 4.177 *The radioisotope bone scan shows increase in uptake laterally, that is, in the areas which are still patent, not fused, but at the site of the stress changes seen in Figure 4.176.*

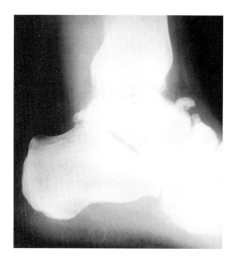

Figure 4.178 *Very prominent spur formation is demonstrated on the talus and navicular of this professional footballer. The posterior process of the talus is also prominent and irregular.*

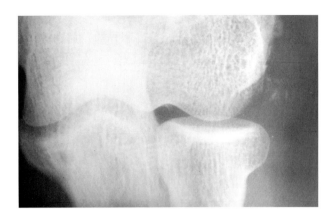

Figure 4.179 *An AP radiograph of the elbow demonstrates irregular soft tissue calcification in the extensor origin.*

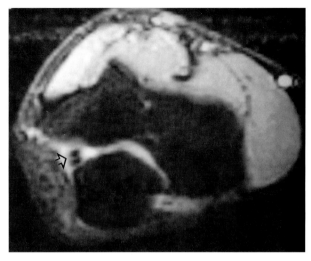

Figure 4.181 *Axial fat suppression MR image through the elbow demonstrates a loose body within the joint (arrow), seen as a low signal mass in the synovial fluid.*

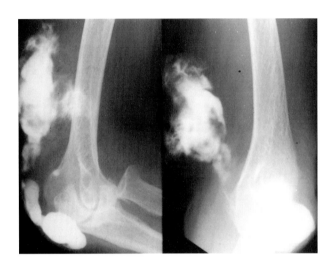

Figure 4.180 *Injection of an inflamed olecranon bursa, which has ruptured superiorly into the triceps. The appearances are analogous to those seen behind the knee from a ruptured Baker's cyst.*

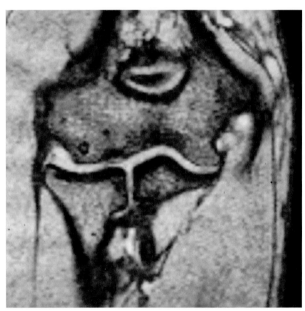

Figure 4.182 *Coronal T$_2$-weighted gradient echo MR sequence showing inflammatory changes in the flexor origin and erosions in the medial epicondyle.*

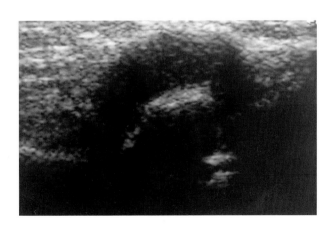

Figure 4.183 *Rheumatoid arthritis of the elbow. Hypoechoic soft tissue surrounds the radial head. This is pannus in a rheumatoid patient.*

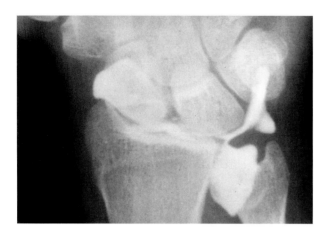

Figure 4.184 *Right wrist arthrogram in a young patient. A defect is demonstrated at the insertion of the triangular fibrocartilage into the radius, with filling of the distal radio-ulnar joint. No filling of the mid-carpal joint space is shown.*

Arthrography: this is used to confirm the integrity of the triangular fibrocartilage and the interosseous ligaments.

Injection of contrast medium into the radiocarpal joint is facilitated by opening up of the radiocarpal joint space with the hand in ulnar deviation. An intact triangular fibrocartilage does not usually allow contrast medium to pass to the distal radio-ulnar joint. Defects are usually post-traumatic in young patients (Figure 4.184) but come to exist as a normal variant in 20–30% of elderly patients.

The radiocarpal joint is limited distally by the scaphoid, lunate and triquetral bones and their intervening ligaments. There is a communication with the triquetral–pisiform joint space.

Proximal carpal ligamentous disruption, such as occurs between scaphoid and lunate, allows contrast to enter the mid-carpal space. Similarly, an injection here should not extend proximally or distally, but again because of naturally occurring ligamentous defects, especially in the elderly, false positive results may occur.

Arthrography may be more convincing in the demonstration of triangular fibrocartilage tears than MRI (Figure 4.185), where often even using a dedicated coil, the findings may be inconclusive. The radial attachment is thin and the ulnar attachment to the ulnar styloid broad. There is a high signal zone at the central portion of the attachment to the ulnar styloid, possibly related to local fat. The articular cartilage of the distal radius into which the triangular

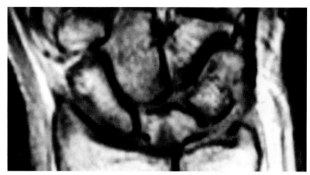

a

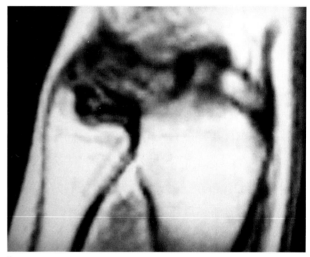

b

Figure 4.185 *(a, b) Coronal T$_1$-weighted MR images in two different patients showing defects in the normally low signal triangular fibrocartilage.*

fibrocartilage inserts also shows up as a brighter signal zone than the triangular fibrocartilage itself, simulating a gap at the insertion.

Ultrasound (Figure 4.186) is again useful for assessment of the tendons in this region.

Carpal tunnel syndrome

Compression of the median nerve in the carpal tunnel especially affects elderly women and is bilateral in 30%. MRI and ultrasound are of value in allowing the diagnosis to be made, complementing clinical signs (Figure 4.187). The flexor retinaculum, normally straight, is bowed palmarly. The median nerve is normally a round structure of intermediate signal lying on the flexor digitorum superficialis. In disease it is compressed and flattened beneath the

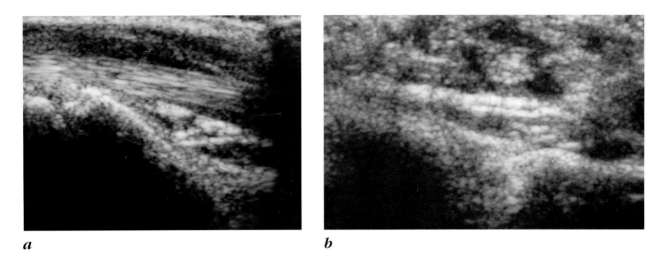

a   *b*

Figure 4.186 *(a) Longitudinal and (b) transverse ultrasound scans of the volar aspect of the wrist. The flexor digitorum tendons lie surrounded by low echogenicity soft tissue and some fluid.*

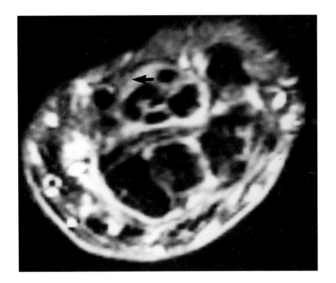

Figure 4.187 *Carpal tunnel syndrome. Axial fat suppression MR sequence through the tunnel shows bowing of the flexor retinaculum with poor visualization of the median nerve (arrow).*

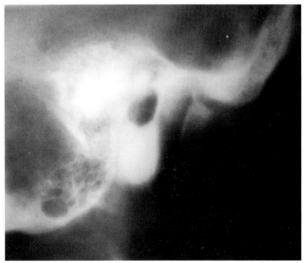

Figure 4.188 *Osteoarthritis of the temporomandibular joint. Degeneration with an osteophyte on the condylar head are shown on this linear tomogram.*

retinaculum at the level of the hamate, and may show local increase in signal on T_2-weighted images. It is swollen posteriorly, at the level of the pisiform. There may be oedema in the tunnel as a whole.

THE TEMPOROMANDIBULAR JOINT

Transpharyngeal and transcranial plain films are used to demonstrate the shape of the condyle and fossa.

The joint space is of even thickness. The condyle moves forward over the articular eminence when the mouth is opened.

Dislocation is unusual because the fossae are obliquely aligned to the coronal plane and to each other; it is usually associated with fracture of the condylar neck.

The temporomandibular joint may be the site of osteoarthritis (Figure 4.188), rheumatoid and seronegative arthritis (Figure 4.189). Changes can then be seen on plain films, at tomography (including orthopantomography) (Figures 4.188 and 4.189), radionuclide bone scanning (Figure 4.190), CT (Figure 4.191) and arthrography (Figure 4.192).

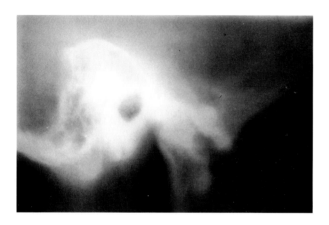

Figure 4.189 *Ankylosing spondylitis. Erosive change at the temporomandibular joint seen at tomography. The joint space is narrowed, indicating disruption of the meniscus. The condylar head is subluxed anteriorly and is eroded.*

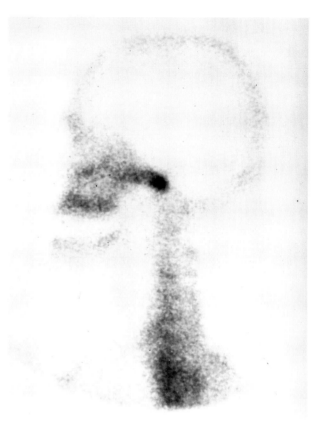

Figure 4.190 *Rheumatoid arthritis. The radionuclide bone scan is strongly positive at the temporomandibular joint in this patient with chronic rheumatoid arthritis.*

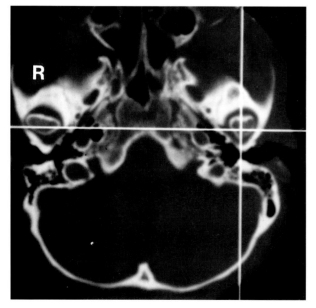

a

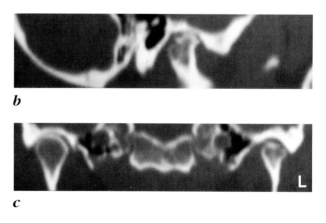

b

c

Figure 4.191 *Osteoarthritis of the temporomandibular joint. (a) The axial CT scan shows the normal oblique alignment of the right condyle in the fossa. (b) Sagittal and (c) coronal reconstructions in the indicated plane show narrowing of the left joint space with irregularity of the condylar head.*

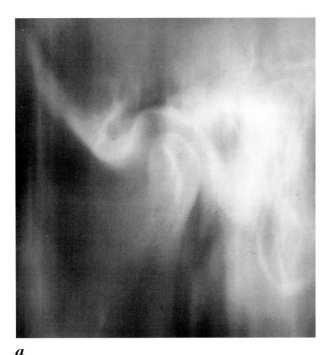

a

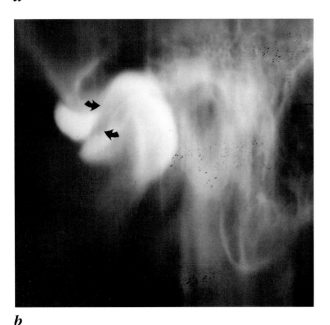

b

Figure 4.192 *Temporomandibular joint malfunction syndrome with an anteriorly displaced meniscus. (a) The initial tomogram in the sagittal plane shows widening of the anterior joint space and narrowing of the posterior. Normally there should be perfect symmetry. (b) After injection of both superior and inferior compartments, a large anterior filling defect is demonstrated (arrows). This represents the thickened and anteriorly displaced mass over which the condylar head cannot pass.*

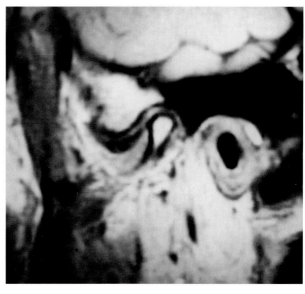

Figure 4.193 *MR image showing an anteriorly displaced meniscal mass. This technique has largely superseded arthrography.*

Temporomandibular joint malfunction syndrome

This syndrome is usually seen in young women, often cheek biters or those with bruxism. The patient has restriction of forward condylar movement with 'clunking', locking or 'grinding'. These symptoms are related to anterior displacement of the intra-articular meniscus. As a result, the condyle is displaced backwards at rest. Symptoms result from an abnormal relationship of the condyle to the anterior meniscal mass. Changes are demonstrated at arthrography (Figure 4.192) and at MRI (Figure 4.193).

BIBLIOGRAPHY

Beltran J, Caudill JL, Herman LA et al (1987) Rheumatoid arthritis. MR imaging manifestations. *Radiology* **165**: 153–7.

Bizarro AH (1921) On the sesamoid and supernumerary bones of the limbs. *J Anat (Cambridge)* **55**: 256.

Brower AC, Kransdorf MJ (1990) Imaging of hip disorders. *Radiol Clin North Am* **28**: 955–74.

Brown TR, Quinn SF (1993) Evaluation of chondromalacia of the patellofemoral compartment with axial magnetic resonance imaging. *Skeletal Radiol* **22**: 325–8.

Burk DL Jr, Dalinka MK, Karal E et al (1988) Meniscal and ganglion cysts of the knee: MR evaluation. *Am J Roentgenol* **150**: 331–6.

Chan WP, Lang P, Stevens MP et al (1991) Osteoarthritis of the knee. Comparison of radiography, CT and MR imaging to assess extent and severity. *Am J Roentgenol* **157**: 799–806.

Gilkeson G, Polisson R, Sinclair H et al (1988) Early detection of carpal erosions in patients with rheumatoid arthritis: a pilot study of magnetic resonance imaging. *J Rheumatol* **15**: 1361–6.

Gold RH, Seeger LL, Yao L (1993) Imaging shoulder impingement. *Skeletal Radiol* **27**: 555–61.

Gompels BM, Darlington LG (1982) Evaluation of popliteal cysts and painful calves with ultrasonography. Comparison with arthrography. *Ann Rheum Dis* **41**: 355–9.

Iannotti JP, Zlatkin MB, Esterhai JL et al (1991) Magnetic resonance imaging of the shoulder. *J Bone Joint Surg* **73A**: 17–29.

Jelinek JS, Kransdorf MJ, Utz JA, Berrey BH Jr (1989) Imaging of pigmented villonodular synovitis with emphasis on magnetic resonance imaging. *Am J Roentgenol* **153**: 337–42.

Kaplan PA, Nelson NL, Garvin KL, Brown DE (1991) MR of the knee. The significance of high signal in the meniscus that does not clearly extend to the surface. *Am J Roentgenol* **156**: 333–6.

Kaye JJ (ed) (1990) Imaging of joints. *Radiologic Clinics of North America* **28** (5).

Kieft GJ, Bloem JL, Rozing PM, Obermann WR (1988) MR imaging of recurrent anterior dislocation of the shoulder.

Comparison with CT arthrography. *Am J Roentgenol* **150**: 1083–7.

Lindblom K (1939) Arthrography and roentgenography in ruptures of tendons of the shoulder joint. *Acta Radiologica* **20**: 548.

Mink JH, Levy T, Crues JV (1988) Tears of the anterior cruciate ligament and menisci of the knee. MR imaging evaluation. *Radiology* **167**: 769–74.

Neer CS (1983) Impingement lesions. *Clin Orthop* **173**: 70–79.

Poleksic L, Zdravkovic D, Jablanovic D et al (1993) Magnetic resonance imaging of bone destruction in rheumatoid arthritis. Comparison with radiography. *Skeletal Radiol* **22**: 577–80.

Renton P (1991) Arthrography. In: *Surgical Disorders of the Shoulder* (ed. M Watson), pp 97–117. Edinburgh: Churchill Livingstone.

Renton P (1991) Radiology of the foot. In: *The Foot and Its Disorders* (ed. L Klenerman), 3rd edn, pp 239–346. Oxford: Blackwell Scientific Publications.

Rosenthall L (1991) Nuclear medicine techniques in arthritis. *Rheum Dis Clin North Am* **17**: 585–97.

Smith JH, Pugh DG (1962) Roentgenographic aspects of articular pigmented villonodular synovitis. *Am J Roentgenol* **87**: 1146.

Stoller DW, Martin C, Crues JV III et al (1987) Meniscal tears: pathologic correlation with MR imaging. *Radiology* **163**: 731–5.

Weissman BN (ed) (1991) Imaging of rheumatic diseases. *Rheum Dis Clin North Am* **17**: 457–816.

Chapter 5 Abnormalities in the region of the metaphysis

The metaphysis is the part of the immature skeleton which is just adjacent to the growth plate, where it is generally transverse opposite the epiphysis, at right angles to long axis of the shaft, and is occasionally curved, for example, beneath the iliac crest apophysis. The contour matches that of the epiphysis and is slightly undulant. The margin at the growth plate is sharply defined, sclerotic and usually less than 1 mm wide. This sclerosis represents the zone of provisional calcification. The metaphysis as a whole widens smoothly to the growth plate until it matches the epiphysis in width, and the contours of epiphysis and metaphysis are contiguous.

Metaphyseal changes may be generalized or localized to one, or a few metaphyses. Metaphyseal abnormalities may affect the growth plate and epiphysis and, conversely, changes at epiphyses may affect adjacent parts of the bone. In some conditions, particularly the dysplasias, changes occur in both the epiphyses and metaphyses.

Table 5.1 Generalized transverse bands of metaphyseal lucency.

Normal appearance in neonates
Immobilization
Systemic disease
Leukaemia
Neuroblastoma
Cushing's syndrome
Scurvy
Rickets
Syphilis
Rubella

TRANSVERSE BANDS OF METAPHYSEAL LUCENCY

In all conditions in Table 5.1, many metaphyses are usually affected by a band of radiolucency extending across the entire metaphyseal width.

IMMOBILIZATION AND SYSTEMIC DISEASE

Disuse of part or all of a limb can cause radiologically demonstrable osteoporosis which may be generalized or localized. Patients, particularly children, who are immobilized because of major illness, lose bone density generally, but the appendicular skeleton is more severely affected than the axial. At the metaphysis, a translucent band of demineralization, 2–4 mm deep, develops beneath the zone of provisional calci-

fication, and extends across the entire metaphysis (Figure 5.1). This zone of lucency may be more clearly demarcated than that seen with widespread malignancy in children, which tends to be poorly defined and often associated with marginal cortical erosions.

LEUKAEMIA AND NEUROBLASTOMA

In leukaemia and neuroblastoma, the band of metaphyseal radiolucency tends to be deeper, more irregular and usually associated with a more obviously aggressive osteolytic process elsewhere (Figure 5.2). Focal areas of medullary and cortical destruction, and sutural widening of the skull are seen in these conditions.

SCURVY AND RICKETS

These are often described together but their radiological appearances are dissimilar. In scurvy, a prominent metaphyseal band of lucency is associated with generalized demineralization which makes the cortical margins prominent. This change occurs particularly at the ring epiphyses in infants (Wimberger sign). The zone of translucency (Trümmerfeld zone)

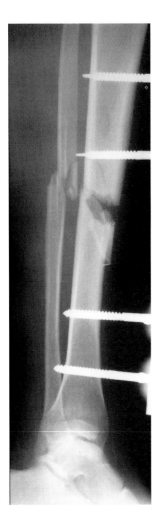

Figure 5.1 *Metaphyseal osteoporosis due to immobilization following a fracture of the mid-shaft of the tibia and fibula. Surgery and immobilization have resulted in a band of lucency at the distal metaphysis of the tibia, extending to the scar of the epiphyseal plate which is rendered more prominent.*

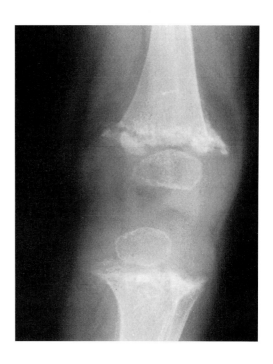

Figure 5.3 *Scurvy. A fracture has occurred through the metaphyseal lucency, leading to marginal spurs and subperiosteal new bone. Osteoporosis is prominent in the epiphyses at the knee.*

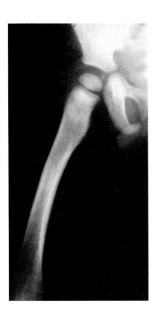

Figure 5.2 *Leukaemia. There is generalized loss of bone density which is accentuated at the metaphyses. A band of lucency extends across the entire metaphyseal region.*

at the metaphysis may fracture transversely, particularly at the distal femur, which bears the child's weight when it is crawling (Figure 5.3). This leaves lateral bone spurs known as Pelkan's spurs.

In rickets, there is loss of metaphyseal density due to the presence of excess non-mineralized osteoid, so that the metaphysis becomes irregular across its entire surface and the epiphyseal plate appears to widen. The metaphysis also becomes splayed because of local softening (Figure 5.4).

CONGENITAL SYPHILIS

Congenital syphilis in the neonate is rare in the UK but involves gross, irregular bone destruction often associated with cortical erosions at the metaphyses, which may fracture. The presence of a periostitis causes an appearance which may resemble leukaemia and neuroblastoma, but bone density in congenital syphilis is often increased (Figure 5.5). In the skull, there is no sutural splaying and the changes are more typically those of a focal osteomyelitis.

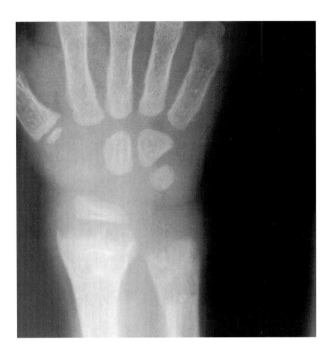

Figure 5.4 *In this patient with rickets, the metaphysis is splayed and irregular and the epiphyseal plate increased in width. Bone density is reduced generally.*

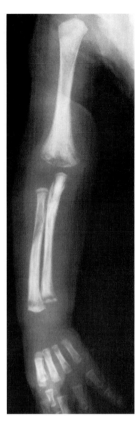

Figure 5.5 *In this patient with congenital syphilis, the shafts of the long bones show increased density and periostitis. The metaphyses are eroded and irregular bands of lucency extend across the entire width of the bone.*

RUBELLA

Rubella as a result of uterine infection in non-immune mothers, produces skeletal changes which are usually maximal around the knee. The metaphysis becomes slightly broadened and frayed, and characteristically shows alternating bands of lucency and density perpendicular to the growth plate—the 'celery stick' appearance (see Figure 2.40). Occasionally, more conventional transverse bands of lucency are found. These changes regress with growth.

FOCAL AREAS OF METAPHYSEAL DESTRUCTION

Destructive metaphyseal lesions do not always traverse the entire width of the bone; occasionally there may be focal destructive lesions, resembling 'bites' (Table 5.2).

Between 1 and 16 years of age, the metaphysis is the site of end-arteries and therefore the focus for septic emboli. In the chronic stage of infection, a well demarcated lytic defect extends to the epiphyseal plate over part of the metaphysis, which is seen as a solitary lesion in simple infections. In children with immune defects, such as the 'lazy leukocyte' syndrome or chronic granulomatous disease, the lesions may be multiple (Figure 5.6). Chronic granulomatous disease eventually results in reactive sclerosis and expansion of bone which extends into the diaphysis. The original metaphyseal focus of destruction may be obscured (Figure 5.7).

Table 5.2 Causes of metaphyseal bites.

Simple osteomyelitis
Tuberculous osteomyelitis
Chronic granulomatous disease
Eosinophilic granuloma and other forms of
    Langerhan's cell histiocytosis

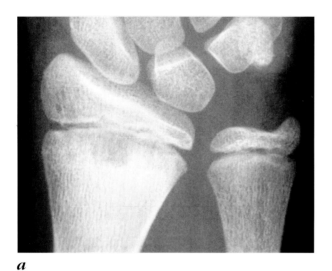

a

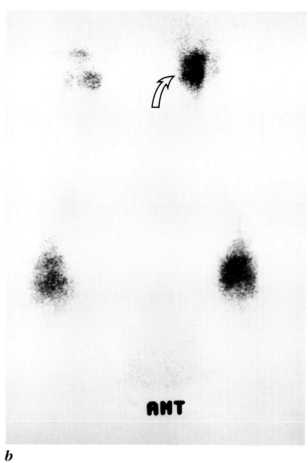

b

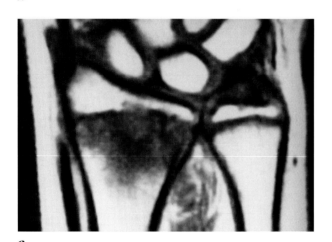

c

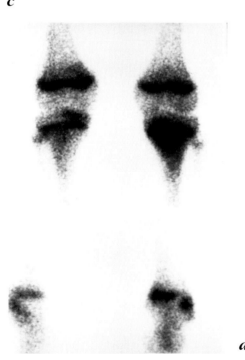

d

Figure 5.6 *Chronic granulomatous disease. (***a***) A discrete metaphyseal focus of destruction is demonstrated at the distal radial metaphysis surrounded by a zone of reactive sclerosis. (***b***) The delayed radionuclide bone scan shows marked increase in uptake at the distal radial metaphysis (arrow) as well as the elbow. (***c***) The T₁-weighted MR sequence shows replacement of bright marrow signal by a low signal zone corresponding to the area of sclerosis seen on the plain film, within which there is an intermediate soft tissue signal mass compatible with chronic inflammation. (***d***) The radioisotope bone scan shows substantial increase in uptake at the left proximal tibial metaphysis as well as the ankle joint. (***e***) Coronal T₁-weighted and (***f***) fat suppression images confirm the presence of chronic metaphyseal inflammatory change and also at the proximal tibial epiphysis. (***g***) Metaphyseal change is seen at the distal fibula. (By courtesy of Dr R Philips, The Whittington Hospital.)*

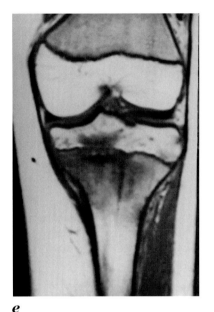

e

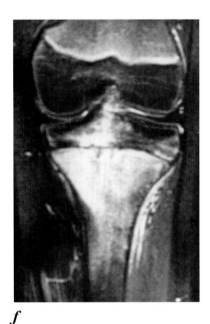

f

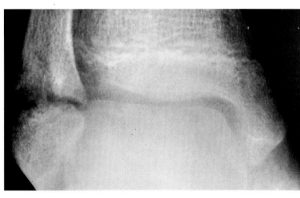

g

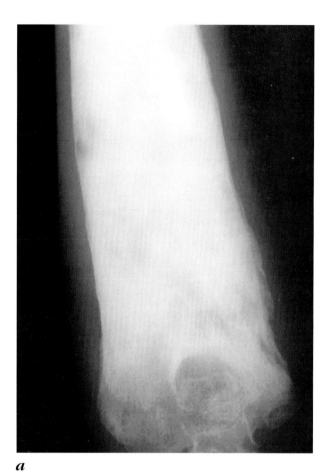

a

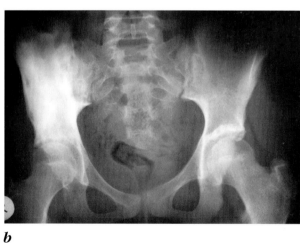

b

Figure 5.7 *In chronic granulomatous disease, the entire bone may become involved. (**a**) In this patient with longstanding disease, the appearances of bone expansion, sclerosis and periostitis in the distal humerus are those of a chronic infection. (**b**) In the pelvis there is sclerosis with expansion of the iliac blade resembling a malignant process. The joint space of the right hip is slightly narrowed.*

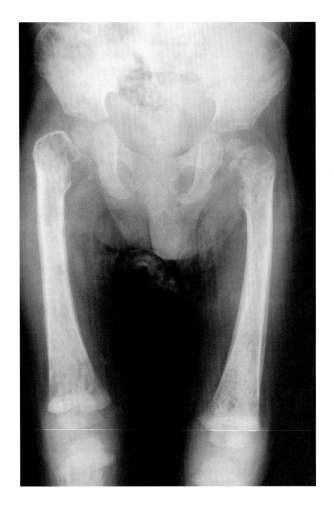

Figure 5.8 *Extensive metaphyseal destruction is demonstrated, resembling the change seen in leukaemia in this patient with Langerhan's cell histiocytosis. (By courtesy of Dr K Walmsley, University College London Hospitals.)*

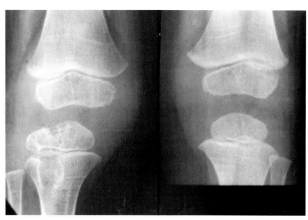

Figure 5.9 *A well demarcated destructive lesion is demonstrated at the proximal tibial metaphysis in this patient with tuberculous disease. There is bony overgrowth compared with the normal left side, and local soft tissue swelling. Growth arrest lines are seen.*

Table 5.3 Causes of metaphyseal density.

Normal in neonates
Growth arrest lines
Hypothyroidism in children
Heavy metal poisoning
Healing rickets
Healing leukaemia
Methotrexate osteopathy
Healing scurvy
Osteopetrosis
Chronic infection and chronic granulomatous disease

Multiple metaphyseal foci of destruction may be seen in eosinophilic granuloma and other forms of Langerhan's cell histiocytosis (Figure 5.8) and tuberculosis which are often associated with lytic defects elsewhere (Figure 5.9).

CONDITIONS CAUSING AN INCREASE IN DENSITY AT THE METAPHYSIS

The normal zone of provisional calcification at the metaphysis is seen as a dense line, less than 1 mm thick. Occasionally the metaphyseal density may be thicker, particularly in the neonate. The conditions causing an increase in density at the metaphysis are listed in Table 5.3.

LEAD POISONING

In the acute phase of lead poisoning in children, the only manifestation may be suture diastasis due to cerebral oedema, and there may be particulate densities in the gut representing ingested paint. However, chronic lead ingestion causes a dense band of metaphyseal density, which is seen at all metaphyses, including that of the proximal fibula, which is not

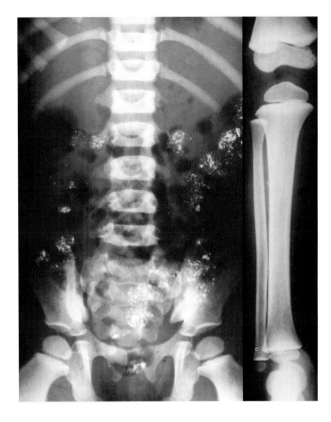

Figure 5.10 *Lead poisoning. Particulate densities are present in the abdomen of this child who was in the habit of eating the paint on his cot. Metaphyseal densities are demonstrated.*

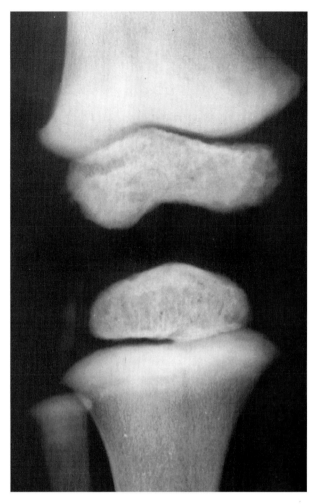

Figure 5.11 *A patient with osteopetrosis has metaphyseal density and broadening.*

usually dense under normal physiological conditions. Inhibition of osteoclastic activity by lead also causes undertubulation of metaphyses (Figure 5.10). Other heavy metals, such as phosphorus, bismuth and arsenic, have a similar effect. Vertebral bodies may be affected, giving a bone-within-a-bone appearance, corresponding to the episodes of heavy metal poisoning.

GROWTH ARREST LINES

These are seen during severe illness and immobilization, when longitudinal growth behind the epiphyseal plate ceases, but local calcium deposition continues, so that the zone of provisional calcification becomes particularly dense. When growth resumes, this dense line is left behind and lies proximally in the shaft. Often a number of these thin transverse bands are seen, indicating separate episodes of growth arrest (Figure 5.9).

OSTEOPETROSIS

Alternating bands of dense and normal bone are seen in the epiphysis, metaphysis and diaphysis. The bands of increased density vary in thickness, but are never as thin as growth arrest lines (Figure 5.11). Longitudinal striations at bone ends are the sites of local blood vessels (see Figure 2.41).

HEALING RICKETS

The poorly mineralized and irregular metaphysis gradually ossifies with treatment, producing an appearance of woven rather than well formed bone (Figure 5.12). The adjacent epiphyseal plate narrows to a more normal width, and the epiphysis and

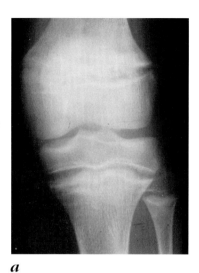

a

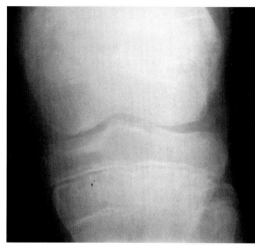

b

Figure 5.12 *(a) Healing rickets. Changes of rickets are shown with widened epiphyseal plates and irregular metaphyses, although healing is taking place. (b) Skeletal fusion at maturity in rickets. Skeletal fusion is not particularly delayed. The metaphysis fills with coarse and irregular woven bone, and the epiphyseal plate then fuses.*

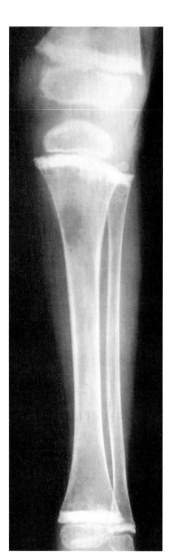

Figure 5.13 *Healing in leukaemia. Marked transverse sclerosis is seen at all the metaphyses.*

subperiosteal region become more clearly defined. When epiphyseal fusion occurs in rachitic patients, the previously widened epiphyseal plate is obliterated by a band of coarsely trabeculated woven bone.

HEALING LEUKAEMIA

In healing leukaemia there is an increase in bone density, and healing may occur in the destructive metaphyseal lesions, occasionally resulting in local sclerosis (Figure 5.13). Ten per cent of leukaemic patients are osteosclerotic in the acute phase.

CONDITIONS CAUSING METAPHYSEAL BROADENING (Table 5.4)

THALASSAEMIA

Thalassaemia is associated with the most severe form of anaemia and therefore presents with the most marked marrow hypertrophy and bone expansion (see Figure 1.87). Bone density is reduced and the cortex thinned, particularly at the metaphyses, where it may be breached by marrow (Figure 5.14), but infarcts do not occur. Elsewhere, changes of marrow hypertrophy are gross, for example, in the skull (see Figure 1.84), spine and hands (see Figure 1.85). The liver and spleen are enlarged and extramedullary haemopoiesis may be seen (Figures 1.83 and 5.15).

Table 5.4 Conditions causing metaphyseal broadening.

Haemolytic anaemias:	Thalassaemia Sickle-cell disease	Associated with marrow hyperplasia Associated with infarcts	Erlenmeyer flask appearance
Storage disease:	Gaucher's disease		

Rickets
Hypophosphatasia—generally more severe in
   appearance than rickets
Metaphyseal dysostosis—generally less   Associated with metaphyseal irregularity
   severe in appearance than rickets

Enchondromatosis
Diaphyseal aclasia   Associated with multiple tumours of cartilaginous origin

Osteopetrosis
Lead poisoning   Associated with increased metaphyseal density

Perthes' disease   At the hip only

SICKLE-CELL DISEASE

In sickle-cell disease, infarcts causing sclerosis, cortical splitting (see Figure 1.82) and avascular necrosis at joints (see Figure 1.92) complicate the marrow hypertrophy which is less marked than in thalassaemia. The spleen is generally small.

GAUCHER'S DISEASE

In Gaucher's disease, marrow infiltration expands the bone and thins the cortex. There are infarcts, avascular necrosis and splenomegaly. Focal areas of osteolysis are seen due to local aggregations of Gaucher cells (Figure 5.16).

ENCHONDROMATOSIS

In enchondromatosis, multiple radiolucent cartilaginous tumours are present in the diaphyses and metaphyses of tubular bones. The lesions show characteristic punctate calcification, have thin, well defined margins, scallop the cortices from within, and expand the bone. Smaller bones, such as those in the hand, have the greatest relative enlargement and deformity. The enchondromatous lesions may abut onto the growth plate but do not cross it until after epiphyseal fusion. Occasionally, long strands of lucent cartilage stream backwards from the growth plate in parallel strands (see Figure 1.59). Abnormalities of growth also occur in enchondromatosis at the wrist, with ulnar shortening (see Figure 1.59), and similar dysplastic changes are seen at the distal radius and ulna in diaphyseal aclasia.

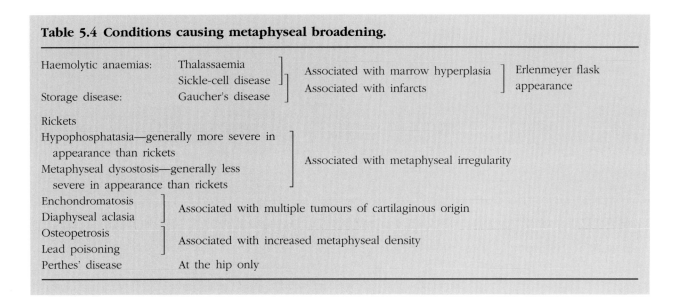

Figure 5.14 *Thalassaemia. A close-up view of the metaphysis shows a soft tissue mass of marrow breaking through the cortex (arrows).*

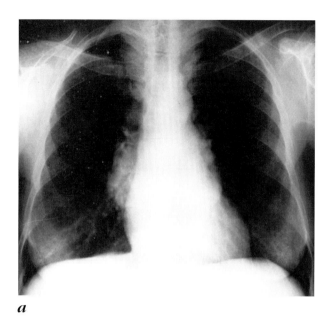

a

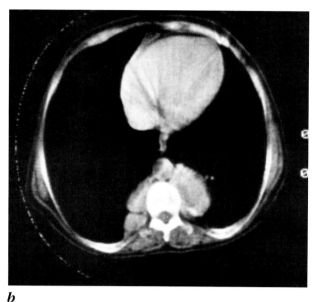

b

Figure 5.15 *Thalassaemia.* (**a**) *The bones are expanded, the cortices thinned, and trabeculation is sparse. These features are particularly prominent in the clavicles; Hilar masses are also seen.* (**b**) *The CT scan confirms the presence of extramedullary haemopoiesis.*

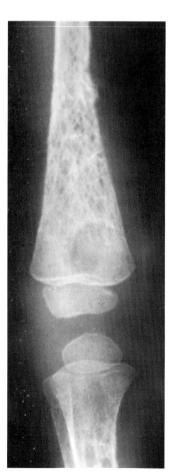

Figure 5.16 *In this patient with Gaucher's disease, there is widespread marrow infiltration due to deposition of Gaucher cells. The cortex is broken through in places. An Erlenmeyer flask appearance of the distal femur is present.*

DIAPHYSEAL ACLASIA (MULTIPLE EXOSTOSES)

In this condition, the metaphyses of the long bones, particularly at the shoulders, hips, knees and ankles, become progressively irregularly expanded and club-like. Exostoses arise on the expanded metaphyseal regions, grow in size (Figure 5.17), and finally point away from the adjacent joint. The exostosis is surrounded by a lucent cartilaginous cap which ossifies progressively during growth, becoming completely ossified at the time of skeletal maturity (Figure 5.18), (see Chapter 7, page 345). The marrow of the exostosis is contiguous with that of the underlying bone. Similarly, the cortex of the shaft merges with that of the exostosis.

In bizarre parosteal osseous proliferation (BPOP) (see Chapter 3, page 130), however, there is a band of cortex separating the exostosis from the underlying bone (Figure 5.19).

OSTEOPETROSIS

Osteopetrosis is the result of failed resorption of bone by vascular mesenchyme during growth, which results in the persistence of dense fetal bone and abnormal modelling, particularly at the metaphyses, which show undertubulation (Figure 5.20).

LEAD POISONING

In lead poisoning, inhibition of osteoclastic activity also results in broadening of metaphyses in association with local dense lead lines (Figure 5.10).

RICKETS

Rickets is the most common form of metaphyseal broadening with irregularity (Figure 5.4), which results from excess, localized, soft, non-mineralized osteoid.

HYPOPHOSPHATASIA

This resembles rickets but radiologically the disease presents with changes of varying severity. Neonates are most severely affected with marked rickets-like changes at metaphyses and minimal general

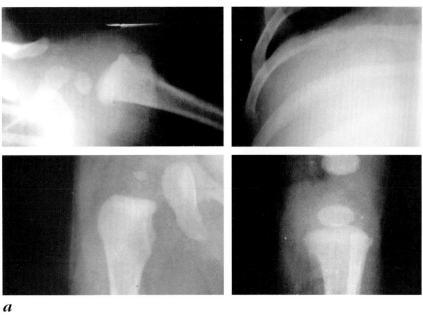

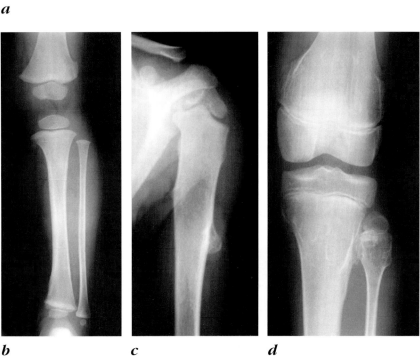

a

b   *c*   *d*

Figure 5.17 *Growing lesions in multiple exostoses (diaphyseal aclasia). (***a***) An initial radiograph taken at 3 months of age shows small metaphyseal spurs. (***b***) At 13 months of age, metaphyseal broadening and spurring is more evident. (***c***) At 40 months, the disease is now gross. (***d***) In the same patient at 10 years of age, modelling defects are now prominent.*

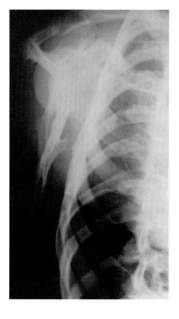

Figure 5.18 *Multiple exostoses. Exostoses often arise on the scapula, and patients complain of pain when using the arm.*

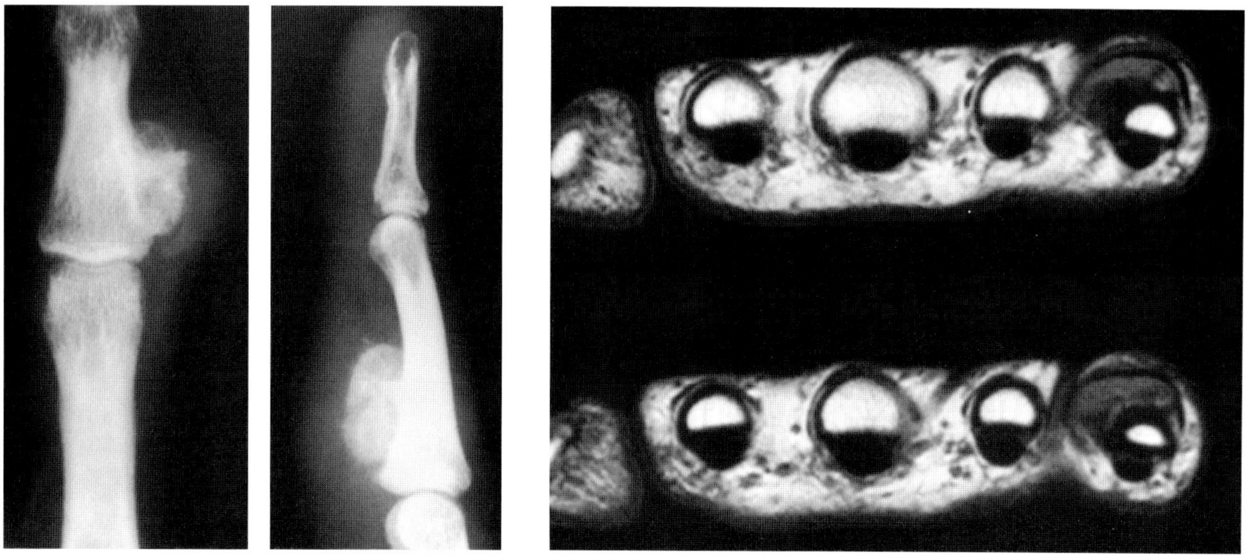

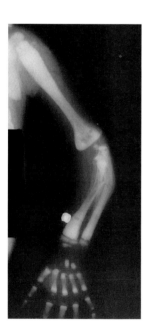

Figure 5.19 *Bizarre parosteal osteochondromatous proliferation (BPOP). (**a**) The plain film demonstrates an osseous mass sitting upon the middle phalanx of a finger. (**b**) The axial T₁-weighted MR image shows separation of the lesion from the underlying marrow.*

Figure 5.20
Osteopetrosis. Metaphyseal broadening is associated with increased density; alternating bands of dense and normal bone can be seen, producing a bone-within-a-bone appearance. Pathological fractures have occurred in the mid-shafts of the radius and ulna, and at the distal humerus.

ossification. The skull vault particularly shows non-mineralization. In infant and adolescent patients, severe rickets-like changes are seen, particularly affecting metaphyses (Figure 5.21). In the adult, an Erlenmeyer flask appearance is seen. All groups show pathological fractures and demineralization.

METAPHYSEAL DYSOSTOSIS

Metaphyseal dysostosis is rare and only the Schmid form is seen relatively often. The metaphyses are splayed, irregular and dense. The epiphyses are normal, which is not true of rickets and hypophosphatasia. The long bones are often shortened (Figure 5.22).

PERTHES' DISEASE

Perthes' disease is the eponymous term for avascular necrosis of the femoral head during childhood. Flattening and fragmentation of the epiphysis is associated with broadening and shortening of the femoral neck. The metaphysis shows cystic changes adjacent to the epiphyseal plate (Figure 5.23; see also Chapter 4, page 235).

METAPHYSEAL TRAUMA

Although trauma is generally not discussed in this book, two conditions involving metaphyseal trauma are of interest. In non-accidental injury, the only indication of an acute lesion may be a chip fracture,

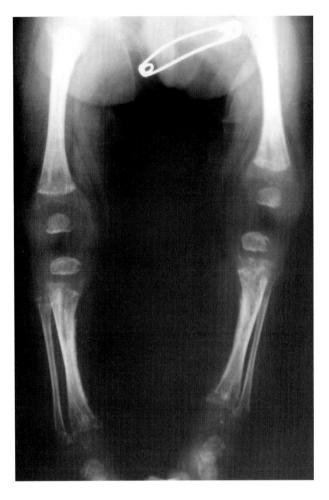

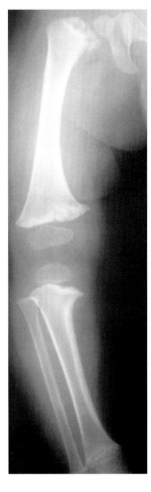

Figure 5.22 *In this patient with metaphyseal dysostosis, type Schmid, there is irregularity and broadening of the metaphyses but the epiphyseal plates are not generally widened. The bones are much more dense and sharply defined than in rickets.*

Figure 5.21 *Hypophosphatasia. The changes are like rickets but are more gross. There is quite marked irregularity of the metaphyses but the changes extend into the shafts. The epiphyses are also irregular.*

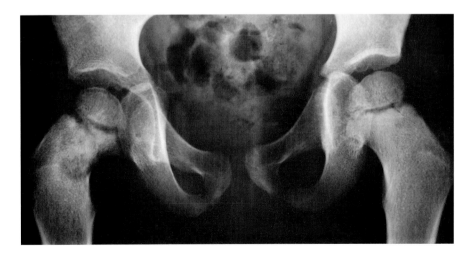

Figure 5.23 *Perthes' disease. There is irregularity of the right femoral neck, which is broadened with loss of cortical definition medially, extending to the region of the epiphyseal plate. The epiphysis shows a necrotic cortex and a subjacent crescentic lucency. The left femoral head also shows early signs of articular collapse.*

or flake of bone, at the metaphysis, which arises because of the firm local attachment of the periosteum. The loosely applied diaphyseal periosteum is easily stripped with violent twisting of the limb

(Figures 5.24 and 5.25), and this later results in gross periostitis. However, at the metaphysis, the underlying cortical bone is locally elevated. There may also be epiphyseal malalignment.

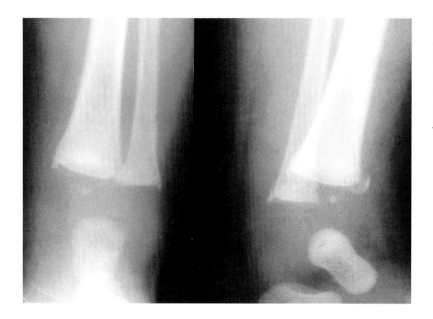

Figure 5.24 *Non-accidental injury. Metaphyseal chip fractures are often the only indication of acute trauma. The flakes of bone are avulsed because of the firm local attachment of the underlying periosteum.*

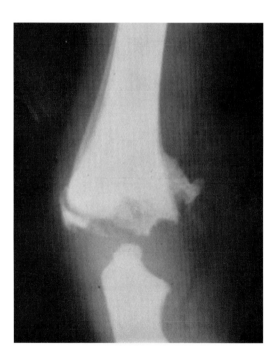

Figure 5.25 *Non-accidental injury. In this battered baby, further stripping of the periosteum results in subperiosteal new bone formation at the metaphysis.*

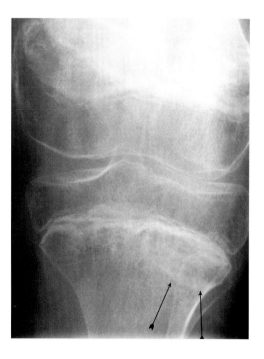

Figure 5.26 *Idiopathic juvenile osteoporosis. There is widespread loss of bone density, and areas of increased density at the metaphyses. These are the result of metaphyseal impaction fractures.*

Idiopathic juvenile osteoporosis (IJO) (see Chapter 1, page 25) is associated with metaphyseal fractures, which distinguishes this lesion from osteogenesis imperfecta at adolescence, in which fractures tend to be diaphyseal. The shaft impacts into the metaphysis, where the cortex is deficient and almost absent (Figure 5.26).

Tumours arising in the metaphyses are listed in Table 5.5.

Table 5.5 Solitary tumours arising in the metaphysis.

Simple bone cyst Aneurysmal bone cyst Enchondroma Fibrous dysplasia	Benign
Chondroblastoma Giant-cell tumour	Only occasionally metaphyseal
Osteosarcoma Metastasis	Malignant

Chapter 6 Periosteal reactions

Elevation of the periosteum is followed by the laying down of new bone by osteoprogenitor cells. The periosteum may be elevated by malignant or benign processes but, occasionally, the cause of periosteal elevation and new bone formation is unknown. Some authors (Edeiken et al, 1966) have attempted to demonstrate that the radiological appearance of the new bone is often an indicator of the underlying disease process.

The two main types of periosteal new bone either lie parallel to the cortex or at right angles to it (Figures 6.1 and 6.2). Edeiken et al (1966) further divide those lying parallel to the cortex into solid or lamellar types. A solid periostitis is totally applied to the underlying cortex with no intervening lucent zone (Figure 6.3). When the thickness of the new bone exceeds 1 mm, which it does in most solid periosteal reactions, the underlying lesion is benign. Lamellar periosteal reactions may be benign or malignant in origin.

According to Edeiken et al, a solid periostitis occurs in the following conditions:

- Eosinophilic granuloma
- Fractures
- Osteomyelitis
- Hypertrophic osteoarthropathy
- Osteoid osteoma
- Vascular and storage diseases

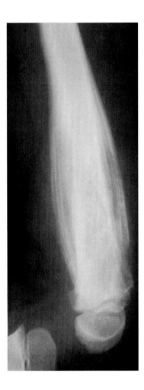

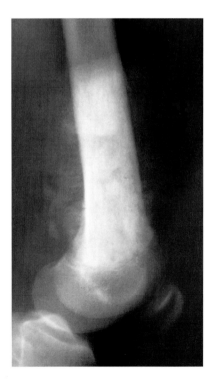

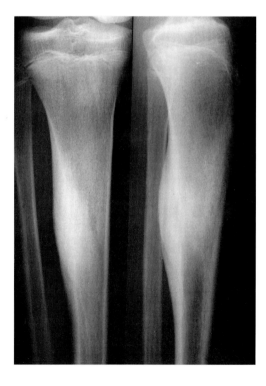

Figure 6.1 *Ewing's sarcoma. A fine lamellar periosteal reaction lies parallel to the cortex.*

Figure 6.2 *Osteogenic sarcoma. In this patient the periostitis is perpendicular to the shaft.*

Figure 6.3 *Solid periostosis—osteoid osteoma. The osteoid osteoma is not visible and is obscured by a solid layer of locally applied periosteal new bone.*

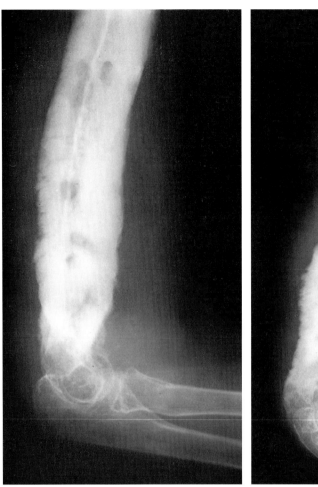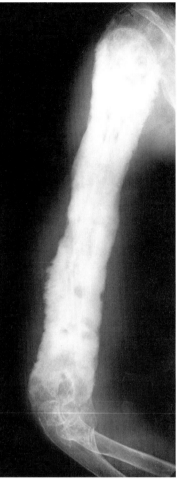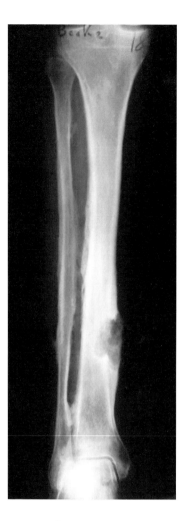

Figure 6.4 *Osteomyelitis. The nature of the underlying process is evident from the extensive cortical sequestrum buried deep in the bone. The periostitis itself is undulant and irregular, but solid.*

Figure 6.5 *Osteomyelitis. A shaggy lamellar periostitis is seen on the tibia and fibula, and apparent fusion is progressing between the two bones. In places the periostitis is solid.*

The contour of both solid and lamellar periostitis may be smooth, undulant or very irregular (Figures 6.4 and 6.5). Lamellar lesions may have as many as five or six layers of new bone external to the cortex. Lamellations are thought to be due to intermittent changes in growth rates in the underlying lesion. If the lesion temporarily stops growing, the elevated periosteum has time to form new bone beneath itself which is initially woven, but then becomes more mature (Figure 6.6).

The periosteum is loosely applied to the diaphysis in children and so periostitis is often much more florid. This is particularly marked in infections resulting in a florid involucrum (Figure 6.7).

Perpendicular spiculation occurs when new bone is laid down upon stretched subperiosteal blood vessels and upon the Sharpey's fibres, which tether periosteum to bone (Figures 6.8 and 6.9).

Most periosteal reactions are the result of subperiosteal pathology, but soft tissue lesions can also cause new bone to be laid down by the underlying periosteum (Figure 6.10). With tumours, periosteal new bone may be present in conjunction with new bone formed within the tumour itself (Figure 6.2), while in infections, sequestra may be associated with the periostitis (Figure 6.4 and Table 6.1).

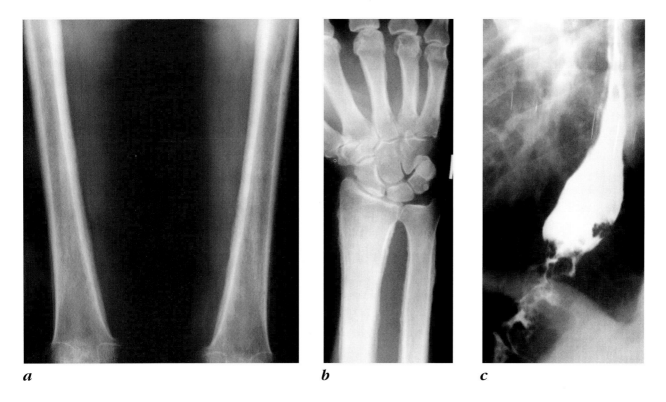

a   *b*   *c*

Figure 6.6 *Hypertrophic osteoarthropathy. (**a**) In this patient, the new bone has united in places with the underlying cortex. (**b**, **c**) In this patient, a more usual form of lamellar periostitis is due to an oesophageal carcinoma.*

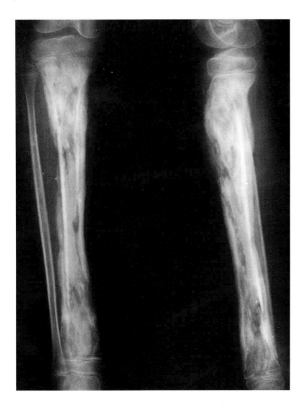

Figure 6.7 *Osteomyelitis. There is a florid involucrum. The original cortex has died and now presents as a linear density lying within the involucrum. This is another example of cortical splitting.*

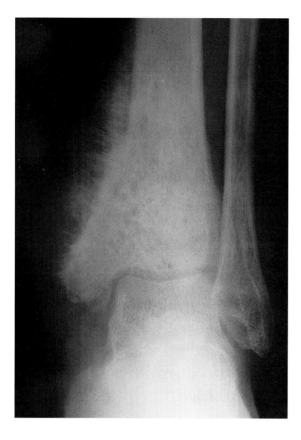

Figure 6.8 *Mycetoma. Perpendicular spiculation or a hair-on-end appearance in a fungal infection which is a variety of Madura foot. The patchy defects in the region of the medial malleolus are related to osteomyelitis.*

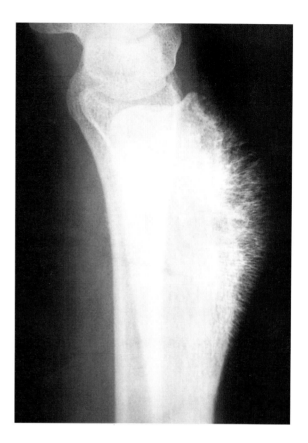

Figure 6.9 *Sunray spiculation in an angioma associated with expansion of bone. In this case the lesion is a solitary one, but such lesions may also be multiple.*

Table 6.1 Causes of local periostitis.

Arthritides	Adjacent to affected synovium. Less common in rheumatoid arthritis and juvenile chronic arthritis. More common in psoriasis and Reiter's syndrome Osteoarthritis at the hip
Fractures	Following major injury, or stress fractures
Osteomyelitis	Usually localized unless associated with immune defects Florid in children
Following haemorrhage	
Vascular stasis	Usually in the lower limb associated with varicose veins, occasionally with lymphatic obstruction, with or without local ulceration

Tumours	1 Benign, such as osteoid osteoma
	2 Malignant:
	  Osteosarcoma ⎡ central
	                    ⎢ periosteal
	                    ⎣ parosteal
	  Ewing's sarcoma
	  Chondrosarcoma
	  Fibrosarcoma

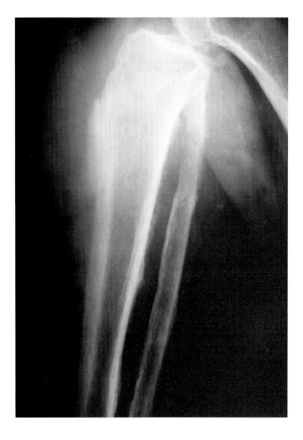

Figure 6.10 *In this patient with liposarcoma, periostitis is related to an overlying tumour. The soft tissue swelling is visible although its nature is not evident. Translucency is not a feature of liposarcoma. The tumour has caused a florid hair-on-end periostitis at the proximal tibia and fibula.*

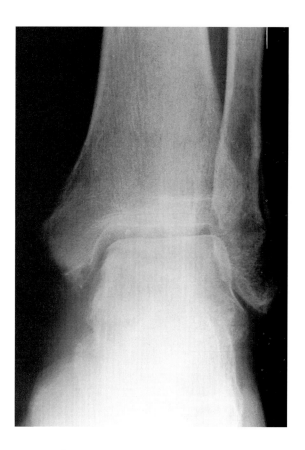

Figure 6.11 *Psoriasis. Irregularity with fluffy new bone formation is present, particularly on the medial malleolus.*

CAUSES OF LOCAL PERIOSTITIS

ARTHRITIDES

Periosteal new bone is unusual in rheumatoid arthritis, but can occur along the shafts of the tubular bones of the hands and feet. Erosions may be visible locally, but often the change is associated with a synovitis in the local tendon sheath causing soft tissue swelling and osteoporosis. Fine, lamellar new bone is laid down at the metaphysis or diaphysis, as shown in Figure 4.16. A similar situation occurs in Still's disease (juvenile chronic arthritis). Seronegative arthritides in adults are associated with a much more florid and generalized form of periosteal reaction. Patients with

Reiter's syndrome and psoriasis have erosions with a distribution different to those seen in rheumatoid arthritis (see Chapter 4, pages 218–220), and bone density is usually preserved. Erosions are frequently associated with a florid, often shaggy, perpendicular periostitis in the same area, for example around the calcaneus (Figure 4.37) and malleoli (Figure 6.11), and along phalangeal shafts, resulting in an increase in bony density (Figure 6.12).

Degenerative disease is often associated with florid new bone formation at disc and joint margins, but a true periostitis is seen at the medial aspect of the femoral neck in osteoarthritis, probably due to a buttressing phenomenon following altered local stresses (Figure 4.40).

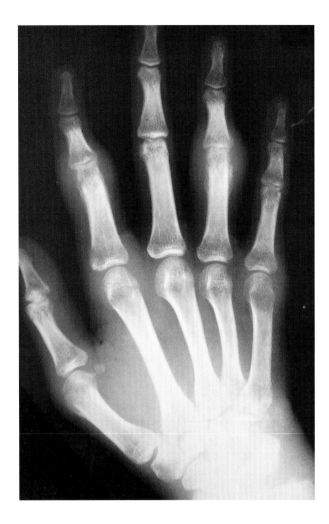

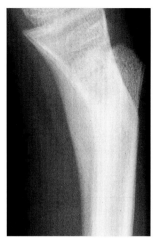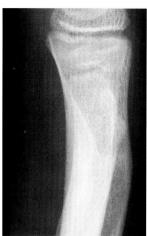

Figure 6.13 *New bone formation following a fracture. A distal radial fracture has resulted in the laying down of new bone on the concavity of the fracture (left) resulting in eventual remodelling, even in the absence of initial reduction of the fracture (right).*

Figure 6.12 *Reiter's syndrome—sausage digits. Soft tissue swelling is present over the proximal phalanges of the index and ring fingers. This is associated with an increase in density, partly due to an overlying shaggy periostitis and partly to soft tissue thickening.*

FRACTURES

Bleeding at a fracture elevates the periosteum, and within 7 to 14 days amorphous new bone, known as callus, begins to form. Generally, the amount of callus is greater at fractures immobilized in plaster than at those fixed by nail or plate, where less local movement can occur. With a greenstick fracture, new bone formation at the concave surface results in a lamellar buttress, while bone is resorbed on the opposite convexity, so that the periostitis is part of a remodelling phenomenon (Figure 6.13).

STRESS FRACTURES

Stress fractures are the result of normal activity on abnormal bone, or regular, repeated subliminal trauma to normal bone. Particular sports or occupations produce stress lesions at characteristic sites, as shown in Table 1.9. For example, common sites for stress fractures in an athlete are the proximal tibia and fibula (Figure 6.14) and the second or third metatarsal neck (Figure 6.15). These painful lesions are often bilateral and symmetrical and initially not visible on a radiograph, but will show up on a radioisotope bone scan (Figure 6.16).

Characteristically, a stress fracture appears as a poorly defined transverse band of lucency surrounded by sclerosis extending through the medulla to a cortical surface, which shows a localized area of subperiosteal new bone formation (Figures 1.62 and 6.17), which is initially hazy and then becomes well defined. A smooth local mass of bone is produced, which is eventually resorbed into the cortex (Figure 6.18).

A similar appearance may be seen around an osteoid osteoma (Figure 6.3), in chronic osteomyelitis (Figure 6.19), in a Looser's zone in osteomalacia (Figure 6.20), in an insufficiency fracture in Paget's disease (Figure 2.13) and, occasionally, with other

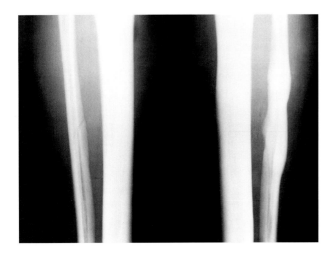

Figure 6.14 *Stress fractures may be seen on both left and right tibia and fibula of a professional footballer. On the left a more longstanding lesion is associated with a solid periostitis of the mid-shaft of the fibula, while on the right, the more recent stress fracture is seen.*

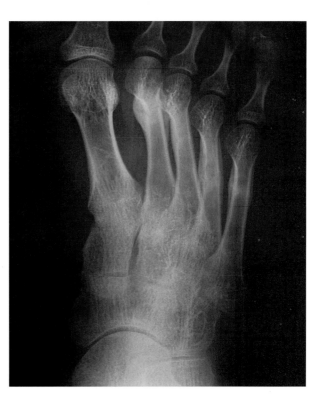

Figure 6.15 *Stress fractures. Typical healing fractures of the second, third, fourth and fifth metatarsal necks are visible. Fracture lines can still be seen and are transverse. Both a lamellar and a solid periostitis are present.*

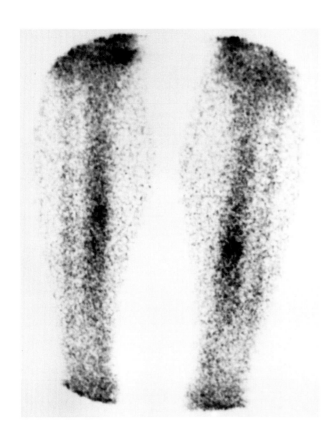

Figure 6.16 *Stress fractures. Radioisotope bone scan showing stress fractures of the mid-shafts of the tibiae in an athlete.*

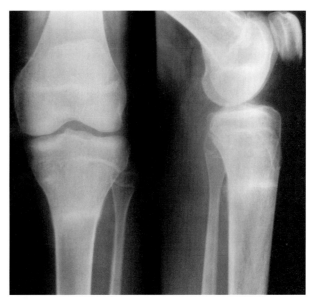

Figure 6.17 *Stress fracture. A typical transverse density is seen in the proximal tibia associated with a localized lamellar periostitis.*

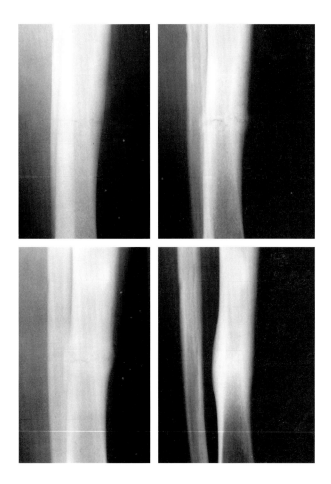

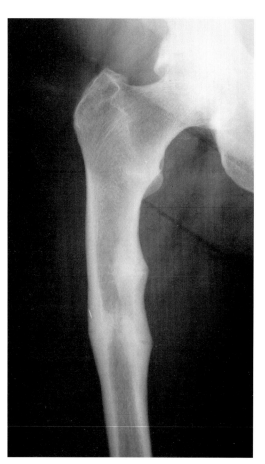

Figure 6.18 *Progression of a stress fracture. The initial lesion across the mid-shaft of the tibia is barely visible. Progressive films show the formation of callus and finally the fracture line becomes poorly defined with a surrounding solid localized periostitis.*

Figure 6.20 *In this patient with osteomalacia there are Looser's zones which are a characteristic feature of the disease. Transverse bands of lucency are associated with local areas of solid periostitis in the healing phase.*

Figure 6.19 *Osteomyelitis. There is thickening of the cortex, both endosteally and superficially, with obliteration of the medullary cavity. The external periosteal reaction is solid.*

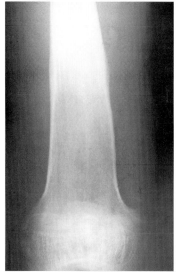
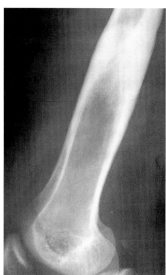

bone-forming tumours including osteosarcoma. In these lesions a small, usually smooth, cortical exostosis formed by a localized focus of subperiosteal new bone is associated with a central zone of endosteal sclerosis or lysis, which may be observed radiologically but is often better defined with conventional or computed tomography.

SUBPERIOSTEAL HAEMATOMA

A subperiosteal haematoma is the result of trauma, often without a frank fracture, although a fracture line may be visible eventually. In children, the loose

application of periosteum to bone can result in avulsion, for example by a twisting motion. The elevated periosteum forms a localized bony protrusion which eventually amalgamates with the underlying cortex (Figure 6.21).

OSTEOMYELITIS

The basic features of osteomyelitis have been described previously (page 151). Pus breaches the cortex through cloacae and elevates the periosteum (Figure 6.22). This occurs to a greater extent in children than in adults, when the entire periosteum

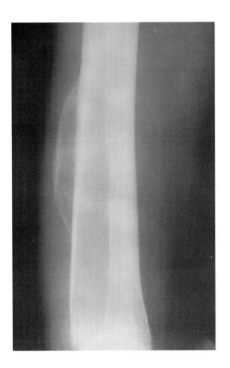

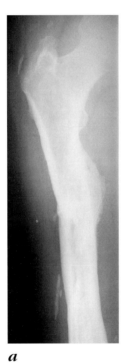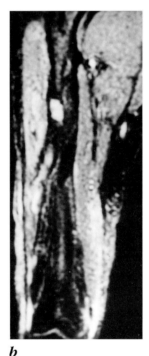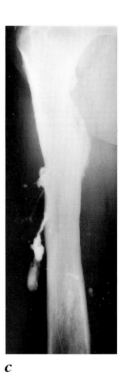

a   *b*   *c*

Figure 6.21 *Subperiosteal haematoma. A smooth and well defined exostosis is present, which is well corticated on its external surface and closely applied to the underlying bone.*

Figure 6.22 *Chronic osteomyelitis. (**a**) The preliminary radiograph shows a deformed right femur. There is cortical thickening with evidence of intramedullary cavitation and angulation. Linear calcified densities in the soft tissues may represent extruded sequestra. (**b**) Coronal fat suppression MR images show muscle wasting; the deformity of the bone is again demonstrated. There is extensive increase in signal within the medulla, indicating a fluid collection. A band of high signal can be seen extending from the medulla superiorly, through the cortex laterally and into the adjacent soft tissues. There is an effusion in the knee joint and oedema of the subcutaneous soft tissues. (**c**) The sinogram shows contrast medium in the same distribution as the fluid in (**b**) above.*

of a long bone may be stripped off. In infants a thick, wavy involucrum forms, which often sheaths the entire shaft of a long bone, but is clearly separated from it, as shown in Figure 6.7. The underlying sequestra and necrotic tissue become absorbed beneath the involucrum and, with growth, a normal shape of bone results. In adolescents and adults, the changes at the periosteum are more localized and bony expansion less marked (Figure 6.19).

In adults the tubular bones are not usually the site of blood-borne infection, which is generally confined to the spine and pelvis. Infection of the small bones of the hands and feet is usually due to direct inoculation.

There is no specific type of periostitis in osteomyelitis. A solid, perhaps wavy periostitis may be formed which is typically benign (Figure 6.23). Fine lamellar periostitis, of one or more layers, may also be seen (Figure 6.24) and the lesion may

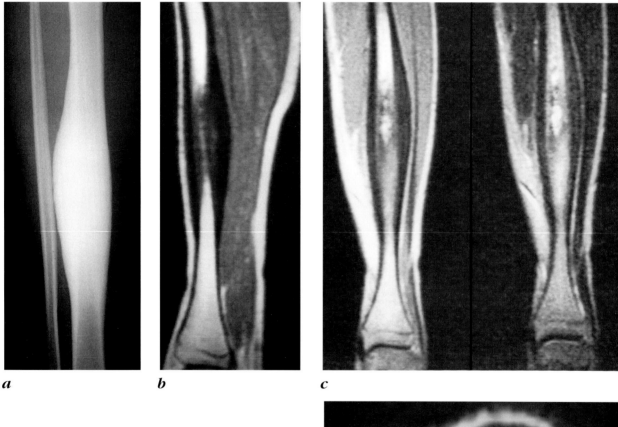

a   *b*   *c*

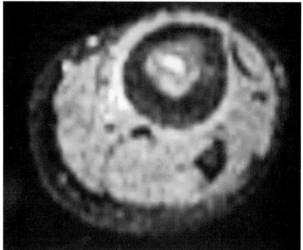

d

Figure 6.23 *Osteomyelitis—solitary periosteal reaction. (**a**) So dense is the periosteal reaction that any change in the underlying bone is obliterated. (**b**) The sagittal T$_1$-weighted MR image demonstrates an extensive periosteal reaction which is solid and incorporates into the underlying cortex. A marginal Codman's triangle is seen. (**c**) On the coronal T$_1$- (left) and T$_2$-weighted (right) MR sequences a central cavity is seen within the bone, as well as the solid periosteal reaction. (**d**) On the axial fat suppression MR image solid cortical thickening is demonstrated, together with the central cavity in the bone and also oedema around the tibia.*

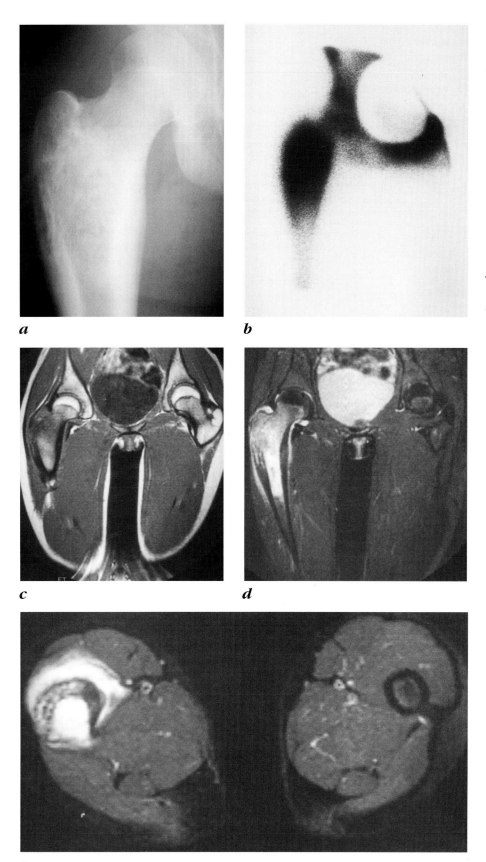

Figure 6.24 *Osteomyelitis of the femur. (**a**) The plain film shows expansion, medullary lysis and cortical thickening. (**b**) The radioisotope bone scan confirms the extent of the disease. (**c**) On the coronal T$_1$-weighted MR image the area of decreased signal in bone corresponds to the infected area. There is cortical breakthrough laterally and a Codman's triangle is formed inferiorly; a lamellar periostitis is present. (**d**, **e**) Coronal and axial fat suppression MR sequences show the inflammatory change and a lamellar periostitis.*

a

b

c

d

e

resemble Ewing's sarcoma (see page 320) (Figure 6.25). In addition, the periostitis may be diaphyseal and widespread along the shaft.

With unusual infections, more bizarre patterns of periosteal new bone are seen. Brucellosis and mycetomal lesions are associated with sclerosis and coarse, vertical spiculation of the sunray type (Figures 6.8 and 6.26).

Soft tissue infections such as decubitus ulcers can also cause change in the underlying bone. The bone beneath varicose ulcers at the ankle may show a local lamellar or florid sunray periostitis although a periostitis occurs in varicose disease in the absence of ulceration.

A small, dome-like exostosis occurs beneath tropical ulcers which is rarely seen in temperate climes

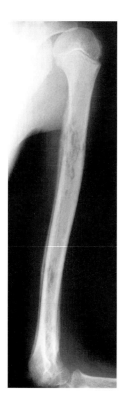

Figure 6.25 *In this patient with osteomyelitis there is patchy destruction of bone associated with sequestrum formation. The cortex of the bone is breached, giving a cloaca. The periostitis in this patient is delicate and lamellar.*

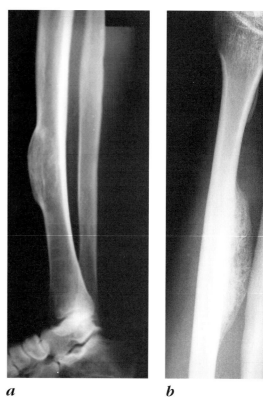

a   *b*

Figure 6.27 *(a) A small dome-like exostosis is produced beneath this tropical ulcer. (b) A similar lesion beneath a chronically infected ulcer.*

Figure 6.26 *Madura foot. The appearance shown here has been likened to a 'melting snowman's foot'. There is a mixture of bone resorption and destruction, sclerosis and cystic change, with overlying soft tissue swelling. The appearances are those of secondary bacterial infection superimposed upon a pre-existing mycetomal or fungal infection of bone, representing the end-stage lesion.*

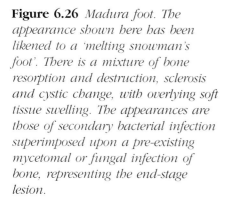

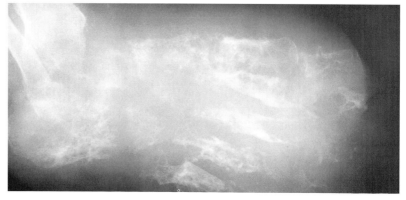

(Figure 6.27a). A similar appearance is shown beneath a chronic ulcer in an intravenous drug abuser (Figure 6.27b).

VASCULAR STASIS

Longstanding varicose veins in the lower limbs are associated with periosteal new bone formation along the diaphysis and metaphysis of the tibia and fibula, and in the small bones of the foot. The periostitis may be lamellar but is usually solid and applied to the cortex, with an outer irregular or undulant margin (Figure 6.28). Its presence is not dependent upon a varicose ulcer. Varicosities may be visible in subcutaneous fat and the soft tissues are generally thickened and oedematous. Phleboliths are often present. Similar changes occur with lymphatic obstruction and arterial insufficiency.

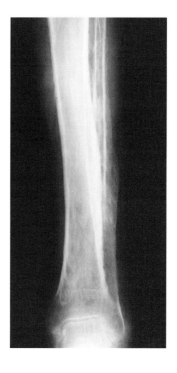

Figure 6.28
Vascular stasis. Patients with chronic varicose disease develop a very profuse, shaggy periostitis. In this patient, it has incorporated into the underlying bones.

PERIOSTEAL REACTIONS ASSOCIATED WITH TUMOURS

The important criteria for distinguishing between benign and malignant lesions have already been listed (see Chapter 3, page 107). A solid periosteal reaction is almost always indicative of a benign lesion, while a lamellar periostitis may be due to an underlying benign or malignant lesion. Malignancy cannot be diagnosed on the basis of the periosteal pattern alone. All other features must be taken into account.

Aggressive tumours break through the cortex and elevate the periosteum beneath which new bone is laid down. Cyclical tumour activity results in a lamellar periostitis which may be fine or coarse, according to the tumour type. If further tumour growth occurs, it may exceed the ability of the periosteum to lay down new bone. The tumour bursts through the periosteum centrally, leaving an elevated triangle of new bone at the tumour margin—Codman's triangle (Figure 6.29). This is radiologically similar to the process of buttressing which occurs at the margin of the periosteal elevation with benign tumours, where new bone fills the angle between cortex and elevated periosteum. This phenomenon is seen with giant-cell tumours and aneurysmal bone cysts (Figure 6.30). Codman's triangles also occur after subperiosteal infection or haemorrhage.

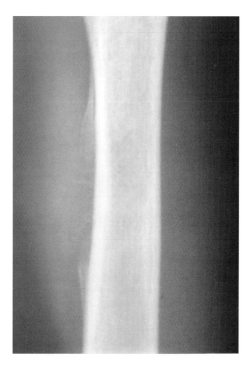

Figure 6.29 *Ewing's sarcoma with a Codman's triangle. There is a very faint and barely perceptible destructive process affecting the cortex and medulla, but sunray spiculation is associated with a soft tissue mass and a peripheral Codman's triangle. The delicate nature of the new bone is typical of Ewing's sarcoma.*

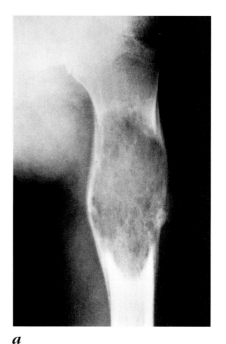
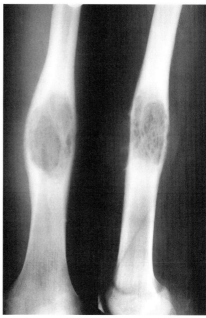

a   *b*

Figure 6.30 *(a) Aneurysmal bone cyst. At the margin of the cyst and the shaft a buttressing or lamellar periostitis is visible. This phenomenon does not occur with simple bone cysts. (b) Telangiectatic osteosarcoma. This highly vascular and aggressive lesion bears a strong resemblance to the benign lesion shown in (a). A lamellar periostitis and well defined Codman's triangle are seen.*

EWING'S SARCOMA AND OSTEOGENIC SARCOMA

Ewing's sarcoma classically infiltrates along the shaft, breaking through the cortex over a considerable distance (see Chapter 3, page 187). The resulting periostitis is usually lamellar, with fine parallel layers of new bone, indicating a cyclic process. The lamellae are delicate and thinner than the tumour-filled spaces between them (Figure 6.31).

In Ewing's sarcoma a perpendicular periostitis is occasionally produced, due to new bone laid down upon stretched subperiosteal Sharpey's fibres and blood vessels. Fine, short, delicate spicules of new bone are laid down perpendicular to the eroded cortex, often over a considerable length of shaft. Again, the new bone spicules formed are often thinner than the spaces between them, producing a hair-on-end appearance (Figures 3.131 and 6.32).

Osteogenic sarcoma does not infiltrate along the shaft but tends to radiate from a central focus through cortex and into soft tissues, producing a large soft tissue mass with irregular, coarse tumour new bone formation. The periosteal lamellations are also coarse, thick and often irregular, with little clear space between them. If a hair-on-end appearance is present, it is coarse and of the sunray type, radiating from a central focus (Figures 3.121c and 6.33).

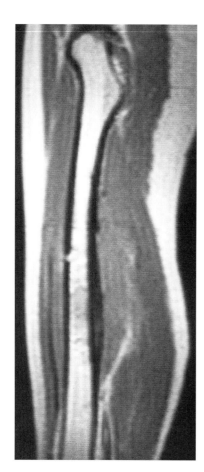

Figure 6.31 *Ewing's sarcoma. At MR imaging the lamellar periostitis is demonstrated on the sagittal T$_1$-weighted sequence. The marrow shows signal change at the level of the periosteal reaction.*

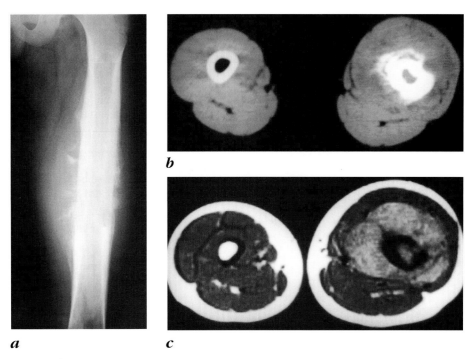

a   *c*

Figure 6.32 *Ewing's sarcoma. (**a**) Cortical thinning is associated with a lamellar periostitis which has broken through centrally. At the margins a Codman's triangle is seen. Centrally, there is vertical hair-on-end periosteal new bone laid down along Sharpey's fibres. Permeation is demonstrated proximally, at least as far as the beginning of the periosteal reaction. (**b**) The CT scan demonstrates cortical thickening with medullary encroachment and alteration of medullary signal. In addition, the lamellar periostitis and sunray spiculation are shown. (**c**) The axial T_1-weighted MR sequence confirms the presence of cortical thickening and replacement of marrow fat. The surrounding muscles show quite marked oedema. (By courtesy of Professor HG Jacobson, MD.)*

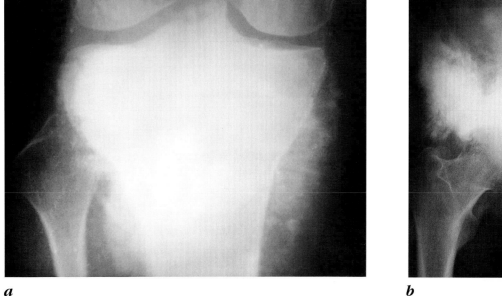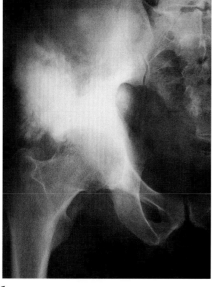

a   *b*

Figure 6.33 *Osteogenic sarcoma. (**a**) In this patient the periostitis is much more coarse than in Ewing's sarcoma. The lesion has caused much sclerosis and sunray spiculation. (**b**) Here, too, in another patient, there is bone expansion and sclerosis, together with a very coarse and shaggy sunray spiculation.*

PAROSTEAL OSTEOSARCOMA

Incidence: 1% of primary malignant tumours of bone and 4% of all osteosarcomas.
Sex: M:F = 1:1.
Age: 60% in the third and fourth decades.
Site: see Figure 6.34.

This uncommon lesion has a better prognosis than the central osteogenic sarcoma. Dense new bone is laid down upon the cortex of the metaphysis of a long bone, usually around the knee or shoulder. The outer margin is undulant. Occasionally, lumps of ossified tumour become detached, presumably because of muscular activity (Figure 6.35).

Characteristically, a lucent plane of cleavage separates the cortex from the tumour. This lesion can closely resemble traumatic myositis ossificans, in which the bony mass often blends with the underlying bone and, occasionally, it is difficult to differentiate between them (see Chapter 9, page 451). In the early stage of

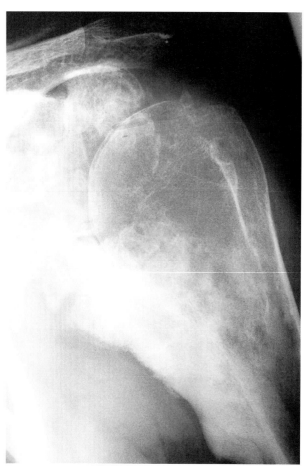

Figure 6.35 *Parosteal osteosarcoma. (a) This radiograph shows a typical parosteal osteosarcoma. There is a well defined dense tumour with undulant margins, closely applied to the cortex of the upper humerus. Because of its close proximity to a joint and intracapsular location, fragments have broken off into the joint and are separating the humeral head from the glenoid. (b) This detail from a chest X-ray taken 8 years previously shows the same shoulder, but the lesion was missed. Its growth can thus be accessed over 8 years. (c) Five years after the initial radiograph some growth has occurred. Again, this is part of a chest X-ray. Maximal growth occurred in the last 3 years.*

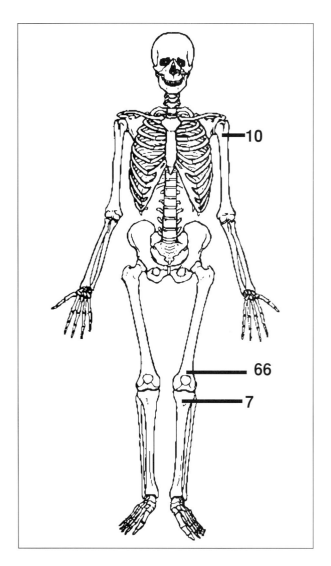

Figure 6.34 *Parosteal osteosarcoma: percentage distribution at major sites only. (After Unni, 1996, with permission.)*

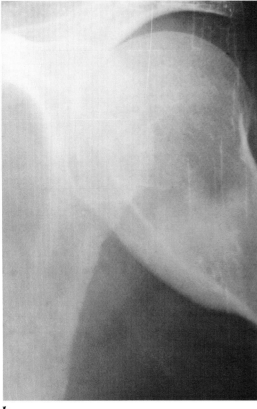

b

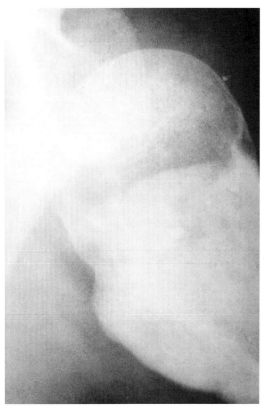

c

this lesion, peripheral definition may be poor. A haematoma ossifies much more rapidly under observation, often peripherally, incorporates into the cortex and eventually often vanishes. Under observation, growth and ossification of the parosteal sarcoma is slow, and years elapse before the underlying medulla is invaded; this lesion therefore metastasizes later. Prognosis following surgery is good.

Computed tomography shows the extent of mineralization in the soft tissues, initially less marked peripherally than at the base (Figure 6.36); subsequently the entire mass becomes densely ossified. The non-mineralized element may be of low attenuation if fat is enclosed. Dedifferentiation may occur within the tumour and is seen as a destructive lesion in the tumour.

MRI demonstrates the soft tissue and ossified element, the latter as a low signal mass, and stages soft tissue extension (Figure 6.36).

PERIOSTEAL OSTEOSARCOMA

Incidence: 1.5% of osteosarcomas.
Sex: M:F = 2:3.
Age: Most cases occur between the ages of 20 and 30 years.
Site: see Figure 6.37.

This rare variant is seen as a short 1–3 cm defect in the cortex associated with a soft tissue mass, having a slightly irregular and perpendicular hair-on-end periostitis (Figures 6.38 and 6.39). Its behaviour and prognosis is between that of parosteal and conventional osteogenic sarcoma.

The soft tissue mass sitting on the cortex is cartilaginous and bony spicules extend into it from the basal cortex. MRI reflects this, with an intermediate signal mass interspersed with low signal spicules, often surrounded by oedema (Figure 6.39).

Primary malignant tumours occurring in the fourth and fifth decades are malignant lymphoma of bone, fibrosarcoma and chondrosarcoma, whose features are discussed in more detail in Chapter 3. Malignant lymphoma of bone resembles Ewing's sarcoma and can cause a lamellar periostitis (Figure 6.40). Malignant fibrous histiocytoma does not cause a marked periosteal reaction but can be associated with irregular new bone formation (Figure 6.41). Chondrosarcoma is a relatively slowly growing malignant tumour which scallops the cortex from within but which allows a thick layer of subperiosteal new bone to form. The cortical margin of the lesion may be thicker than the normal cortex.

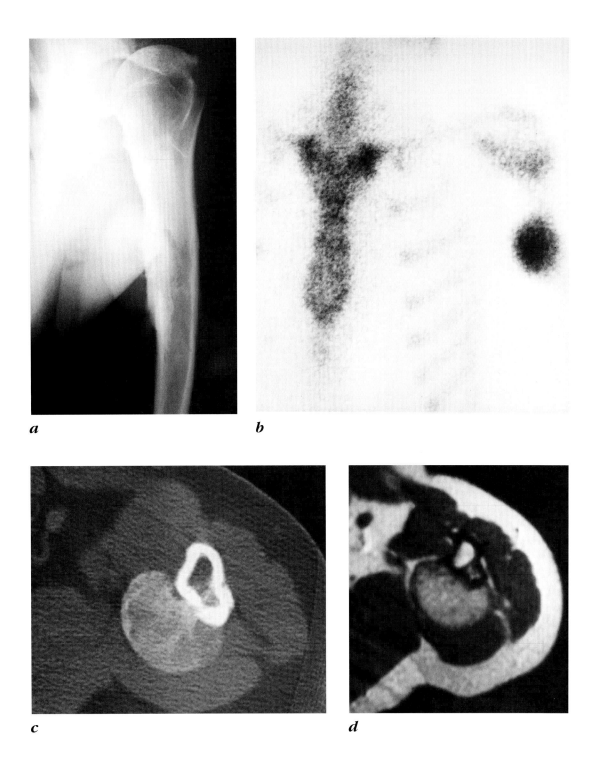

a   *b*

c   *d*

Figure 6.36 *Parosteal osteosarcoma. (**a**) The plain film shows extensive thickening of the medial cortex of the upper and mid-shaft of the humerus. (**b**) The radioisotope bone scan shows a rather more focal increase in uptake corresponding to the soft tissue mass seen on the plain film medial to the area of bony thickening. (**c**) The CT scan demonstrates a faintly mineralizing, higher attenuation, soft tissue mass with a smooth margin based on the cortex. (**d**) The axial T$_1$-weighted MR sequence shows a well demarcated and corticated mass posterior to the humerus and in the area of the soft tissue mass seen on the plain film. It is of intermediate signal density corresponding to the vague mineralization seen on the CT scan.*

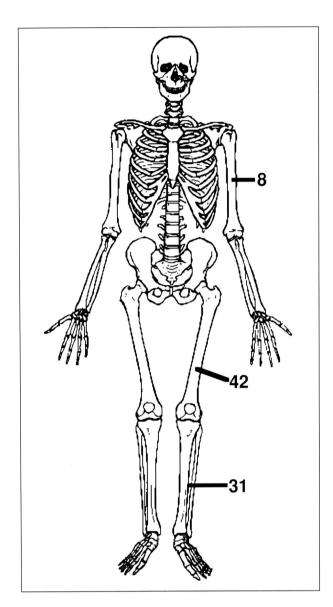

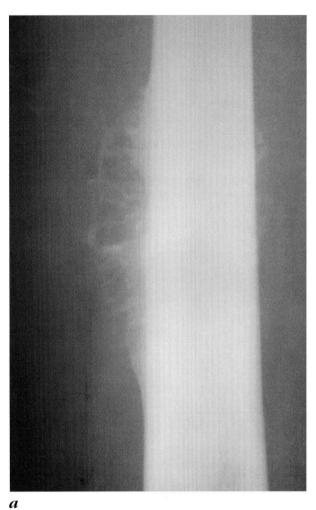

a

Figure 6.37 *Periosteal osteosarcoma: percentage distribution at major sites only. (After Unni, 1996, with permission.)*

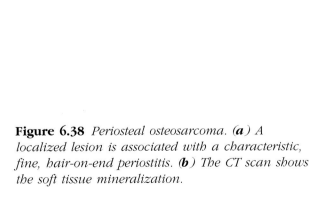

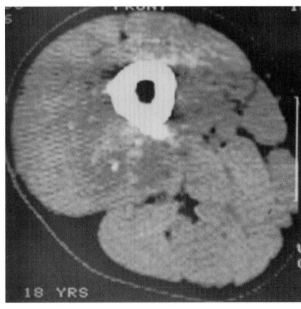

b

Figure 6.38 *Periosteal osteosarcoma. (**a**) A localized lesion is associated with a characteristic, fine, hair-on-end periostitis. (**b**) The CT scan shows the soft tissue mineralization.*

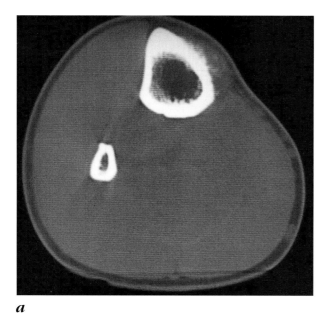

a

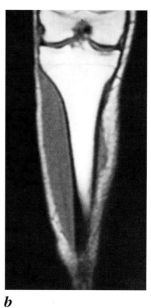

b

Figure 6.39 *Periosteal osteosarcoma. (**a**) The CT scan shows a very fine, mainly hair-on-end periostitis on the anterior tibia. This ossification is within a well defined soft tissue mass. (**b**) On the T$_1$-weighted MR sequence the soft tissue mass is shown and is well defined. The mineralization is not really evident.*

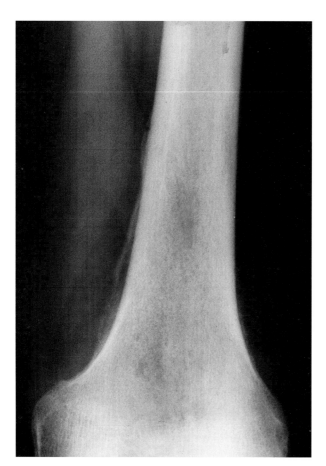

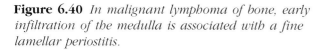

Figure 6.40 *In malignant lymphoma of bone, early infiltration of the medulla is associated with a fine lamellar periostitis.*

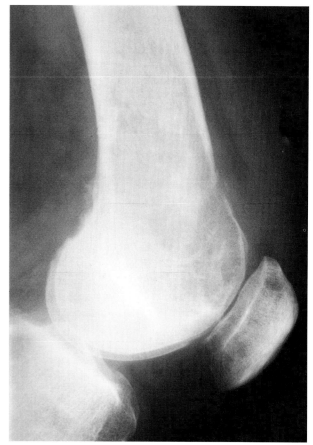

Figure 6.41 *Irregular destruction of the distal femur associated with a delicate periostitis is visible in this patient with malignant fibrous histiocytoma.*

GENERALIZED PERIOSTITIS

Generalized periosteal new bone formation is unusual, and may occasionally be seen with widespread skeletal metastases, for example from the prostate (Figure 6.42) or osteogenic sarcoma, and with widespread angiomatous tumours (Figure 6.43). However, metastatic disease is not commonly associated with florid or even minor periostitis (Table 6.2).

PERIOSTITIS ASSOCIATED WITH SOFT TISSUE SWELLING

HYPERTROPHIC (PULMONARY) OSTEOARTHROPATHY

This is a painful condition in which periosteal new bone is laid down in response to lesions elsewhere,

usually in the lung. The new bone is most commonly found at the distal radius and ulna, distal tibia and

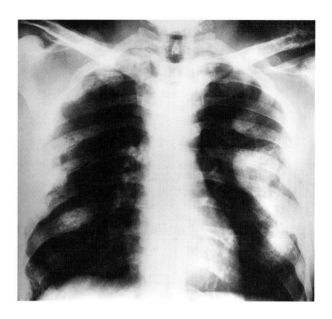

Figure 6.43 *Multiple skeletal angiomas. The appearances vary from a gross hair-on-end periostitis, seen in profile, to an expansile honeycomb change, seen face-on. The two often represent the same appearance viewed from different angles.*

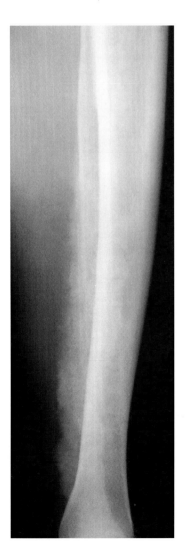

Figure 6.42
Periostitis due to secondary deposits is uncommon but, in this patient, has resulted from a carcinoma of the prostate.

Table 6.2 Generalized periostitis in adults.

Primary or idiopathic pachydermoperiostitis
Hypertrophic osteoarthropathy secondary to benign
  or malignant pulmonary and pleural lesions
  Chronic lung infections, tuberculosis
  Chronic liver disease
  Congenital cyanotic heart disease
  Chronic inflammatory bowel disease
Arthritides
Thyroid acropachy
Polyarteritis nodosa
Myeloma and, occasionally, secondary deposits, e.g.
  from the prostate

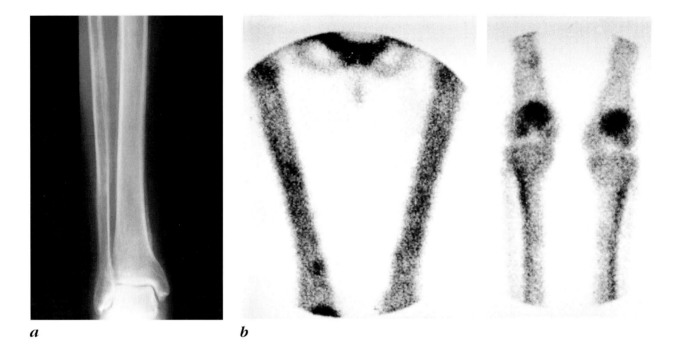

a   *b*

Figure 6.44 *Hypertrophic osteoarthropathy. (a) Fine lamellar periostitis is seen along the diaphysis and metaphysis of the tibia and fibula. The epiphyseal regions are not affected. (b) At radionuclide bone scanning the tubular bones appear broadened and show a diffuse increase in uptake which is maximal in the region of the periosteum and cortex.*

fibula, metatarsals, metacarpals and phalanges. The epiphyseal regions are spared. The periostitis has many forms. A common presentation is of a fine solitary layer of new bone separated from the intact, underlying cortex by a plane of lucency but, occasionally, up to six layers of lamellar new bone may be seen. The new bone may merge with the underlying cortex or may be irregular and, occasionally, hair-on-end (Figure 6.44).

The affected areas of the skeleton show a diffuse or linear peripheral increase in uptake on radioisotope scans (Figure 6.44b). Although epiphyses do not show new bone formation, a non-erosive synovitis is often present and may be the presenting symptom, with pain and soft tissue swelling around joints.

The lesions regress following removal or treatment of the underlying (usually pulmonary) pathology, and even after vagotomy or pleural section.

Clubbing of the fingers is often associated with hypertrophic osteoarthropathy, but the two do not always accompany each other.

PACHYDERMOPERIOSTOSIS

This is an idiopathic form of periostitis which is not associated with an underlying visceral lesion. It is associated with clubbing and gross thickening of the skin of the scalp, face, hands and feet. The disease often starts in adolescence, long before the usual age of onset of lung-related hypertrophic osteoarthropathy, most cases of which are associated with malignant thoracic disease. The periostitis is similar in distribution to hypertrophic osteoarthropathy, but extends to the epiphyses and is shaggy rather than finely lamellar. Gross thickening of the diaphysis may be seen (Figure 6.45).

THYROID ACROPACHY

This occurs in patients who are usually myxoedematous following treatment for thyrotoxicosis. Pretibial myxoedema is present with swelling of hands and feet, associated with a shaggy periostitis of the tubular bones in these areas and, less commonly, the distal tibia and fibula (Figure 6.46).

POLYARTERITIS NODOSA

This can be associated with gross, coarse, symmetrical or velvety new bone formation on the tibia, fibula and tubular bones of the feet. The lesions may be due to arterial insufficiency and, therefore, possibly related to vascular stasis or hypoxia (Figure 6.47).

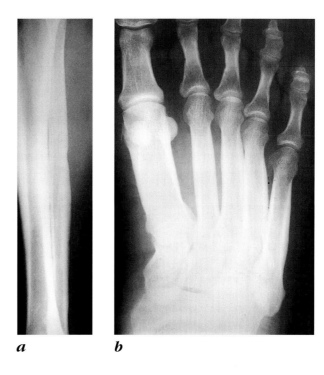

a   **b**

Figure 6.45 *Pachydermoperiostitis. (**a**, **b**) These radiographs illustrate that this condition is similar to hypertrophic osteoarthropathy, but more florid and extensive.*

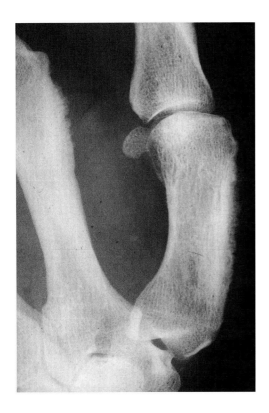

Figure 6.46 *Thyroid acropachy. The extent of periostitis in this disease can vary greatly but, in this patient thickening of the cortices is demonstrated, associated with a hair-on-end appearance at the mid-shafts of the tubular bones.*

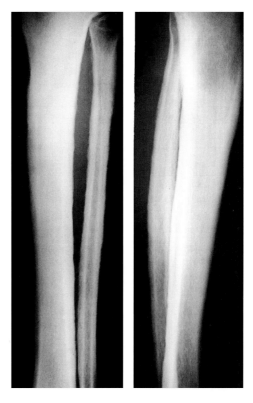

Figure 6.47 *Polyarteritis nodosa. The amount of periostitis in this disease can vary greatly. In this radiograph, a solid periostitis is laid down along the mid-shafts of the paired long bones. Often a hair-on-end appearance results.*

PERIOSTEAL NEW BONE IN CHILDREN (Table 6.3)

CAFFEY'S INFANTILE CORTICAL HYPEROSTOSIS

In this disease periosteal reactions appear before 5 months of age. The affected children are ill with fever, irritability and a raised ESR. Soft tissue masses occur, beneath which new bone formation appears. One or many bones may be involved and, as some lesions heal, others appear. Changes are usually seen in the mandible, scapula and ribs, as well as in the long bones of the limbs (Figure 6.48). A lamellar or coarse periostitis can appear, which may be even thicker than the underlying shaft, and unite the paired long bones (see Figure 1.33bc).

New bone is diaphyseal and metaphyseal but the epiphysis is spared. In the long bones, the lesions are not generally symmetrical. The usual tendency is towards remission but, occasionally, the changes persist into adult life.

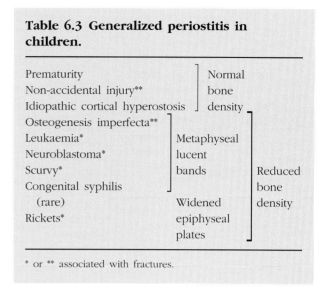

Table 6.3 Generalized periostitis in children.

Prematurity	Normal	
Non-accidental injury**	bone	
Idiopathic cortical hyperostosis	density	
Osteogenesis imperfecta**		
Leukaemia*	Metaphyseal	
Neuroblastoma*	lucent	
Scurvy*	bands	Reduced
Congenital syphilis		bone
(rare)	Widened	density
Rickets*	epiphyseal	
	plates	

* or ** associated with fractures.

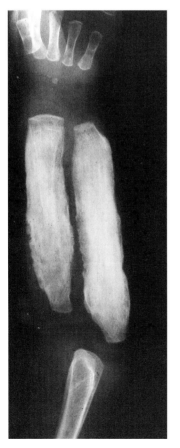

Figure 6.48
Infantile cortical hyperostosis. A florid multilamellar periostitis may be seen, and the underlying bone is hardly visible.

NON-ACCIDENTAL INJURY

Multiple fractures of different generations are classically found together with deformities (see Chapter 5, page 304). The skull, ribs and lower limbs are involved and the changes imply long-term child abuse (Figure 1.36). In an acute case, the only manifestation may be a metaphyseal chip fracture, where the strongly attached periosteum pulls off a small flake of bone. The diaphyseal periosteum, which is not firmly attached to the underlying cortex, is easily stripped and large subperiosteal haematomas may form, which are not necessarily related to an underlying fracture of the shaft. These lesions may be single, or multiple and asymmetrical. Osteoporosis is not usually present (Figure 6.49).

OSTEOGENESIS IMPERFECTA

This can be difficult to differentiate from non-accidental injury (see Chapter 1, page 25). Clinically, blue sclerae are not always present. Diaphyseal fractures, which are usually multiple and of different generations, are associated with deformity. Callus formation is probably more gross than in any other disease associated with fractures (Figures 1.32 and 1.33a) and, in addition, there are features of bone softening such as platybasia and bowing, as well as osteoporosis. The skull vault may be extremely thin and the sutures widened.

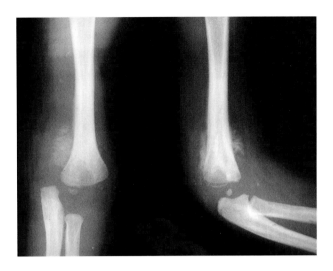

Figure 6.49 *Non-accidental injury. Amorphous new bone is laid down beneath the elevated periosteum following avulsion of a metaphyseal flake. A dislocated elbow is shown.*

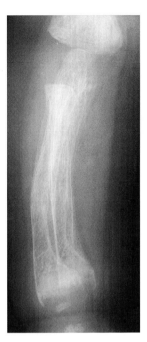

Figure 6.50 *Rickets. The presence of rickets is shown by the broadened and irregular metaphyses. Bone density is reduced. There is bowing of the radius with evidence of a previous mid-shaft fracture or Looser's zone. Quite widespread lamellar periostitis is present, which may follow fracture healing, or ossification of previously non-mineralized osteoid when the patient is treated. Note the amorphous new bone at the distal metaphyses, part of the healing process.*

SCURVY

This is rare in the Western world, is associated with vitamin C deficiency and is occasionally seen in patients on bizarre diets. Defects in collagen result in capillary fragility and bleeding beneath the periosteum. This becomes elevated, and a symmetrical lamellar periostitis is formed along the shafts of affected long bones (see Chapter 1, page 27). Metaphyseal fractures and osteoporosis and ring epiphyses are also present.

RICKETS

In its healing phase this also causes periosteal new bone formation due to ossification of previously non-mineralized osteoid. There is generalized alteration of bone density and texture in epiphyses as well as shafts (Figure 6.50). The epiphyseal plates are widened, which is a feature almost unique to rickets, but they are progressively narrowed during healing (Figure 6.51).

LEUKAEMIA AND NEUROBLASTOMA

Elevation of the periosteum by malignant cells may cause a single, or lamellar, periostitis. Metaphyseal

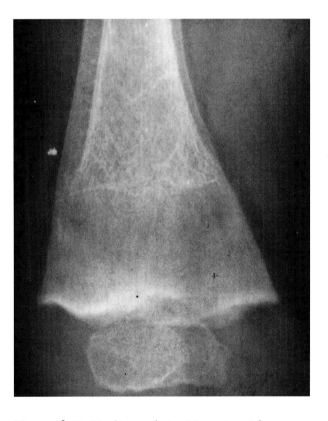

Figure 6.51 *Healing rickets. A prominent bone-within-a-bone appearance is shown at the distal femur. The healing process has initiated new bone formation along the cortex and at the metaphysis, and the epiphyseal plate is now narrow.*

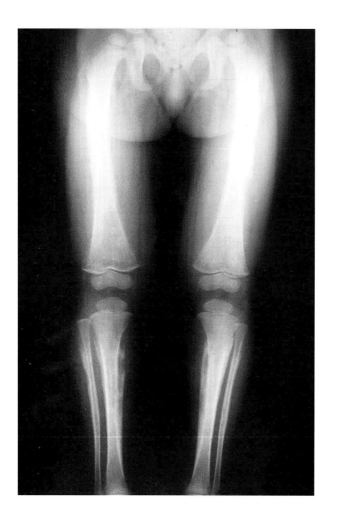

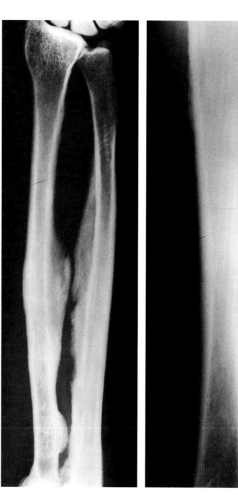

Figure 6.52 *Leukaemia. Bands of metaphyseal lucency are visible which are irregular at the margins of the bone and are accompanied by lamellar periostitis around the mid-shafts.*

Figure 6.53 *In this patient with fluorosis, there is ossification at the interosseous membrane linking the radius and ulna. This disease is another cause of cross-union between paired bones (see Figure 1.33).*

Table 6.4 Causes of generalized hyperostosis.

Ankylosing spondylitis Reiter's syndrome Psoriasis	Seronegative	Associated with erosive change	Bilateral symmetrical sacroiliac fusion
Occasionally rheumatoid arthritis	Seropositive		May be associated with sacroiliac fusion
X-linked hypophosphataemic osteomalacia Fluorosis	Increased bone density		
Diffuse idiopathic skeletal hyperostosis	Occasional increase in bone density		

lucent bands, which are also present in scurvy and generalized osteoporosis, may also be seen but focal areas of bone destruction indicate a malignant infiltrative aetiology (Figure 6.52).

GENERALIZED HYPEROSTOSIS

A number of conditions, some of which are related, have new bone formation at musculotendinous insertions as a common feature. The appearances are those of a generalized hyperostosis often affecting the pelvis, ribs and occasionally hands and feet, as well as the spine (Table 6.4) (see Chapter 8, pages 373–91).

RHEUMATOID ARTHRITIS

Rheumatoid arthritis is less commonly associated with sacroiliac disease and spinal fusion, and erosions only rarely heal with new bone formation.

FLUOROSIS

Irregular cortical thickening is seen with whiskering at musculotendinous insertions (Figure 6.53). The bones show an increase in density.

X-LINKED HYPOPHOSPHATAEMIC OSTEOMALACIA

The bones become thickened with increase in density; bowing of long bones is a characteristic feature. Looser's zones are seen, and whiskering occurs at musculotendinous insertions, as well as paraspinal ossification.

BIBLIOGRAPHY

Edeiken J, Hodes PJ, Caplan LH (1966) New bone production and periosteal reaction. *Am J Roentgenol* **97**: 708–18.

Lindell MM Jr, Shirkhoda A, Raymond AK et al (1987) Parosteal osteosarcoma: radiologic-pathologic correlation with emphasis on CT. *Am J Roentgenol* **148**: 323–8.

Okada K, Frassica FK, Sim FH et al (1994) Parosteal osteosarcoma: a clinicopathological study. *J Bone Joint Surg* **76A**: 366–78.

Chapter 7 Abnormalities in size and modelling of bone

COMMON CAUSES OF SHORT-LIMBED DWARFISM

ACHONDROPLASIA

This is the commonest form of dwarfism which is predominantly due to limb shortening (Table 7.1). Recently, many conditions have been separated from achondroplasia, including hypochondroplasia and thanatophoric dwarfism. Although inherited as a dominant condition, the majority of patients are new mutants.

In the long bones, the shortening is predominantly rhizomelic. The metaphyses are grossly splayed and have a local chevron sign at the knees. This is seen as a central failure of growth resulting in a defect in which the abnormally shaped epiphysis sits. In addition, the metaphyses around the knee are narrow in the sagittal plane, causing the area to appear lucent on anteroposterior films (Figure 7.1).

The pelvis is abnormally shaped with a 'champagne glass' pelvic brim (Figure 7.2). In children the cartilages are prominent, so that the ischiopubic synchondrosis and the triradiate cartilages are wider than normal. The iliac blades in the adult are round and squat, with little waisting above the acetabulum. The spine shows progressive narrowing of the interpedicular distance in the lumbar region (Figure 7.3). The discs further narrow the spinal canal and neurological symptoms are common. Canal stenosis is clearly demonstrated at radiculography and at MRI (Figures 7.4 and 7.5). In addition, an exaggerated lumbar lordosis makes the

Table 7.1 Abnormalities in size and modelling of bone.

Common causes of short-limbed dwarfism
Achondroplasia
  This has been confused in the past with:
    Hypochondroplasia
    Pseudoachondroplasia
    Thanatophoric dwarfism
    Achondrogenesis ⎤ Often fatal

Short-trunked dwarfism
Spondyloepiphyseal dysplasia

Proportionate dwarfism
Mucopolysaccharidoses ⎤ Associated
Hypophosphataemia with diminished
Osteogenesis imperfecta ⎦ bone density — Associated with multiple fractures

Osteopetrosis ⎤ Associated with
Pyknodysostosis increased bone density ⎦ Clavicular hypoplasia;
Cleidocranial dysplasia ⎦ Normal bone density — acro-osteolysis; Wormian bones

Adapted from Wynne-Davies R, *Heritable Disorders in Orthopaedic Practice*, (Blackwell: Oxford, 1973), with permission.

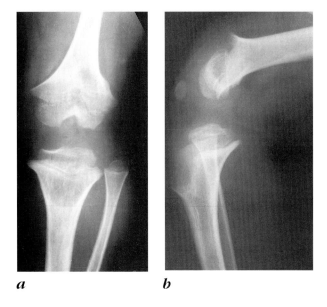

a　　　*b*

Figure 7.1 *Achondroplasia. (**a**) Chevron deformities are present at the metaphyses, and the epiphyses fit into the metaphyseal defects. In addition, there are metaphyseal lucencies. (**b**) The lucencies are due to defects of the anterior tibial and femoral metaphyses.*

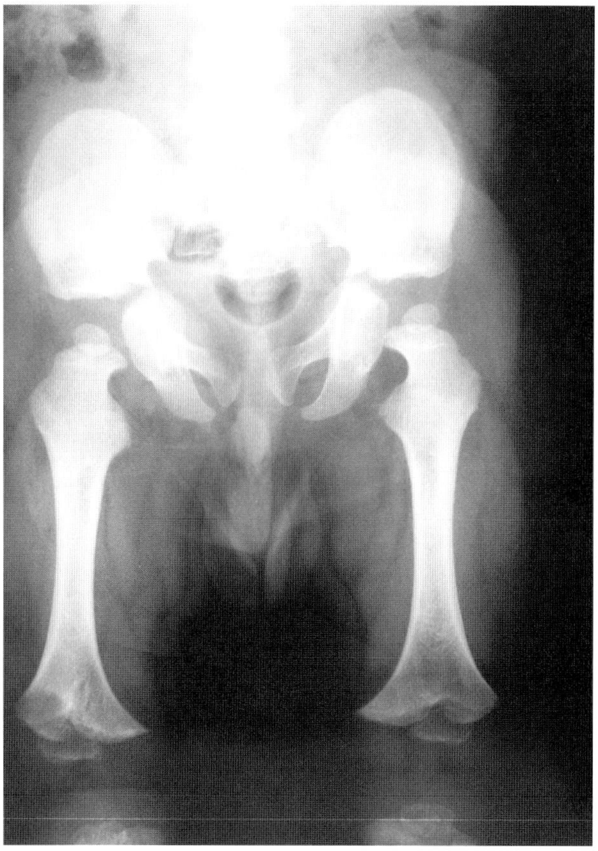

Figure 7.2 *Achondroplasia. The iliac blades are squat and show no constriction above the acetabula, which have horizontal roofs. The pelvic inlet is shaped like a champagne glass. There is rhizomelic dwarfism. The interpedicular distances of the lower lumbar spine are narrow, and the triradiate and ischiopubic cartilages are prominent.*

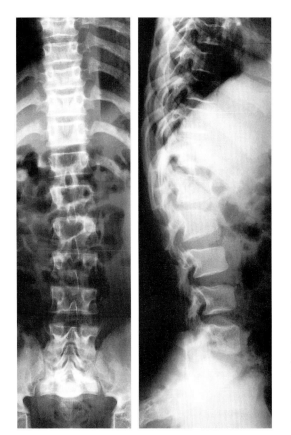

Figure 7.3 *Thoraco-lumbar spine in achondroplasia. There is a moderate degree of platyspondyly. Concavities are demonstrated on the posterior aspects of the vertebral bodies but there are prolongations into the canal at the posterior end-plates. The pedicles are short and the interpedicular distances narrow. Minor wedging at L1 and L2 may be related to local minor instability. The pelvis is noted to be abnormally shaped and the ribs too are broadened posteriorly.*

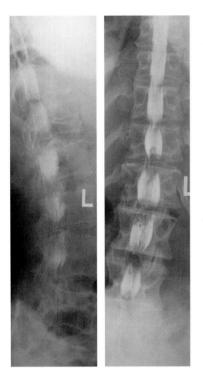

Figure 7.4 *The radiculogram in this achondroplastic patient shows posterior scalloping of vertebral bodies and multiple constrictions related to the intervertebral discs. The interpedicular distances narrow from above downwards in the lumbar region.*

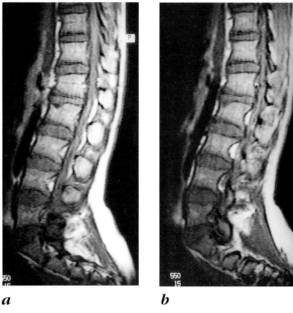

a   *b*

Figure 7.5

Achondroplasia at MR imaging. (a, b). On the sagittal T$_1$-weighted sequences the vertebral bodies have the same shape as demonstrated on the plain radiograph (see Figure 7.3), with marked scalloping posteriorly and bone spurring adjacent to the intervertebral discs. The canal is narrow in the sagittal plane and in the axial T$_1$-weighted images too (c, d). A marked degree of stenosis is shown, worse at L5 than at L1.

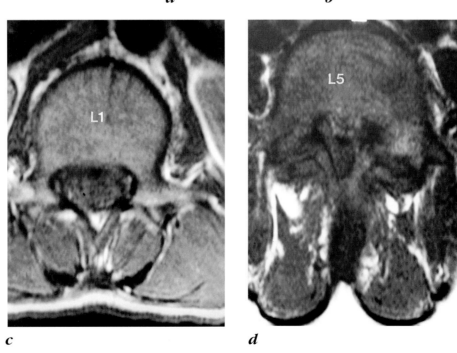

c   *d*

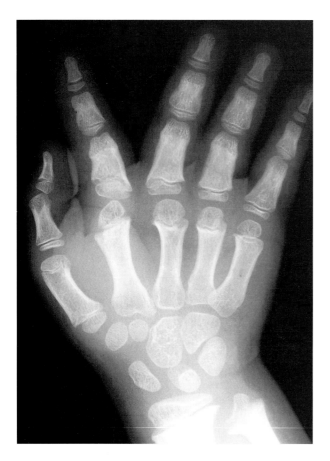

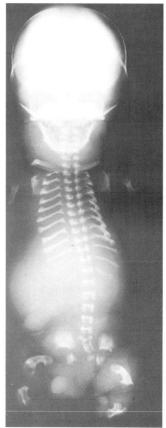

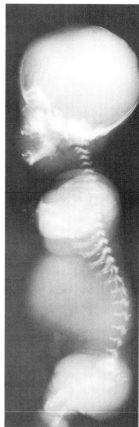

Figure 7.6 *This patient with achondroplasia has a trident hand. There is divergence at the second and third fingers, and all the fingers are similar in length. There are multiple growth anomalies. The distal ulna shows a minor chevron deformity.*

Figure 7.7 *Thanatophoric dwarfism. There is a clover-leaf skull and marked platyspondyly in the lumbar spine with H-shaped vertebrae and short-limbed dwarfism. The major long bones are curved which differentiates thanatophoric dwarfism from achondroplasia, which is not fatal. The child was stillborn.*

buttocks prominent. The hands are 'trident' in type with short tubular bones so that the fingers all appear the same length and diverge from the midline (Figure 7.6).

The skull has a large calvarium with a short base. The narrow foramen magnum causes hydrocephalus, which may further enlarge the skull.

THANATOPHORIC DWARFISM

In the neonate, thanatophoric dwarfism has in the past been confused with achondroplasia but there are marked dissimilarities between these conditions. In thanatophoric dwarfs, the extremely short limbs are

curved (Figure 7.7), which is not a feature of achondroplasia, in which the diaphyses are straight. In addition, there is a severe generalized platyspondyly with more normal posterior elements, so that the vertebrae resemble the letter H. The skull shows a trefoil deformity, known as the *clover-leaf skull*, with prominent temporal bulges. This condition is usually fatal.

ACHONDROGENESIS

This is a rare, fatal dysplasia which is similar to thanatophoric dwarfism. The long bones are extremely short and often curved, but ossification is defective in

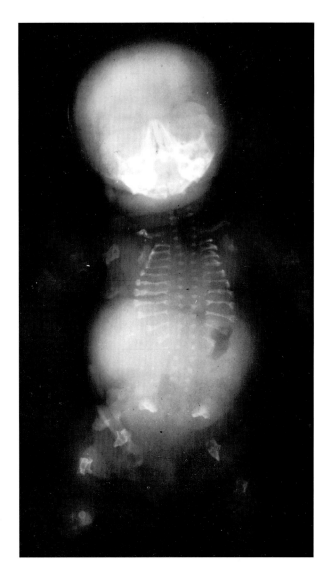

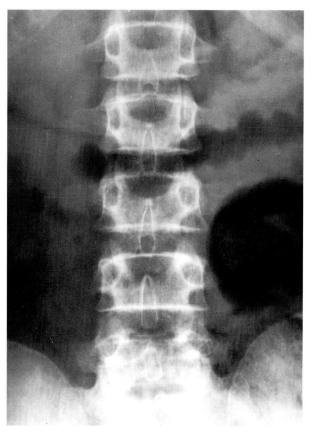

Figure 7.9 *Hypochondroplasia. The interpedicular distance is narrowest at L5.*

Figure 7.8 *Achondrogenesis. The skull vault is barely mineralized in this stillborn child; the ribs are hypoplastic and have suffered multiple fractures. The pedicles in the spine are mineralized but no other parts are seen. There is gross shortening of the long bones, which are curved and irregular. There is hardly any mineralization of the pelvis.*

the lower spine, pelvis and lower limbs, so that often these parts can barely be seen (Figure 7.8).

HYPOCHONDROPLASIA

Hypochondroplasia has also been distinguished from achondroplasia, because hypochondroplasts gener-

ally are not as short as achondroplasts and the skull is normal. The interpedicular distances in the lumbar spine become progressively narrow caudally (Figure 7.9), but limb shortening is not as pronounced and trident hands are not present. The fibula is longer than the tibia at the ankle (Figure 7.10), which is also a feature of achondroplasia, but the metaphyseal splaying and irregularity seen in this disease do not occur in hypochondroplasia, and the epiphyses are not irregular.

PSEUDOACHONDROPLASIA

The pseudoachondroplastic forms of spondyloepiphyseal dysplasia are another group of conditions that resemble achondroplasia. They are not a single entity but a heterogeneous group of diseases with rhizomelic dwarfism inherited in dominant and recessive forms of varying severity. In the most severe

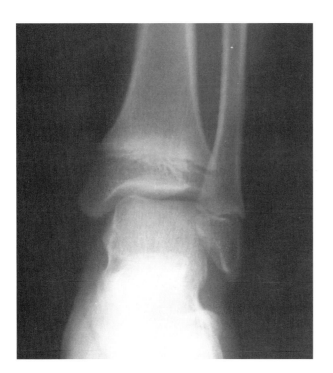

Figure 7.10 *Hypochondroplasia. Overgrowth of the fibula is seen, but the epiphyses are normal in appearance.*

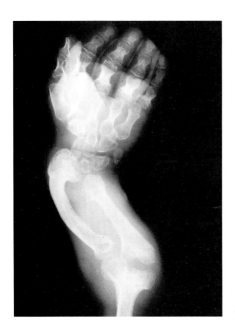

a

Figure 7.11 *This patient has the severe recessive form of pseudoachondroplasia. Gross limb shortening (**a**) with irregularity of the epiphyses (**b**) can be seen. (**c**) The deformities are considerably greater than those seen in achondroplasia.*

form, in adults, joint alignment deformities are prominent (Figure 7.11).

Unlike achondroplasia, changes are not present at birth but become apparent in childhood, and progressively more severe in adolescence. The skull is always normal, as in hypochondroplasia, but metaphyseal flaring may be more gross than in achondroplasia, and the epiphyses may be irregular (Figure 7.11). In contrast to achondroplasia, the spine shows varying degrees of platyspondyly with scoliosis (Figure 7.12), and also anterior beaking in the lumbar vertebral bodies.

Therefore, the pseudoachondroplastic forms of spondyloepiphyseal dysplasia have some features of achondroplasia, particularly rhizomelia, metaphyseal flaring and short hands, but also some features of true *spondyloepiphyseal dysplasias* which do not

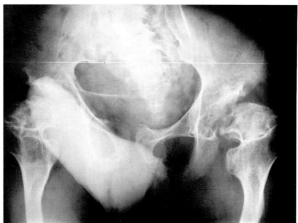

b

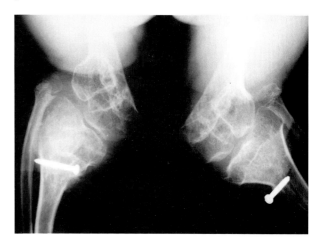

c

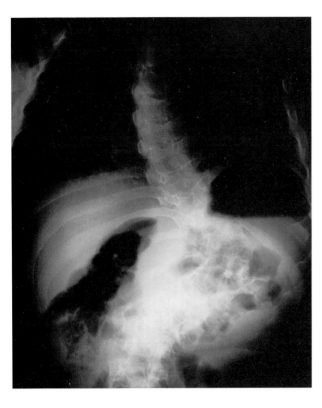

Figure 7.12 *Pseudoachondroplasia. The spine of the patient shown in Figure 7.11 shows a gross kyphoscoliosis and platyspondyly.*

show rhizomelia, have normal skulls and which show a short-trunked, not short-limbed, dwarfism, with abnormal spines (Figure 7.13), platyspondyly and often scoliosis. Spondyloepiphyseal dysplasia tarda has already been mentioned (see page 242).

PROPORTIONATE DWARFISM

MUCOPOLYSACCHARIDOSES (MPS)

Of these uncommon disorders, only MPS I-H (Hurler's syndrome) is seen relatively frequently. Affected children are normal at birth and changes start appearing at around 1–2 years of age. Mental defect progresses and the coarsened face resembles that of a gargoyle. Epiphyses become progressively irregular, metaphyses broaden and the diaphyses thicken. A tibio-talar slant develops at the ankles (Figure 4.92) and a radio-ulnar tilt deformity at the wrists (Figure 4.90).

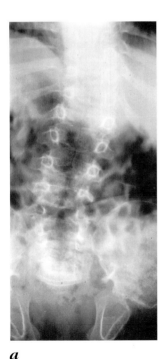
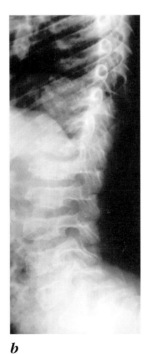

a   *b*

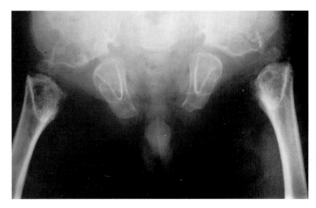

c

Figure 7.13 *Spondyloepiphyseal dysplasia congenita. (**a**, **b**) There is gross platyspondyly with a scoliosis. Some of the vertebral bodies also show anterior beaking. The congenita form does not have the posterior vertebral body humps seen in the tarda type of spondyloepiphyseal dysplasia. (**c**) The acetabular roofs are flat and irregular. The femoral heads are displaced, the metaphyses broad and irregular, and the medial acetabular walls thickened.*

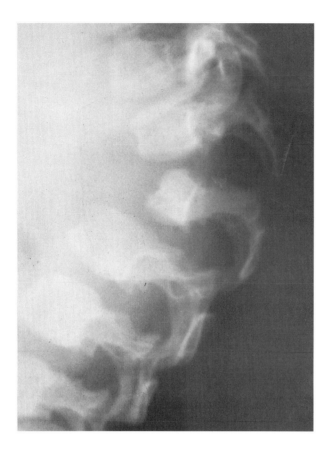

Figure 7.14 *MPS I-H. There is a hypoplastic vertebral body at the thoraco-lumbar junction with a central anterior defect.*

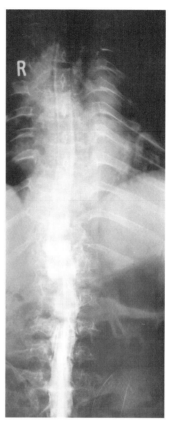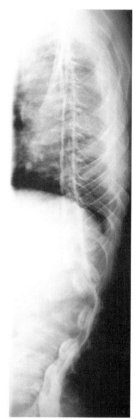

Figure 7.16 *MPS IV. There is an acute kyphos at L1 which shows a prominent anterior beak and hypoplasia of the superior surface. Multiple areas of stenosis are present on the radiculogram. There is platyspondyly with end-plate irregularity and the ribs are abnormal in shape.*

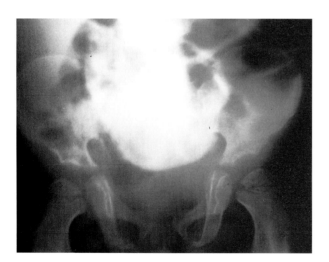

Figure 7.15 *MPS I-H. There is quite marked enlargement of the liver and a large umbilical hernia, with coxa valga and hypoplasia of the ilium in the supra-acetabular region.*

In the hands, the phalanges become bullet-shaped and the metacarpals broaden with proximal pointing (Figure 4.90), which is a characteristic appearance. The skull shows a J-shaped sella, scaphocephaly, odontoid hypoplasia and irregular condyles at the temporomandibular joints (Figure 4.91). In the spine, one or more vertebral bodies in the thoraco-lumbar region show an anterior beak with an associated kyphos (Figure 7.14). The pelvis is abnormally shaped with coxa valga and acetabular dysplasia. In the abdomen, the liver and spleen are grossly enlarged (Figure 7.15).

MPS IV

MPS IV (Morquio–Brailsford disease) is a well recognized, but extremely rare, disease which, unlike MPS

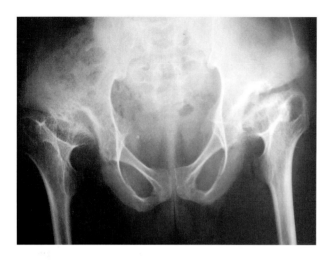

Figure 7.17 *MPS IV. There are very prominent iliac blades with deepened acetabula. The femoral heads are broad and flat, and articulate laterally.*

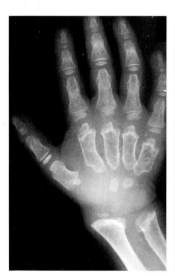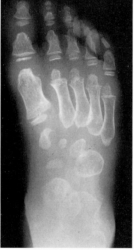

Figure 7.18 *MPS IV. The appearances are those of a mucopolysaccharidosis, with bullet-shaped phalanges and pointed metacarpals in the hand and foot.*

1-H, is not associated with mental defect, and in which the skull is normal, although odontoid hypoplasia is present. Throughout the spine there is irregular platyspondyly with central anterior beaking (Figure 7.16), whereas the beak in MPS I-H tends to be antero-inferior (Figure 7.14). The pelvis shows progressive acetabular dysplasia and the flattened, fragmented epiphyses lie in pseudo-acetabula beneath the iliac blades, which are prominent (Figure

7.17) unlike those seen in achondroplasia. In general, the metaphyses are flared, the epiphyses irregular, the phalanges bullet-shaped, and the metacarpals show proximal pointing (Figure 7.18).

OSTEOGENESIS IMPERFECTA

Osteogenesis imperfecta is described in Chapter 1 as showing osteopenia, multiple fractures which heal with hyperplastic callus, Wormian bones in the skull (Table 4.2) and platyspondyly, resulting from bone softening. Limb shortening and bowing also result from softening and pathological fractures (see Figure 1.24). Thin, gracile, bowed, demineralized long bones are also a feature of this disease; they are also occasionally seen in juvenile chronic arthritis and rickets but, in osteogenesis imperfecta, the metaphyses and epiphyses are more normal in appearance. Often fractures are of different generations and tend to be diaphyseal, unlike those seen in idiopathic juvenile osteoporosis which are characteristically metaphyseal in adolescents (see Figure 1.34).

OSTEOPETROSIS (ALBERS–SCHÖNBERG DISEASE)

This causes limb deformity due to multiple fractures, with shortening. In the recessively inherited congenital form, dwarfism can be severe but, in the dominant, tarda form, it may not be readily apparent. The vertebral bodies do not seem to show collapse (see Chapter 2, page 95).

PYKNODYSOSTOSIS

This rare condition is characterized by severe symmetrical dwarfism, osteosclerosis and pathological fractures, so that it resembles osteopetrosis. However it differs from osteopetrosis because increased density is diffuse rather than in alternating bands. It has many features in common with cleidocranial dysplasia (see also Chapter 2, page 97).

CLEIDOCRANIAL DYSPLASIA

This may be associated with slight shortening, but bone density and the spine are normal. The skull shows Wormian bones and often numerous supernumerary teeth (Figure 7.19). In childhood, there are

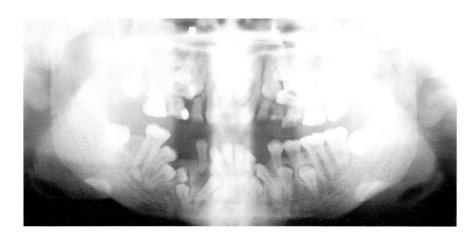

Figure 7.19 *Cleidocranial dysplasia. The orthopantomograph shows failure of shedding of deciduous teeth, failure of eruption of the secondary dentition and numerous supernumerary teeth leading to a crowded dentition. The maxilla is hypoplastic.*

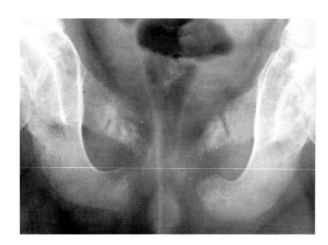

Figure 7.20 *Cleidocranial dysplasia. There is failure of ossification of the symphysis pubis, resulting in an appearance similar to osteomalacia.*

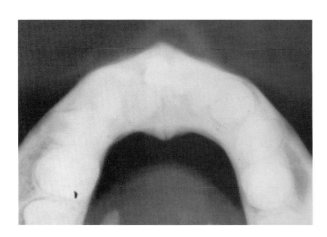

Figure 7.21 *In this patient with cleidocranial dysplasia, a midline defect is seen at the symphysis mentis.*

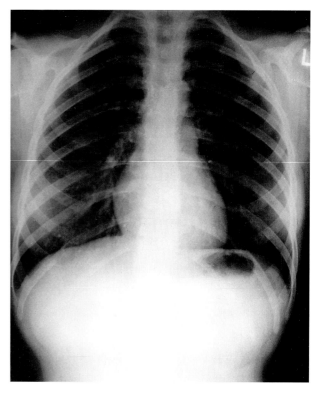

Figure 7.22 *Cleidocranial dysplasia. In this patient the clavicles are absent.*

typically midline defects at the symphysis pubis (Figure 7.20) and symphysis mentis (Figure 7.21), and clavicular aplasia or hypoplasia (Figure 7.22). In the hands, acro-osteolysis may be present, as well as an accessory epiphysis at the base of the second metacarpal (Figure 7.23).

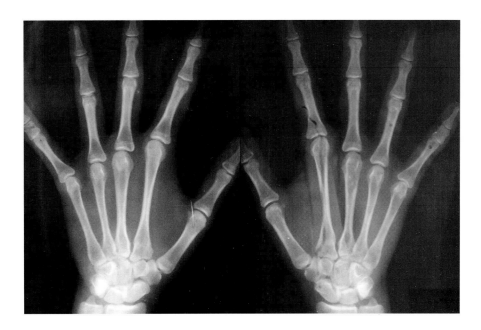

FURTHER CONDITIONS CAUSING SHORTENING OF BONE

ENCHONDROMATOSIS

Masses of immature cartilage remain at the metaphyses, resulting in tumours which have the characteristic features of cartilaginous lesions. They are mainly lucent, ossifying centrally, and have a narrow zone of reactive sclerosis. This produces expansion of the metaphysis with shortening of the shaft.

A characteristic change is seen in the radius and ulna (Figure 7.24). The ulna is short, broad and deformed by an enchondromal mass distally and the radius may then overgrow at the wrist and dislocate proximally. The hands become particularly deformed because of the large, expansile, medullary cartilaginous masses, and function may be severely impaired. Malignant change is uncommon, but is more common in Maffucci's syndrome (enchondromatosis and haemangiomas; Figure 7.25).

DIAPHYSEAL ACLASIA (MULTIPLE EXOSTOSES)

Progressive, eventually gross, metaphyseal expansion with superimposed cartilage-capped exostoses affects major joints (Figures 7.26 and 7.27) as well as the spine and pelvis. Exostoses also arise characteristically

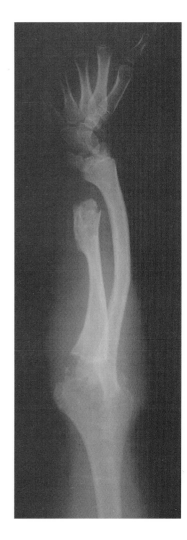

Figure 7.24 *This patient with enchondromatosis has hypoplasia of the ulna with overgrowth of the radius. Islands of cartilage are visible at the distal radial and ulnar metaphyses.*

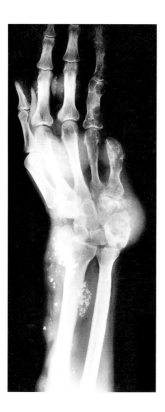

Figure 7.25 *Maffucci's syndrome. There is a combination of multiple enchondromas with haemangiomas, which are seen as large soft tissue masses containing punctate calcification. No malignancy is demonstrated.*

on the scapula, best seen on axial views (see Figure 5.18). There is often limb shortening and shortening of phalanges, metacarpals and metatarsals.

A characteristic lesion affects the radius and ulna, which is similar in appearance to that seen in enchondromatosis. Shortening and deformity of the distal ulna result in overgrowth and deformity of the distal radius and dislocation of the proximal radius (Figure 7.26b).

For lesions of the epiphyseal plate causing shortening, see page 208. For causes of localized discrepancy in length, see Table 7.2. Causes of undertubulation are listed in Table 7.3 and of overtubulation in Table 7.4.

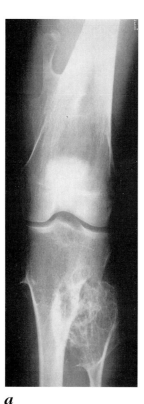

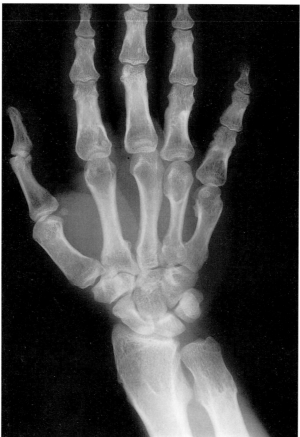

Figure 7.26
(a) Diaphyseal aclasia. Broadening of the metaphyses is associated with 'coat-hanger' exostoses at the distal femur, while the gross expansion of the fibula has resulted in proximal tibio-fibular fusion.
(b) Diaphyseal aclasia. Shortening of the fourth and fifth metacarpals results from a growth anomaly, while the distal radius and ulna show local expansion with exostoses.

a　　　　*b*

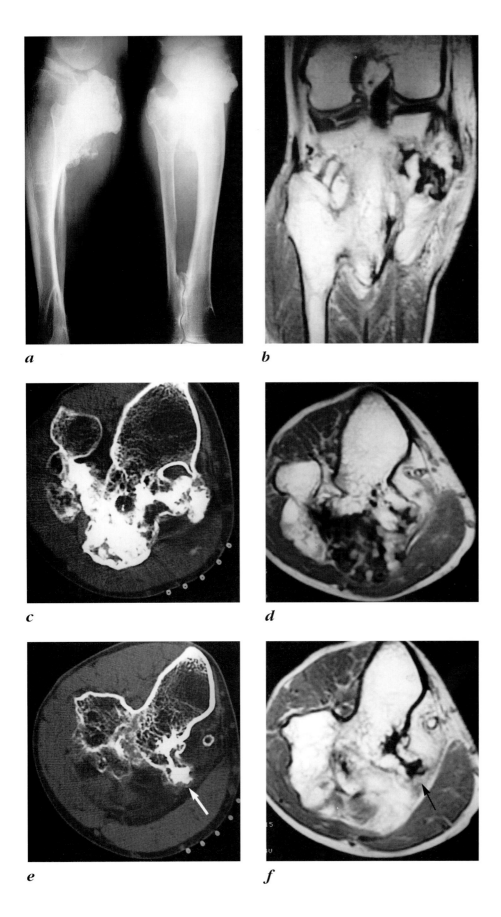

Figure 7.27 *Diaphyseal aclasia. (**a**) A large cartilage-capped exostosis is demonstrated at the proximal tibia. The fibula is dysplastic and the two bones are fused. Typical changes are also seen distally with a talo-tibial slant and a synostosis at the two adjacent exostoses. (**b**) A coronal T₁-weighted MR image showing cross-fusion between the tibia and fibula proximally. (**c**) The CT scan shows mature exostoses fusing posterior to the tibia and fibula. (**d**) An axial T₁-weighted MR image at the same level as (**c**). Extensive low signal posteriorly is related to dense mineralization. (**e**) Slightly further down, a CT scan demonstrates fusion between proximal tibia and fibula and shows the high attenuation mineralized end of the cartilage-capped exostosis (arrow) surrounded by fat, presumably due to local muscle atrophy. (**f**) The axial T₁-weighted MR sequence, taken at the same level as (**e**), again shows the exostosis. This time the cortical bone is of low signal and the fat is bright.*

a

b

c

d

e

f

Table 7.2 Common causes of localized discrepancy in length.

Overgrowth

Arteriovenous malformation		
Haemangioma	Associated with	
Lymphangioma	changes in local	
Macrodystrophia lipomatosa	soft tissues	Associated with
Neurofibromatosis		overgrowth of
Melorheostosis		all or part
Dysplasia epiphysealis hemimelica		of a limb
Fibrous dysplasia		
Tuberculosis	Associated with	
Juvenile chronic arthritis	increased blood	
Haemophilia	flow at joints	
Congenital hemihypertrophy		

Shortening

Infection	
Trauma	
Radiation	
Sickle-cell disease	Damage to the epiphyseal plate
Scurvy	
Thermal injury	
Polio	
Spina bifida	Congenital or acquired defects of motor function
Enchondromatosis	
Diaphyseal aclasia	Growth abnormalities associated with cartilaginous tumours

Table 7.3 Causes of undertubulation.

Sickle-cell disease	Due to marrow	
Thalassaemia	hyperplasia	Erlenmeyer flask appearance
Gaucher's disease	Due to marrow	
	infiltration	
Fibrous dysplasia		
Enchondromatosis	Associated with multiple local tumours	
Diaphyseal aclasia		
Osteopetrosis		
Pyknodysostosis	Gross sclerosis and dwarfism	
Lead poisoning	Metaphyseal sclerosis	Failure of remodelling at metaphyses
Healing rickets		
Healing scurvy	Diaphyseal new bone beneath the periosteum	
Adult X-linked hypophosphataemic osteomalacia		
Mucopolysaccharidoses		
Trauma in children		
Infantile cortical hyperostosis		

Table 7.4 Causes of overtubulation.

Longstanding paralysis, e.g. polio, spina bifida
Muscular dystrophy
Osteogenesis imperfecta
Neurofibromatosis
Juvenile chronic arthritis
Local extrinsic masses—soft tissue tumours, benign
or malignant, e.g. neurofibroma, angioma, lipoma

the limb. The changes in long bones, including the ribs, may be (1) overgrowth, with an increase in length and breadth of an affected bone (Figure 7.28), (2) bone thinning, as in the thin, twisted 'ribbon ribs', which is a dysplastic change (Figure 7.29) (see also Chapter 8, page 413) and (3) defects due to extrinsic pressure by localized neurofibromas, such as those seen on the undersides of ribs (Figures 7.30 and 7.31). Defects due to neurofibromas also enlarge spinal exit foramina, thin pedicles and laminae (Figure 7.32a) and may be seen as soft tissue masses

OVERGROWTH OF BONE

NEUROFIBROMATOSIS

Overgrowth of all or part of a limb is a feature of this disease. The overgrowth is often related to a plexiform neurofibroma and hyperplasia of local blood vessels and lymphatics supplying the enlarged part of

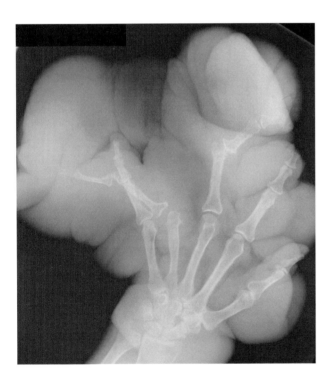

Figure 7.28 *Neurofibromatosis. Gross soft tissue abnormality is seen, and some of the bones are overgrown. The proximal phalanges are elongated. Many of the bones are scalloped due to soft tissue masses causing extrinsic erosion of bone. (By courtesy of Dr R Grant.)*

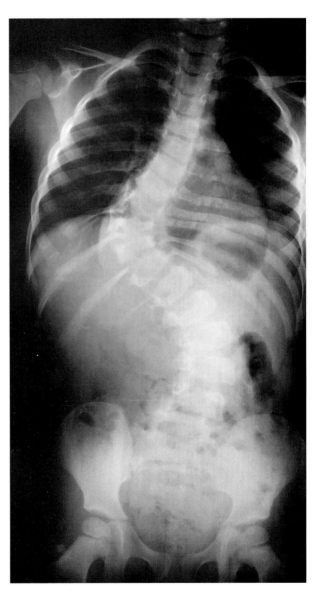

Figure 7.29 *Neurofibromatosis. There is an acute angled kyphos associated with a local soft tissue mass and thin, twisted, ribbon ribs.*

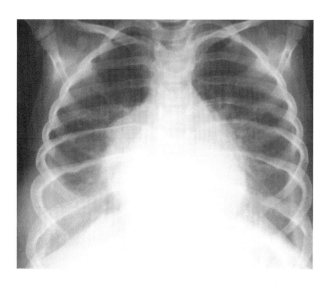

Table 7.5 Causes of posterior vertebral scalloping.

Normal variant
Achondroplasia
Neurofibromatosis
Intraspinal tumour
Acromegaly
Marfan's syndrome
Syringomyelia
Mucopolysaccharidoses
Pyknodysostosis

Figure 7.30 *In this patient with neurofibromatosis, thin, twisted, ribbon ribs are associated with defects due to neurofibromas on the intercostal nerves. However there is also a rather dense shadow behind the heart, caused by a large plexiform neurofibroma, associated with pedicular destruction and expansion of the spinal canal in the thoracic region. There are also neurofibromas related to the pleura and the chest wall in the axillae on both sides.*

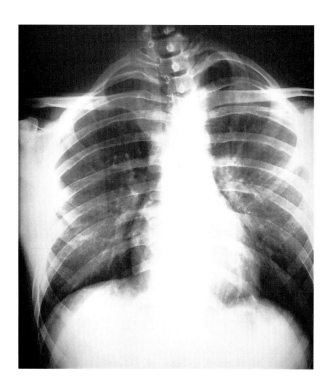

Figure 7.31 *Neurofibromatosis. The chest X-ray shows a scoliosis and inferior rib notching.*

at radiculography (Figure 7.32b) and CT and MR scanning. Often these spinal changes, as well as posterior scalloping of vertebral bodies (Figure 7.32) are not due to tumours but are caused by dural ectasia and meningocoeles (Figure 7.33; Table 7.5). In the spine, the characteristic deformity is an acute kyphosis or scoliosis, which is not necessarily associated with a local tumour (Figure 7.29), but is a dysplastic change.

In the skull, there are orbital and occipital defects which are not necessarily associated with local tumours, but are true manifestations of a local dysplasia (Figure 7.34). A neurofibroma of the inferior dental nerve causes the inferior dental canal to expand, as well as the hemi-mandible supplied by that nerve (Figure 7.35). Neurofibromas may arise anywhere in the body and cause local bone erosion (Figure 7.36).

The paired bones, usually of the lower limbs, show abnormalities of texture in childhood which result in softening and bowing deformities and, finally, fractures which do not heal, producing pseudarthrosis and shortening (Figure 7.37). A similar change is described in fibrous dysplasia. The two diseases have other common features, including skin pigmentation, associated endocrine anomalies, sarcomatous degeneration of tumours and tumoural osteomalacia (see Chapter 1, page 43).

MACRODYSTROPHIA LIPOMATOSA

Marked overgrowth of the digits is associated with gross proliferation of new bone around the affected joints and accumulation of fat in local soft tissues (Figure 7.38).

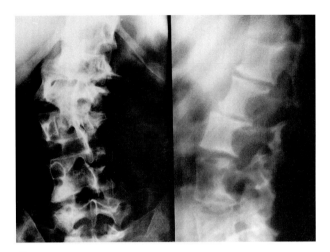

a

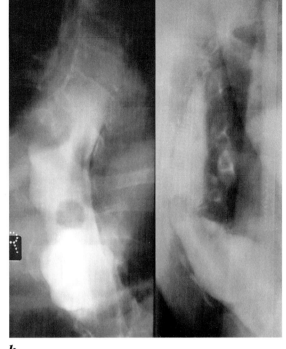

b

c

Figure 7.32 *Neurofibromatosis—dural ectasia.* (**a**) *Posterior scalloping of the vertebral bodies may be seen in this patient. The AP view of the spine shows a scoliosis with erosion of pedicles and transverse processes, as well as vertebral hypoplasia on the concavity.* (**b**) *The radiculogram demonstrates marked widening of the spinal canal in the thoracic region and associated intradural extramedullary neurofibromas displacing the spinal cord. In addition, there are sacular dilatations of the meninges, known as* dural ectasia. *A kyphoscoliosis is present and the ribs differ in shape.* (**c**) *Anterior vertebral scalloping may also be found.*

MELORHEOSTOSIS

The areas of increased bone density which lie in the distribution of the sclerotomes are also increased in length in this condition resulting in, for example, curvature of digits (Figure 7.39; see Chapter 2, page 87).

DYSPLASIA EPIPHYSEALIS HEMIMELICA

In this condition the affected epiphyses are overgrown in toto, not just in the region from which the osteochondroma originates. Also, other bones locally may be enlarged.

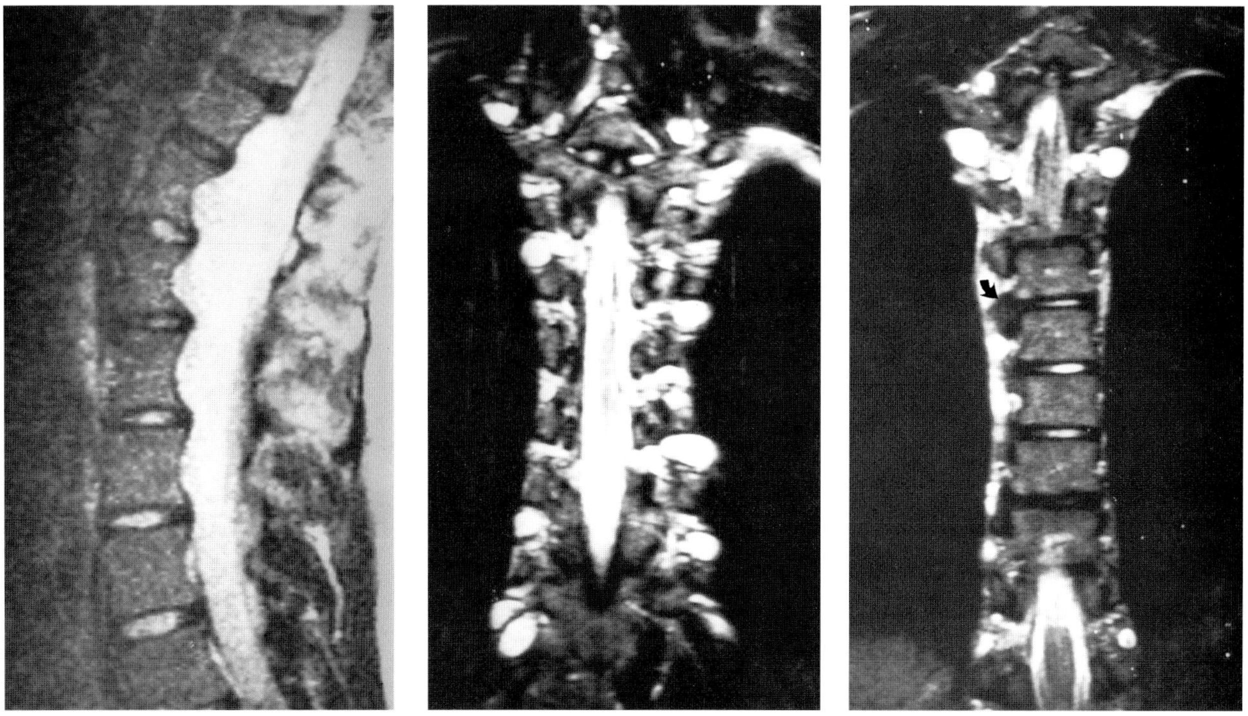

a   *b*   *c*

Figure 7.33 *Neurofibromatosis. (**a**) A T$_2$-weighted MR sequence showing dural ectasia, rather than a soft tissue mass, causing posterior scalloping. (**b**, **c**) Coronal fat suppression MR studies demonstrate multiple lateral thoracic meningoceles containing CSF; a right-sided tumour is present (arrow).*

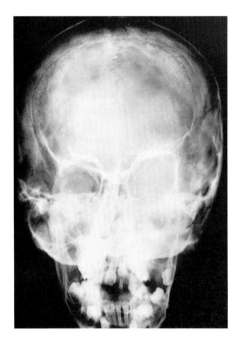

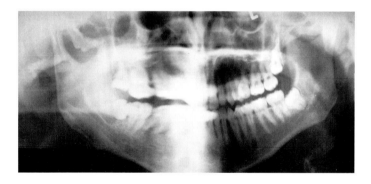

Figure 7.35 *Neurofibromatosis. Expansion of the mandible, deepening of the intercondylar notch and expansion of the inferior dental canal are all demonstrated in this patient with right-sided neurofibromatosis affecting the inferior dental nerve.*

Figure 7.34 *Neurofibromatosis. The left orbit is expanded and no markings are visible within it. This is the 'empty orbit' sign.*

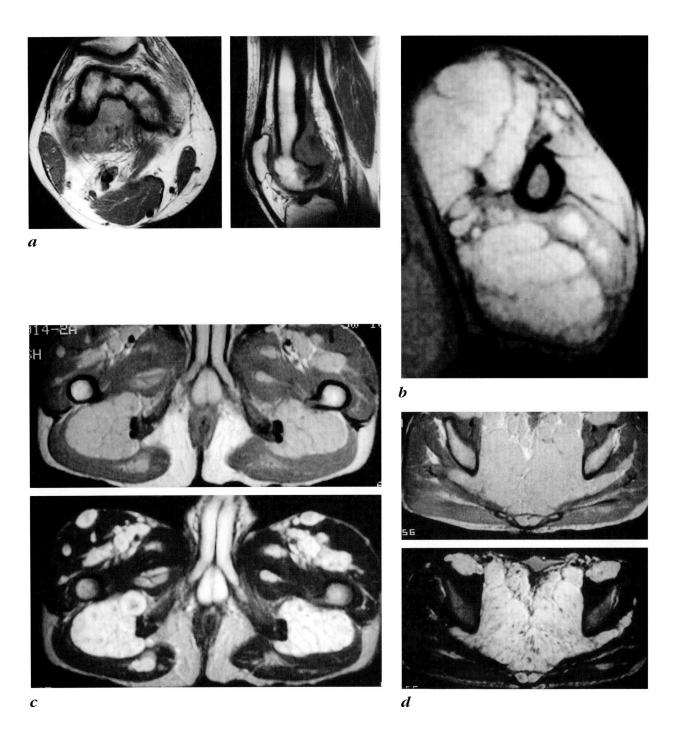

Figure 7.36 *Neurofibromatosis at MR imaging.* (**a**) *At the knee, axial and sagittal* T_1*-weighted sequences show well defined bone erosion by tumour.* (**b**) *Neurofibromas in the deep nerves of the proximal forearm (axial* T_1*-weighting).* (**c, d**) *The sacral plexus, sciatic nerve and femoral nerves are all replaced by large neurofibromatous tumours of intermediate signal on axial* T_1*-weighted MR images* (top); *they are slightly brighter on* T_2*-weighted unenhanced images* (bottom).

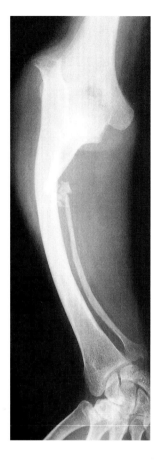

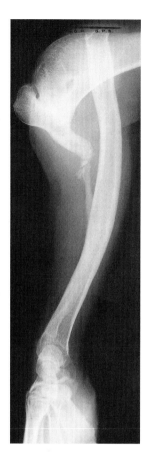

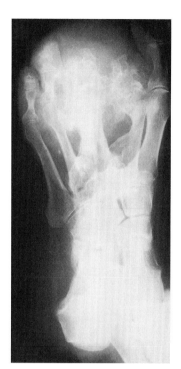

Figure 7.38
Macrodystrophia lipomatosa. It is difficult to see the radiolucent fat in the soft tissues but there is obvious abnormality of growth of many of the metatarsals and phalanges, and huge osseous excrescences resulting in deformity.

Figure 7.37 *Pseudarthroses in neurofibromatosis. Fractures are followed by resorption of bone. The radius has dislocated proximally and is bowed. There appears to be fusion between the distal humerus and the proximal ulna.*

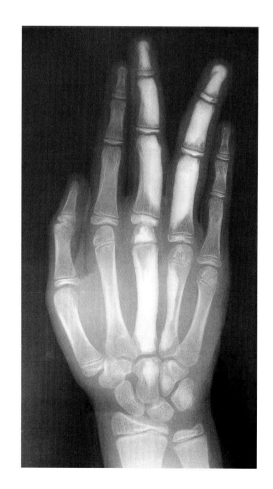

Figure 7.39 *In this patient with melorheostosis, the abnormal bone shows an increase in size which expands the bone cortically and obliterates the medulla. The third and fourth fingers are separated because of the position of the new bone and these fingers are probably elongated.*

Chapter 8 Imaging of the spine

THE LUMBAR SPINE

ANATOMY

On the lateral radiograph, the lumbar spine is lordotic, and concave posteriorly. This is partly because the lower lumbar vertebral bodies are less tall posteriorly than anteriorly. The lower lumbar discs are also thicker anteriorly, further contributing to the lordotic curve.

In the upper lumbar and lower thoracic regions the reverse is true and, at T12 or L1, the body is taller posteriorly than anteriorly; 'wedging' is normal, provided the difference in height is not greater than 1–2 mm (see Figure 1.8a).

The L3/4 disc is inclined horizontally. On the lateral radiograph, the discs increase in height down to L4/5, but the L5/S1 disc is often, but not inevitably, up to half the height of the disc above; some may actually be thicker than the disc above.

The shape of the disc is reflected in the contour of the overlying end-plate, with end-plate depressions at the site of the nucleus (see Figure 1.11). However, the L5 and S1 end-plates are often flat and parallel, reflecting the often flat shape of the L5/S1 nucleus.

The upper surface of the body of S1 is angled disto-anteriorly. With an increased lordosis, this angle is increased and, if the lordosis is diminished, the angle approaches the horizontal.

Lines drawn along the anterior and posterior surfaces of the vertebral bodies are continuous curves, interrupted for instance in spondylolisthesis. Nonetheless, tangents along the front of each body are not continuous, unless the lordosis is lost. This occurs for instance with pain or spasm.

On the anteroposterior radiograph, the body of L3 may be identified as its transverse processes are usually the most inferior with a horizontally inclined lower surface; below this they are inclined obliquely upward (Figure 8.1). The transverse processes at L5 are the bulkiest, and they may approach or even articulate with the upper surface of S1 in 15–30%. A degenerate pseudarthrosis may result at the lateral

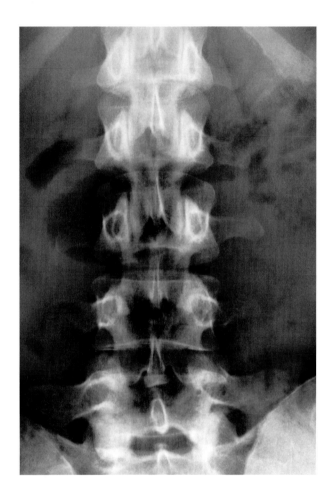

Figure 8.1 *Anatomy of the lower lumbar transverse processes. The transverse process of L3 has a horizontally inclined lower border. At L4 the lower border of the transverse process inclines upwards. The transverse processes at L5 are the broadest; they may articulate with the sacrum.*

articulation with partial or total sacralization of L5 (Figure 8.2). With this lateral buttressing, especially if unilateral, the intervening disc may be narrow but is 'protected' and often will not degenerate. Similarly, an S1/2 disc may form with varying degrees of lumbarization of S1. In any case, if the lowest free

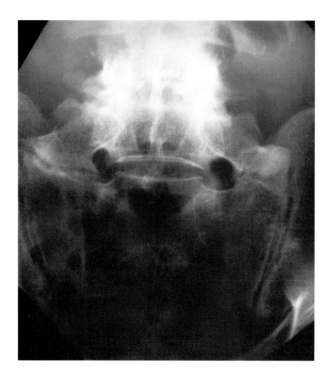

Figure 8.2 *Lateral pseudarthroses. The pseudarthroses may be degenerate, and this is the case here on the right.*

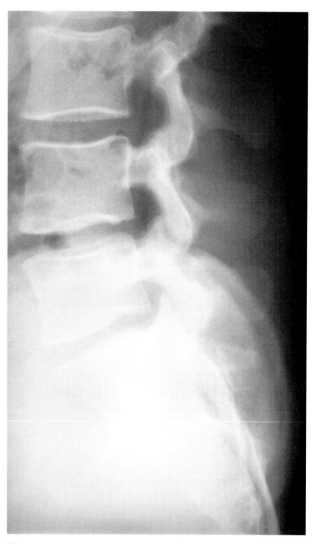

a

Figure 8.3 *Transitional lumbosacral junction. (a) On the lateral view the lowest disc seen on the plain film is that protected by the transverse processes at a transition. The disc above it, however, the lowest free disc, is obviously narrowed and degenerate, associated with retrolisthesis. (b) On the sagittal T₁- and T₂-weighted MR images the lowest disc is the transitional disc and it is normal, but the disc above, which is the lowest free disc, is degenerate, with a loss of height and signal and a dorsal discal protrusion. A high intensity zone is seen posteriorly. (Reproduced from O'Driscoll CM, Irwin A, Saifuddin A (1996) Variations in morphology of the lumbosacral junction on sagittal MRI: correlation with plain radiography. Skeletal Radiol **25**: 225–301, by kind permission of the authors and publishers.)*

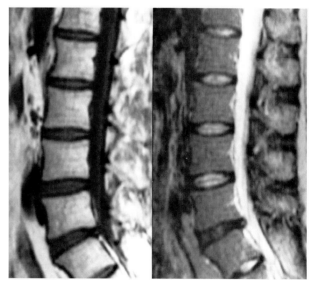

b

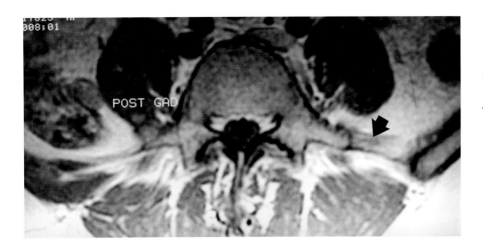

Figure 8.4 *Localization of the L5 vertebral body at axial imaging by the presence of the ilio-lumbar ligament (arrow). This leads from the transverse process of L5 to the adjacent iliac blade.*

disc lies above the level of the iliac crest, it is vulnerable to degeneration irrespective of how it is numbered (Figure 8.3).

On an AP view of the spine, a minor degree of scoliosis, often unknown to the patient, is seen in up to 15% of spines.

The ilio-lumbar ligament connects the transverse process of L5 to the iliac blade (Figure 8.4); L5 can thus be identified on axial imaging. It apparently never originates from a transitional S1, although occasionally has been seen to originate from L4.

The motion segment

The motion segment consists of the disc, vertebral end-plates and facets, together with the surrounding soft tissues. The nucleus is situated just behind the coronal mid-plane and the end-plates are concave just over it, especially in the young. The annulus surrounds it, with concentric onion-skin-like lamellae. The outer annulus has a rich multilevel sensory nerve supply (Figure 8.5), as do the facets (Figure 8.6) and the vertebral body. The sympathetic chain lying alongside vertebral bodies and discs also has sensory pain fibres, while at each level the anterior and posterior longitudinal ligaments have a sensory innervation derived from the level above. Patterns of pain are complicated by multiple levels of innervation at each site (Figure 8.7).

Facet joints vary in orientation. Asymmetry is not normal but is seen in around 30% of the population. This change is greatest at L5/S1. A correlation is reported between the side of greatest asymmetry and facet rotation, and disc protrusion with sciatica.

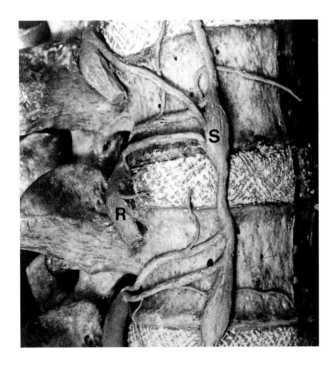

Figure 8.5 *Superficial view of lumbar spine demonstrating the nerve supply of the disc. Note the close proximity of the sympathetic chain to the disc and vertebral margin and also the communication between the nerve root and sympathetic chain just above the level of the disc. R, nerve root; S, sympathetic trunk. (Reproduced from* Textbook of Pain, *by courtesy of Mr JP O'Brien, FRCS, and Churchill Livingstone.)*

These changes are best assessed at axial imaging. The facet joints are orientated sagitally in the lumbar spine, and towards the coronal plane in the thoracic spine.

DISC DEGENERATION

Disc degeneration and narrowing are an inevitable concomitant of ageing and take place at sites of maximal movement in the spine. In the cervical spine degeneration is maximal at C5/6 and in the lumbar spine at L4/5.

Loss of disc height follows disc dehydration and protrusion. As a result, the vertebral end-plates approximate to each other. Facet alignment then alters and degenerative changes occur at the facet joints. Exit foraminal encroachment results, compounded by thickening and redundancy of the yellow ligaments (Figure 8.8; Table 8.1).

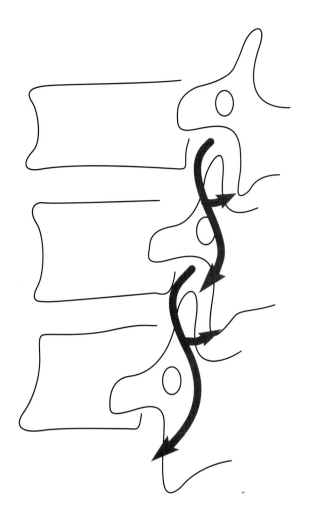

Figure 8.6 *Innervation of the facet joints. Note the nerve branches supplying the facet joint at both the level of the nerve root and the one below. (Reproduced from Griffiths HJ (1991)* Imaging of the Lumbar Spine, *Aspen Publications, by courtesy of the author and the publishers.)*

Table 8.1 Summary of plain film change associated with disc degeneration.

Discal narrowing
Marginal new bone formation
Reactive sclerosis at end-plates
Vacuum phenomena
Facet hypertrophy, slip and resulting vertebral
   malalignment on lateral views
Exit foraminal encroachment

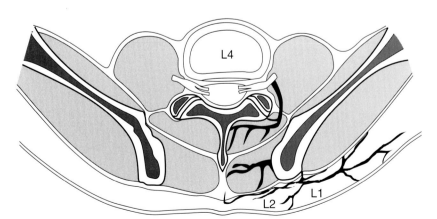

Figure 8.7 *Axial section of the spine and associated structures at L4 to illustrate the different innervations at the same anatomical level. (Reproduced from* Textbook of Pain, *by courtesy of Mr JP O'Brien, FRCS, and Churchill Livingstone.)*

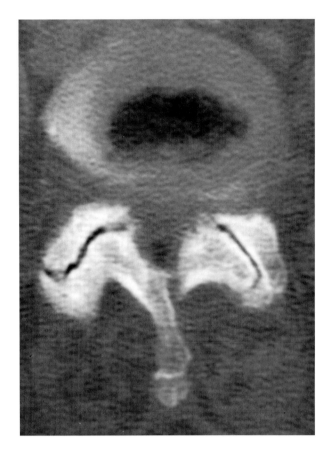

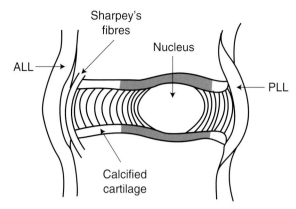

Figure 8.9 *Anatomy of the discovertebral junction (after Resnick, 1995). The nucleus pulposus is situated posteriorly and is associated with a depression on the adjacent end-plate. The nucleus lies within the annulus. This has concentric fibres. The outer fibres of the annulus, or perivertebral ligaments, are attached to the cortex of the vertebral body by Sharpey's fibres. The anterior longitudinal ligament (ALL) is less well attached to the disc than is the posterior longitudinal ligament (PLL).*

Figure 8.8 *Degenerative facet disease in the lower lumbar spine at CT scanning. There is narrowing and irregularity of the facet joints associated with new bone formation at the joint margins. Vacuum phenomena are shown in both joints. In addition, there is vacuum phenomenon in the adjacent disc. Note that the facet joints are situated at the level of the intervertebral disc.*

Posterior circumferential fissures in the annulus occur naturally in the lower lumbar spine in the second decade. Subsequently, the nucleus starts to dehydrate and radial annular tears arise. Discal loading results in further annular fissuring, nuclear protrusion and end-plate fractures, not to be confused with Schmorl's nodes which are smoothly corticated defects in end-plates through which blood vessels passed in infancy.

The inner majority of fibres of the annulus are attached to the cartilaginous end-plate above and below; the stronger outer fibres, also called perivertebral ligaments, run more vertically and are attached to the vertebral body cortex by Sharpey's fibres (Figure 8.9). There is in addition, according to Griffiths (1991), a local interosseous ligament originating 1–2 mm above the disc, on the anterior aspect of the vertebral body, and inserting 1–2 mm below the disc, this running outside Sharpey's fibres (Figure 8.9).

There is some confusion in the literature as to the aetiology and situation of the peridiscal ossification occurring in various diseases. It seems to be accepted that it is the Sharpey's fibres which ossify vertically at the margin of the disc in anklylosing spondylitis, while the new bone formation in psoriasis, Reiter's syndrome and diffuse idiopathic skeletal hyperostosis (DISH) (Table 8.2) is in connective tissue peripheral to the annular margin and, indeed, this change is confirmed at radiology. What is undoubtedly the case radiologically is that the claw or traction spurs in degenerative disease originate 1–2 mm away from the vertebrodiscal margin, have an initially horizontal and subsequently vertical orientation, and lie in ligamentous structures which are displaced by bulging of the disc. The bulging of the disc is itself a consequence of annular tearing, degeneration and instability. The resulting stress causes spurs to form 1–2 mm above or below the vertebrodiscal margin; these subsequently enlarge to become 'claws' (Figure 8.10).

Table 8.2 Causes of paraspinal ossification.

Ankylosing spondylitis
Diffuse idiopathic skeletal hyperostosis
Fluorosis
Hyperparathyroidism
Hypoparathyroidism
Infection
Neuropathy
Ochronosis
Osteoarthritis
Pseudohypoparathyroidism
Psoriasis
Reiter's syndrome
Trauma
X-linked hypophosphataemic osteomalacia

Marginal spurs seen on the plain film are associated with annular tears at discography (qv), where contrast passes from the nucleus towards the spur, often coming to lie over the upper surface of the spur, usually on the superior end-plate of the body below the affected disc.

Reactive sclerosis beneath the end-plates

New bone formation in degenerative disease is more prominent in males than in the elderly, often osteoporotic, female. Buttressing osteophytosis occurs on the concavity of a degenerative scoliosis (Figure 8.11) rather than on the convexity, as a result of the deformity but also preventing further deformity.

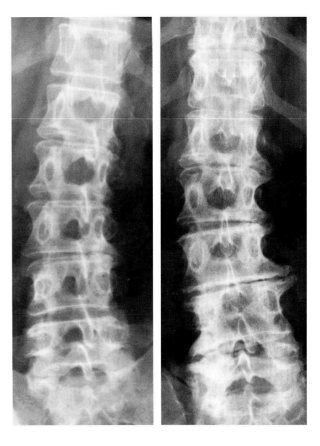

Figure 8.11 *Osteophytes in osteoarthritis. A scoliosis concave to the left and buttressing osteophytes on the concavity are demonstrated in these two radiographs taken over an 11-year period. The osteophytes are well corticated, rather thick structures which are horizontally directed. Syndesmophytes are more vertically directed.*

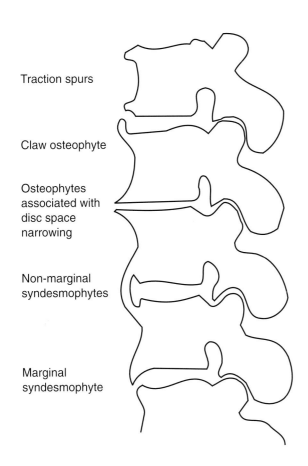

Traction spurs

Claw osteophyte

Osteophytes associated with disc space narrowing

Non-marginal syndesmophytes

Marginal syndesmophyte

Figure 8.10 *Traction spurs, osteophytes and syndesmophytes.*

Table 8.3 Causes of reactive sclerosis around the vertebro-discal margins.

Secondary to disc degeneration*
Infection
Metastases
Ankylosing spondylitis (the Andersson lesion)*
Neuropathic spine*

*May be secondary to local hypermobility.

Quite intense sclerosis may develop around severely degenerative discs, that is, in association with discal narrowing. There is little or no associated bone destruction and no local soft tissue mass, as might be seen with infection, and the bone margins are sharp and well defined. There should be no abnormal clini-

cal features of infection or of seropositive or seronegative spondylarthritis at haematological investigation. Malignant deposits, especially from the prostate or occasionally breast, may cause a similar appearance with bone sclerosis, but a bone scan will usually show widespread change and haematological changes are found (Table 8.3).

Subend-plate sclerosis can be seen on the plain films (Figure 8.12a), and at CT scanning as areas of high attenuation (Figure 8.12b). At MRI scanning, cortical bone has a low signal (Figure 8.12c) and reactive changes in the subend-plate marrow have been classified by Modic et al (1988) (Table 8.4).

The vacuum phenomenon

Dehydration and fissuring within the degenerating disc may be associated with the presence of gas in

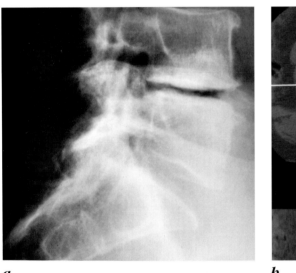

a

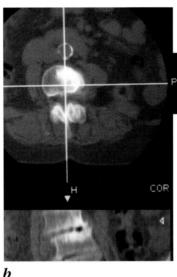

b

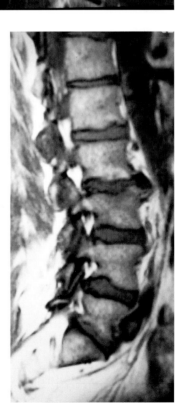

c

Figure 8.12 *Lumbar spine degeneration. (**a**) The lateral radiograph shows a grossly degenerate L4/5 disc with a vacuum phenomenon and surrounding reactive sclerosis in the overlying bone. Anterior claw spurs are also demonstrated. There is facet slip with exit foraminal encroachment. (**b**) End-plate sclerosis at disc degeneration. The CT scan with sagittal and coronal reconstructions demonstrates disc narrowing, marginal new bone formation, vacuum phenomena and reactive sclerosis in the adjacent vertebral bodies. (**c**) Degenerative disease of the lumbar spine in another patient (sagittal T$_1$-weighted MR sequence). Here, the L2/3 disc is affected. There is discal narrowing, anterior claw formation with an anterior discal bulge and reactive changes in the overlying bone. Only a minor dorsal bulge is shown.*

Table 8.4 Disc degeneration: reactive changes in subend-plate marrow at MRI.

Modic Type	Increased signal	Decreased signal
I	T_2W*	T_1W**
II	T_1W and T_2W	—
III	—	T_1W and T_2W

*T_2-weighting
**T_1-weighting
(After Modic MT, Steinberg PM, Ross JS et al (1988) Degenerative disk disease: assessment of changes in vertebral body marrow with MR imaging. *Radiology* **166**: 193–9.)

the disc—the vacuum phenomenon (Figures 8.8 and 8.12b). It is these clefts which presumably fill with contrast medium at discography. A vacuum phenomenon may even be seen in a discal prolapse, in the canal. The gas, which is mainly nitrogen, arises when negative pressure occurs in the disc, allowing nitrogen to leave the adjacent fluid, the rather more soluble O_2 and CO_2 rapidly going back into solution. The presence of gas in the disc effectively rules out infective discitis, as products of inflammation would then fill the crevices. In extension, the cleft fills with gas (Figure 8.13). Occasionally, avulsion of the disc from the vertebral end-plate occurs after trauma. At discography, contrast medium passes between the end-plate and avulsed disc (Figure 8.14).

Gas may be seen *in* vertebral bodies following collapse in avascular necrosis. This excludes malignancy and infection. The gas vanishes if the patient is left in the recumbent position.

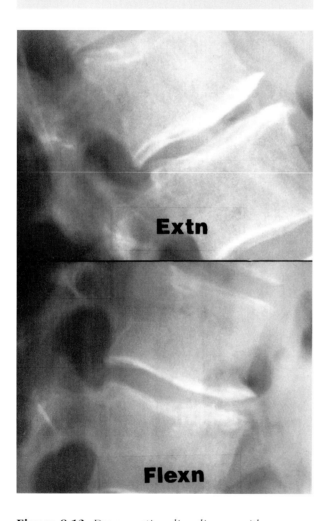

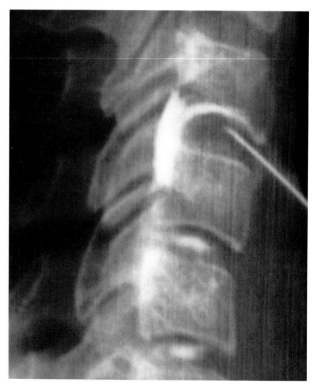

Figure 8.13 *Degenerative disc disease with a vacuum phenomenon in extension. There is discal narrowing with some reactive sclerosis. Anterior traction spurs are demonstrated. The vacuum phenomenon anteriorly is apparent in extension but is less evident in flexion.*

Figure 8.14 *Cervical discography following an acute whiplash injury. Contrast medium passes in a plane between the superior aspect of the disc and the adjacent end-plate and leaks into an extrathecal position. The nuclei below are normal.*

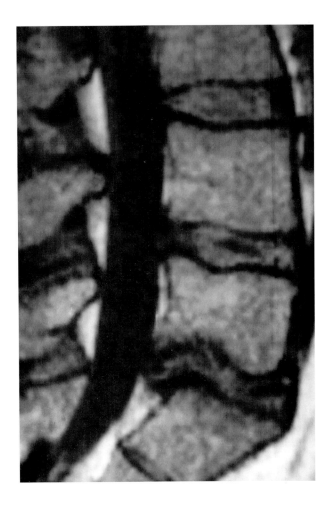

Figure 8.15 *Vacuum phenomenon at MRI (sagittal T₁-weighted sequence). There is retrolisthesis of L5 on S1 and this is associated with a dorsal discal bulge. A vacuum phenomenon is seen anteriorly in this disc. The disc above is also slightly narrowed in height and a vacuum phenomenon is seen here as a band of low signal in the middle of the disc. Here, too, there is a minor dorsal disc protrusion.*

Facet osteoarthritis may also result in a vacuum phenomenon in these small joints (Figure 8.8).

The vacuum phenomenon is also seen at CT as a low attenuation phenomenon (Figures 8.8 and 8.12) and at MR as a low signal area in the disc space (Figure 8.15).

RADICULOGRAPHY

The interior of the spinal canal has long been investigated by introducing contrast medium into the thecal space. Air, oil-based iodinized media, ionic and nonionic water-soluble media have all been used. Nonionic media were latterly used extensively, often in association with CT prior to the advent of MRI, since which the radiculogram is infrequently performed.

Radiculography was used to show cord and root compression and to demonstrate whether a mass lesion was:

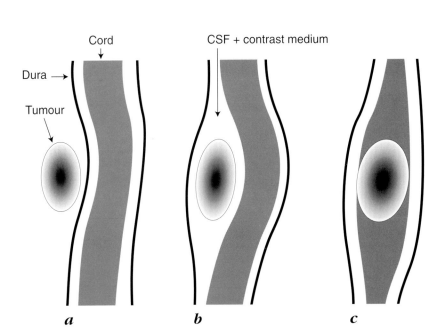

Figure 8.16 *Differentiation at radiculography between (**a**) extradural, (**b**) intradural extramedullary and (**c**) intramedullary mass lesions.*

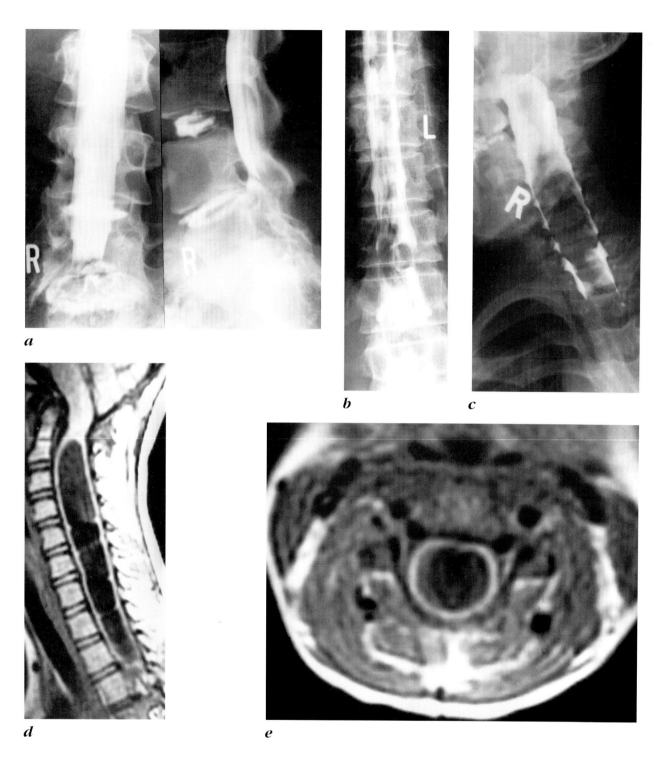

Figure 8.17 (**a**) *Extradural tumour—extradural thecal compression (discoradiculogram). An opacified discal prolapse is demonstrated, compressing the theca from without.* (**b**) *Intradural extramedullary tumour (radiculogram); metastases from a melanoma within the theca displace the cord.* (**c**) *Intramedullary tumour—astrocytoma of the spinal canal demonstrated at myelography. The cord is expanded and occupies most of the cervical canal.* (**d**, **e**) *Intramedullary tumour at MRI—cervicothoracic syringomyelia secondary to cerebellar herniation. This 10-year-old child presented with a painless scoliosis but was neurologically abnormal. Sagittal (**d**) and axial (**e**) T$_1$-weighted MR sequences show the syrinx with cord atrophy.*

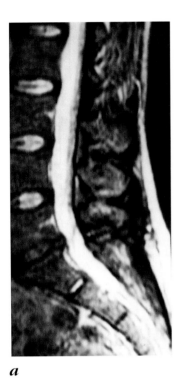
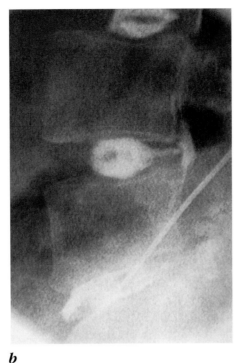

a   *b*

Figure 8.18 *Normal MR; abnormal disc.* (***a***) *The sagittal T₂-weighted MR sequence shows a degenerate L5/S1 disc with signal loss and a dorsal discal protrusion. The L4/5 disc appears entirely normal.* (***b***) *The discogram demonstrates a posterior annular tear at L5/S1 with protrusion of opacified nuclear material into the canal, as shown on the MR image, but also demonstrates a presumably fresh posterior annular tear at L4/5 associated with extrathecal leak of contrast medium tracking down, and up behind L3. The L3/4 disc is normal. The annular tear is presumably too discrete to be seen on MR imaging, while changes of degeneration have not yet arisen.*

(1) *extradural*—such as a prolapsed disc (Figures 8.16 and 8.17a) or vertebral mass, following tumour, trauma or infection
(2) *intradural but extramedullary*—such as neurofibromatosis and meningiomas (see Figure 7.32b) or intradural metastatic seedlings (Figure 8.17b);
(3) *intramedullary*—syrinx or tumour (Figure 8.17c, d, e).

In practice, discal herniation and nerve root compression were the most common indication for radiculography. Arachnoiditis was also well displayed. Lateral disc protrusion could not be shown, but can be seen at CT and MRI.

Currently, CT radiculography is still in use to show lateral recess bone and soft tissue stenosis, and also in dynamic studies e.g. after fusion, in flexion and extension.

If CT or MRI cannot be employed because metal is present around the spine, radiculography is used to show nerve impingement (see below).

MAGNETIC RESONANCE IMAGING AND DISCOGRAPHY

MRI is currently being used as a primary investigation for discogenic and radicular pain. Visualization of unsuspected changes of loss of discal signal and height, and disc protrusion, are often demonstrated at levels removed from the clinical symptoms. There has been a resulting increase in spinal surgery, which may be unnecessary. Disc protrusions can regress spontaneously with time and conservative therapy.

A degenerate disc need not be symptomatic, while a disc that is normal at MRI, at least with current technology, may be abnormal at discography (Figure 8.18). Discography provides an image of normal

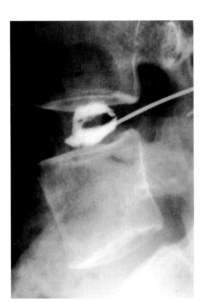

Figure 8.19 *Normal lumbar discogram. Note the 'hamburger' sign with nonopacification of a central nuclear band due to accentuation of fibrous tissue locally.*

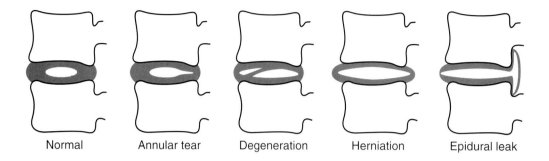

Normal   Annular tear   Degeneration   Herniation   Epidural leak

Figure 8.20 *Disc degeneration—diagrammatic representation of progression of degenerative changes in a lumbar disc, as shown at discography. For an example of a normal discogram see Figure 8.19, a posterior annular tear Figure 8.18b, discal degeneration Figure 8.23b, discal herniation Figures 8.23b and 8.26, and for an epidural leak Figures 8.18b and 8.24a.*

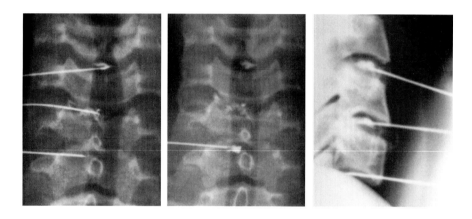

Figure 8.21 *(a) Normal and abnormal cervical discography. Normal nuclei are demonstrated at C4/5 and C6/7 at discography as small, well-localized central collections of contrast, not associated with pain on injection. A degenerative disc shows no central collection of contrast in the nucleus, but rather a diffuse irregular opacification of discal material extending into the adjacent soft tissues.*

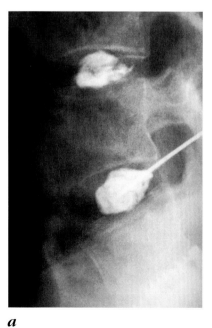

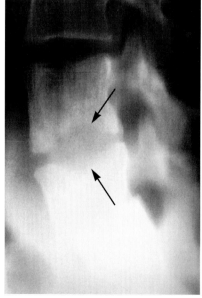

a   *b*

Figure 8.22 *Percutaneous inoculation at discography. (a) The initial radiograph is a discogram showing a normal nucleus and end-plates. (b) The patient subsequently complained of back pain and tomography was performed. This shows end-plate destruction around an infected disc (arrows).*

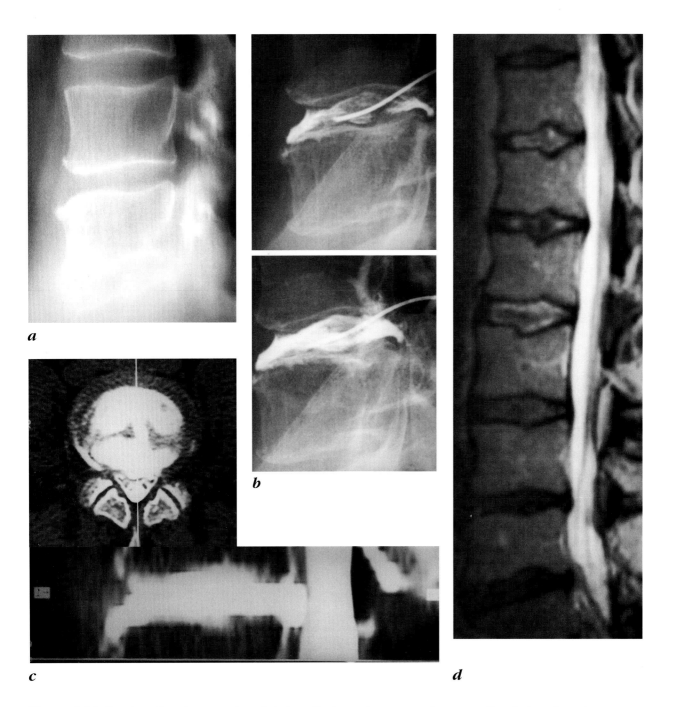

Figure 8.23 *Lumbar disc degeneration. (**a**) A preliminary tomogram shows small anterior claw spurs around the narrowed L4/5 disc, associated with minor retrolisthesis of L4. (**b**) The discogram demonstrates a large anterior annular tear with contrast medium extending to, and sitting upon, the lower claw. There is also a posterior annular tear with a herniation. Vascular filling occurs. This implies inflammatory change around the disc. (**c**) CT discoradiculography confirms the posterior disc protrusion with anterior impression upon the opacified thecal space, seen both on the true axial image and also on the sagittal reconstruction. Here, in addition, the contrast medium passes down antero-inferiorly to the claw spur, and also leaks into the adjacent end-plates. (**d**) On the sagittal T$_2$-weighted MR sequence, the lowest three discs show loss of height and signal, with dorsal discal protrusion at the lowest two levels.*

nuclear anatomy (Figure 8.19) and of discal pathology in disease (Figure 8.20). Discal injection also confirms a particular disc as the pain source (or excludes it), and shows whether adjacent discs are normal or abnormal prior to surgery, and also sources of pain (Figure 8.21). Discography may be complicated by anaphylaxis or spondylodiscitis (Figure 8.22), even when prophylactic antibiotics are used. It is also necessarily painful.

MRI demonstrates spinal anatomy and pathology clearly. Extradiscal structures can be seen and whole areas of the spine can be imaged in one study. The investigation is essentially risk-free.

A plain radiograph is essential prior to discography. Even minor changes on the film—small osteo-phytes (Figure 8.23), retrolisthesis (Figures 8.3 and 8.23) and loss of the lordosis—may be associated with early discal abnormalities. Bone changes reflect disease in the disc.

Simple partial annular tears are not necessarily seen on the MR scan and occur before subsequent changes of dehydration and protrusion (Figure 8.18). In fact, discography mirrors all the discal changes seen at MRI with the possible exception of disc prolapse if the prolapse is not opacified by contrast. Full thickness annular tears allow contrast to pass behind the protruding disc, opacifying it from behind in the extradural space. Contrast also passes into local blood vessels and lymphatics, indicating local vascular invasion of discs and vertebral bone (Figure 8.23c). At

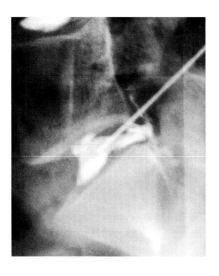

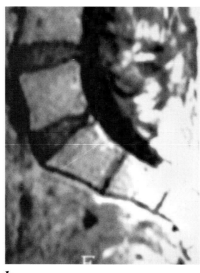

a *b*

Figure 8.24 *The high-intensity zone (HIZ) sign. (**a**) The discogram shows a normal L4/5 disc and, at L5/S1, a posterior annular tear with bulge and leak. (**b**) The sagittal T$_1$-weighted MR sequence demonstrates a high intensity zone in the posterior aspect of the torn L5/S1 disc.*

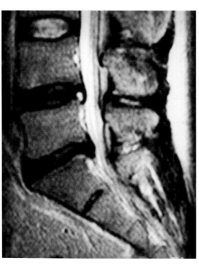

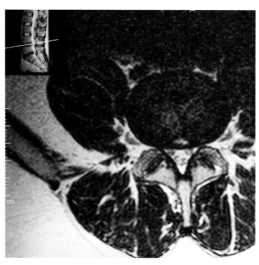

a *b*

Figure 8.25 *The HIZ sign. Sagittal (**a**) and axial (**b**) T$_2$-weighted MR sequences showing the posterior high intensity zone.*

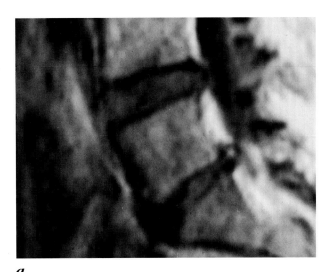

a

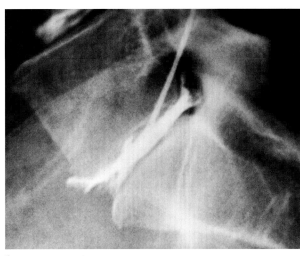

b

Figure 8.26 *The HIZ sign demonstrated on a sagittal T$_1$-weighted MR image (**a**). At discography (**b**), the posterior part of the prolapsed disc corresponding to the high-intensity zone does not opacify.*

MRI the high-intensity zone (HIZ) sign at a discal margin is an uncommon indicator of an annular tear (Figures 8.24, 8.25 and 8.26).

INVESTIGATION OF THE POST-OPERATIVE SPINE

Lateral mass or discal fusions are often best seen with linear tomography, but this is falling into disuse. Detail is better than with coronal or sagittal CT reconstructions. Pseudarthroses after fusion may be demonstrated on radionuclide bone scans as foci of increase in uptake, especially at SPECT imaging.

While recurrent discal or soft tissue masses can be seen with CT, MRI is the investigation of choice after the plain film. Recurrent discal or fibrous masses causing root entrapment are clearly seen. Vascular masses enhance with intravenous gadolinium (Figure 8.27); nonvascular fibrous masses do not. If MRI is not available or is contraindicated, radiculography is valuable, especially in the presence of radicular signs, in conjunction with CT scanning.

SPONDYLOLYSIS AND SPONDYLOLISTHESIS

Pars defects can occur without vertebral slip, and slip can occur without pars defects.

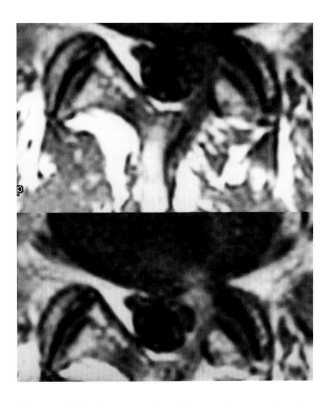

Figure 8.27 *Post-operative MR imaging pre- (top) and (bottom) post-gadolinium enhancement demonstrates the presence of vascular granulation tissue in the left lateral recess. Deep enhancement indicates an annular tear.*

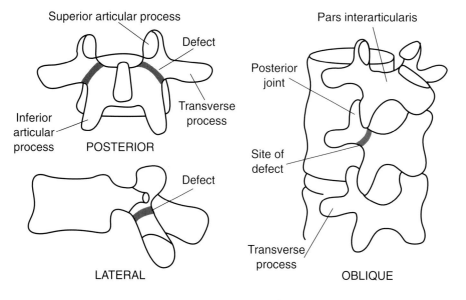

a

b

Figure 8.28
*Spondylolysis.
Diagrammatic represen-
tation of a lumbar
vertebral body in posterior
and lateral projections
(**a**) and of the spine in
an oblique projection (**b**)
to show the pars defect.*

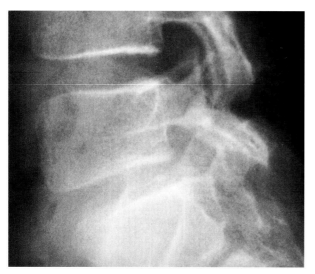

a

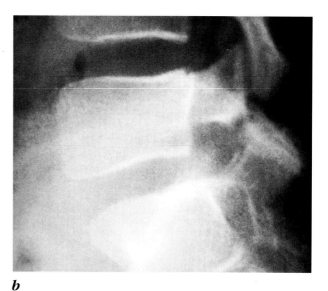

b

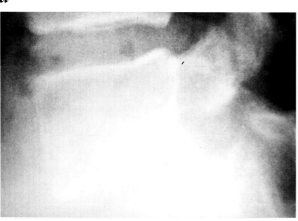

c

Figure 8.29 *Development of spondylolisthesis in a
teenage cricketer. (**a**) The initial radiograph was
passed as normal. No radioisotope bone scan was
undertaken at the time. (**b**) A subsequent
radiograph obtained 6 months later shows that a
pars defect has developed at L5, the margins of
which are already sclerosed. There is minimal
forward slip of L5 on S1. (**c**) Two years later the
defect has widened and the forward slip has
increased. The margins of the pars defect are
sclerosed.*

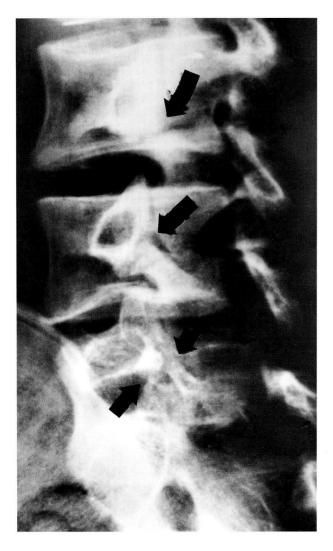

Figure 8.30 *Spondylolysis. Oblique radiograph showing pars defects at L3, L4 and L5.*

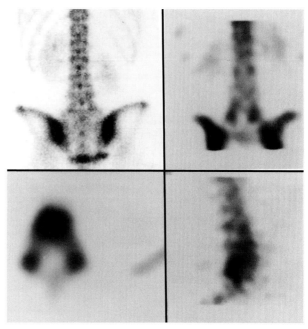

Figure 8.31 *Bilateral pars defects imaged at SPECT. Symmetrical posterior foci of increased uptake are demonstrated at L5 (by courtesy of Dr A Saifuddin).*

Most cases of spondylolysis occur at L5, the fewest at L2 or L3. The latter are often associated with abnormal bone, e.g. osteomalacia or osteopetrosis, or with unusual stresses—trampolining or fast bowling in cricket (Figures 8.28 and 8.29).

Some defects may be congenital, most presumably are acquired stress lesions. Lesions often never heal and pseudarthroses, often painful, are found. Local pain provocation injection confirms the pain source. Lesions may be unilateral or bilateral.

Often seen on AP and lateral plain films, the oblique view clearly shows the pars defect (Figure 8.30). Radionuclide bone scanning is often strongly positive in the presence of a painful defect, presum-

ably where local movement takes place, often associated with bone sclerosis around the defect. SPECT demonstrates the posterior location of the focus of increase in uptake (Figure 8.31). Sclerotic unilateral lesions may resemble an osteoid osteoma on plain films and radionuclide bone scanning.

CT is probably the most effective technique for identifying a pars defect, but the facets are often a cause of confusion. Generally, the facet joints are oblique, symmetrically smooth and well corticated. They lie at the level of the *disc* and just below it. Pars defects are irregular, fragmented and poorly corticated. There may be loose adjacent flakes of bone. They lie at the level of the *transverse processes*, just above the upper level of the exit foramen (Figure 8.32).

MRI is less helpful in showing pars defects than CT, which generally is better at demonstrating bone (Figure 8.33). Slip at pars defects—*spondylolisthesis*—occurs in younger, male patients. The degree of slip is graded in fourths of the lower vertebral body end-plate. Slip may occur in the absence of a defect, if degeneration is present, usually at L4. The slip can occur at facet joints, or the pars may become thinned and elongated. A classification exists (Wiltse et al 1976).

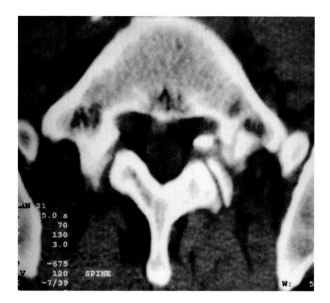

Figure 8.32 *CT of the lumbar spine with a pars defect clearly separate from the left facet joint. The facet joint is well defined, the pars defect irregular and associated with anterior fragmentation of bone.*

Degenerative changes are inevitably present in the intervening disc at MRI and discography, and spurs are seen anteriorly on the vertebral bodies. With chronic slip, the displaced body is often deformed and hypoplastic posteriorly. This is usually not the case with a recent slip in adult life.

The theca and nerve roots are angled over the lower body. This is seen at radiculography and at MR imaging (Figure 8.34). Axial CT and MR images show an elongated sagittal diameter of the canal above the affected disc (Figure 8.33b), then a discal bulge or pseudobulge, often surprisingly minor, and a narrowed canal below the disc. Facet joints contain synovial fluid on T_2-weighted MR sequences.

Nerve roots are identified at radiculography and at axial CT or MR imaging.

RETROLISTHESIS

This is commonly seen on plain films, often in association with posterior annular tears at discography, even in the absence of significant discal degeneration.

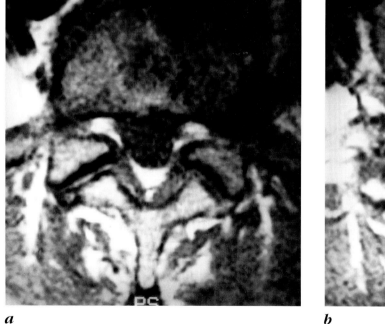

a

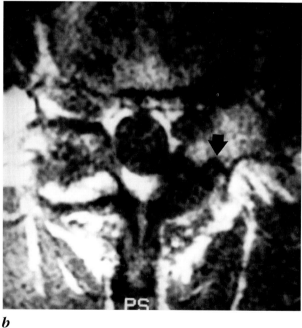

b

Figure 8.33 *Facet joints and pars defects at MR imaging. Axial T_1-weighted MR sequences showing (**a**) normal facet joints and (**b**) pars defects (arrow). (**a**) The facet joints are smooth, obliquely situated and well corticated. (**b**) Pars defects are less well-defined at MR imaging than at CT. The canal is elongated at the level of the slip. The pars defects are seen as irregular low signal bands crossing the laminae.*

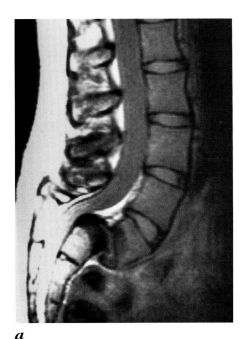 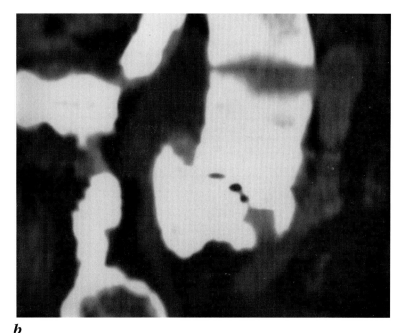

a   *b*

Figure 8.34 *(a) Sagittal proton density weighted MR sequence (midline scan) showing a dysplastic spondylolisthesis with modelling changes on the adjacent vertebral body surfaces, reflecting the chronicity of the disease. (b) Sagittal CT reconstruction showing degeneration of the intervening disc with local claw formation (By courtesy of Dr A Saifuddin).*

SPONDYLARTHROPATHIES

RHEUMATOID ARTHRITIS IN THE SPINE

Cervical spine

Involvement of the cervical spine is of the greatest clinical significance in rheumatoid arthritis. In patients with chronic disease, up to 80% develop disease in the cervical spine.

Changes at the C1/2 level are the most important and reflect the local anatomy. A synovial sac is present between the front of the odontoid peg and the back of the arch of atlas. Proliferative synovitis erodes the adjacent articular surfaces (Figure 8.35). Erosions are seen on the lateral and open mouth AP views, on tomography and on CT scans (Figure 8.36). The anatomy is also demonstrated at MR imaging and pannus is especially well shown by this technique (Figures 8.37 and 8.38). The C1/2 facet joints may also erode (Figure 8.35).

Local hyperaemia results in laxity of the transverse ligament of the atlas which passes behind the dens. An apical ligament extends from the tip of the dens to the anterior margin of the foramen magnum, and this too may be weakened. Instability occurs in up to 40% of rheumatoid patients and is seen in flexion, when a gap of more than 2.5 mm between peg and arch is said to be pathological. Cord compression by the peg may result after ligamentous disruption (Figure 8.37). In infants, up to 4.5 mm is allowed.

The peg may sublux superiorly towards or through the foramen magnum, resulting in brain stem compression. Lateral subluxation may follow erosive disease at the lateral masses between C1 and C2 and the occiput and C1 (Figure 8.35).

In rheumatoid arthritis, vertebro-discal changes are more proximal than is the case in osteoarthritis. Disc space narrowing, end-plate irregularity, overall osteopenia and relative absence of marginal osteophytosis differentiate this change from osteoarthritis (Figures 8.37 and 8.39). Multiple levels are involved

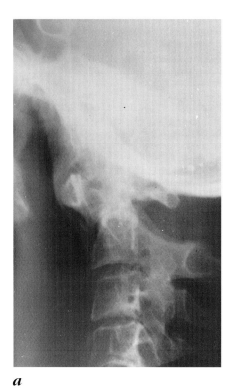

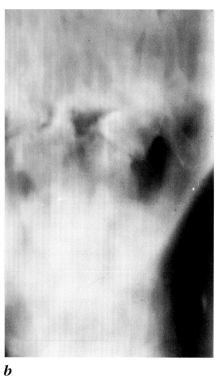

a   *b*

Figure 8.35 *Rheumatoid arthritis. (**a**) The lateral view shows an increase in the space between the odontoid peg and the arch of the atlas. In this patient it is greater than the normal 2.5 mm. The peg is barely visible on this radiograph. (**b**) An AP tomogram shows upward subluxation of a very eroded peg together with irregularity at the C1/2 facets. The odontoid peg is displaced to the right.*

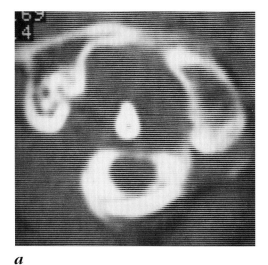

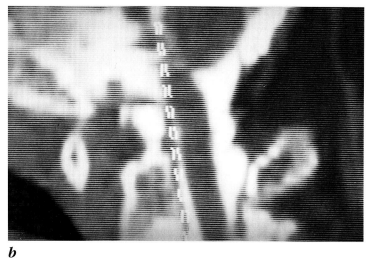

a   *b*

Figure 8.36 *Rheumatoid arthritis at CT radiculography. (**a**) The axial image shows a thinned and narrowed odontoid peg substantially separated from the arch of the atlas by a soft tissue mass. (**b**) The sagittal reconstruction shows a thinned and eroded odontoid peg separated from the arch of the atlas and upwardly subluxed; its tip reaches the foramen magnum.*

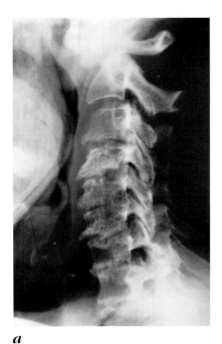

a

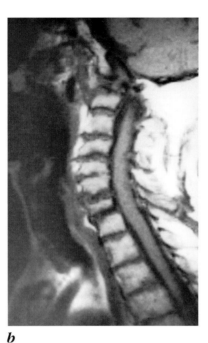

b

Figure 8.37 *Rheumatoid arthritis. (**a**) The plain film shows marked forward subluxation of C1 upon C2. The peg is barely visible but would lie halfway between the anterior and posterior arches of C1. This is associated with osteoporosis and subsequent bony ankylosis across the discs. There is secondary osteoarthritic change with anterior new bone formation. The irregularity of the end-plates in the upper cervical region is a characteristic feature of rheumatoid arthritis, distinguishing it, together with the fusion, from osteoarthritis, where change is inferior and fusion does not occur. (**b**) On this sagittal* T$_1$-*weighted MR sequence the odontoid peg is barely visible. Its remnant protrudes upwards surrounded by pannus. The cord is compressed behind C2. There is end-plate irregularity, as shown on the plain film. Fusion is occurring across discs.*

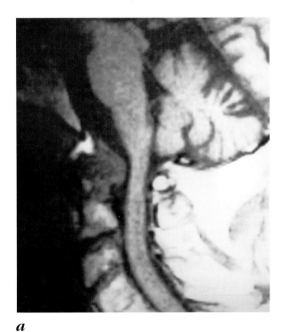

a

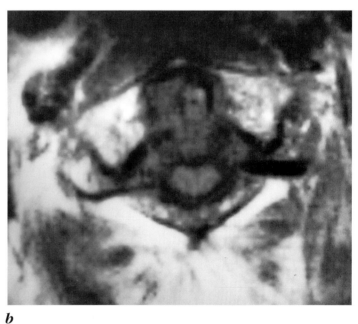

b

Figure 8.38 *Rheumatoid arthritis. (**a**) On the sagittal* T$_1$-*weighted MR image, the hypertrophied pannus is seen as a large soft tissue mass eroding the odontoid peg and compressing the cord. (**b**) The axial* T$_1$-*weighted MR sequence shows pannus and erosion with displacement of the peg.*

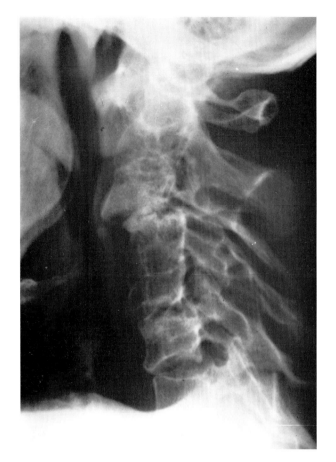

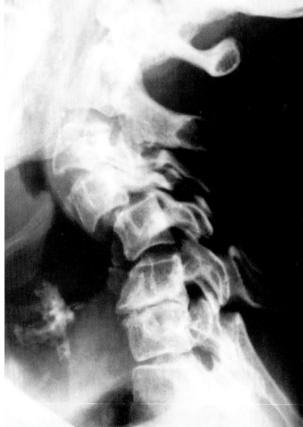

Figure 8.39 *Cervical spine in rheumatoid arthritis. The space between the odontoid peg and the arch of the atlas is increased. Disc spaces are narrow and irregular from C2 downwards. Subluxation is present. The facet joints are eroded and the spinous processes thin and tapered. Vertebral body fusion is also present in the mid-cervical spine.*

Figure 8.40 *Rheumatoid arthritis. There is instability with forward slip of C3 on C4 and C4 on C5. The facets are elongated and subluxed at those levels. The spinous processes are thinned posteriorly.*

but local soft tissue swelling is not conspicuous, unlike infection.

Erosion of the cervical spinous processes occurs; this is an enthesopathy and not the result of synovial proliferation (Figure 8.40).

Thoracic and lumbar spine

Changes in the lower spine are less usual than in ankylosing spondylitis. Patients with rheumatoid arthritis may develop infections; disc narrowing, end-plate sclerosis and fragmentation and a soft tissue mass in the absence of a vacuum phenomenon should raise the possibility of vertebro-discitis. Sacro-iliac joint changes are unilateral, erosive and do not usually result in fusion.

SERONEGATIVE SPONDYLARTHROPATHIES

The seronegative spondylarthropathies, including ankylosing spondylitis, psoriasis and Reiter's syndrome, have distinguishing features, but also many features in common.

ANKYLOSING SPONDYLITIS (Figure 8.41)

In ankylosing spondylitis, the vertebral bodies should be inspected for signs of erosion followed by healing at the margins of the upper and lower end-plates, initially at the thoraco-lumbar junction, but eventually throughout the spine. Syndesmophytes form as vertically directed spurs of new bone in the annulus (see pages 359–60), which bridge the normal disc spaces, and eventually unite (Figure 8.42a). This change follows erosion at the vertebro-discal margin (Figure

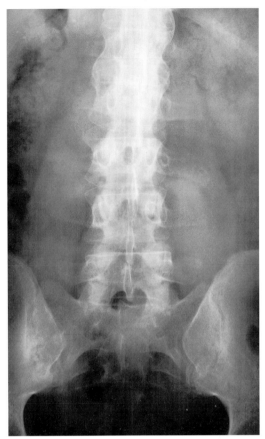

a

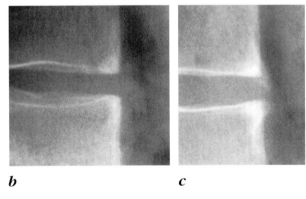

b   *c*

Figure 8.42 *Ankylosing spondylitis. (**a**) There is an early sacro-iliitis, worse on the right than on the left. Syndesmophytes are established at the thoraco-lumbar junction. An early syndesmophyte may be seen on the right on the upper surface of L3. (**b**) In the same patient, there is early erosion followed by sclerosis at the vertebrodiscal margin (Romanus lesion). Squaring is also evident with filling of the space beneath the anterior longitudinal ligament. (**c**) Subsequently a syndesmophyte develops. This change took 4 years to develop.*

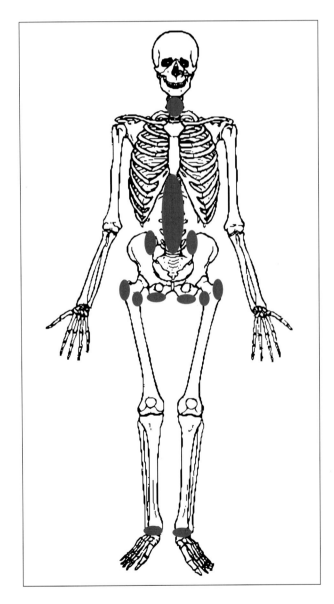

Figure 8.41 *The major sites of involvement of ankylosing spondylitis (shaded areas).*

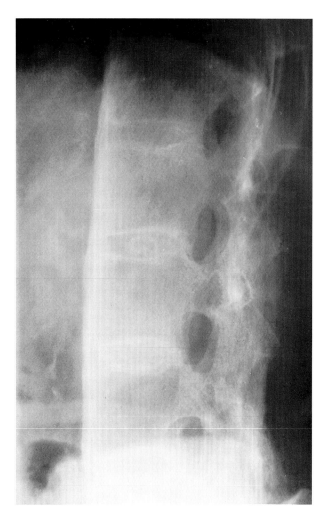

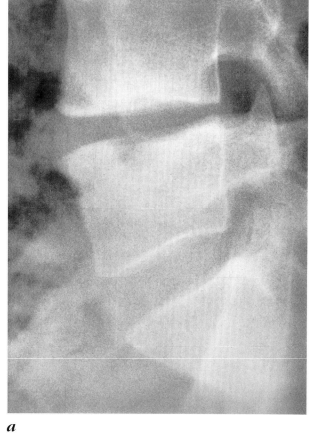

a

Figure 8.43 *Ankylosing spondylitis. There is loss of normal curvature with squaring of vertebral bodies and ossification of the anterior longitudinal ligament. Nuclear calcification occurs in vertebral fusion.*

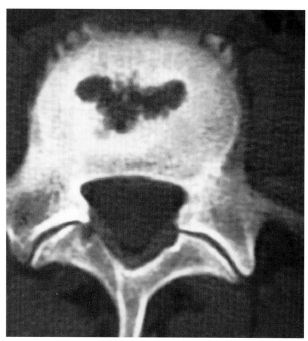

b

Figure 8.44 *Andersson lesion. (**a**) The plain film shows end-plate irregularity around the narrowed L4/5 disc associated with reactive sclerosis. There is vertebral squaring with new bone forming on the anterior aspect of L4. (**b**) The CT scan of L5 shows the vertebral end-plate defect with reactive sclerosis and new bone formation on the anterior aspect of the vertebral body.*

8.42b,c). In rheumatoid disease, erosions occasionally become corticated but only infrequently heal with proliferative new bone formation and 'whiskering'.

Romanus lesions

Vertebro-discal marginal erosions in ankylosing spondylitis may subsequently sclerose; these are the Romanus lesions (Figure 8.42b,c). In any case, vertebral 'squaring' results. Squaring also results when new bone is laid down beneath the anterior longitudinal ligament (Figures 8.43 and 8.44a).

Andersson lesions

Reactive sclerosis is seen at end-plates in the spine in ankylosing spondylitis. The degree of sclerosis varies in extent across the surfaces of the vertebral bodies. Reactive sclerosis may be seen centrally, marginally or across the entire end-plate. The sclerosis may extend into the body for a considerable extent, and the articular surfaces may be irregular (Figure 8.44).

The appearances thus resemble an infective spondylitis (Table 8.3). The disc space may be narrowed or obliterated and vertebral alignment may be abnormal. There should, however, be no significant soft tissue mass.

Other spinal changes

Adjacent marginal syndesmophytes in the outer annular fibres meet at the margin of the usually intact disc and are convex outwards, so that when they meet, a bamboo stick is mimicked in appearance (Figure 8.45). They should be distinguished from osteophytes, which are a feature of degeneration, are horizontally directed and associated with discal narrowing (Figure 8.10).

Paraspinal syndesmophyte formation also occurs in X-linked hypophosphataemic osteomalacia (Figure 8.46), often accompanied by sacroiliac joint fusion, and without such fusion in pseudohypoparathyroidism and, rarely, in hyperparathyroidism as well as seronegative spondylarthropathies.

In the cervical spine, changes occur from C2 down in continuity, and may indeed be the presenting symptom in the juvenile form of the disease (Figure 8.47).

In the thoracic spine, a smooth kyphoscoliosis is often seen in adult life in association with osteoporosis. Fusion is demonstrated at costotransverse joints and between spinous processes. Discal calcification is shown, as well as annular ossification.

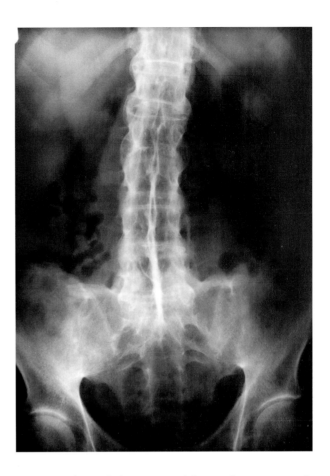

Figure 8.45 *Ankylosing spondylitis with symmetrical fusion of the sacroiliac joints. A bamboo spine is present. There is paraspinal ossification, which is marginal in some places and nonmarginal in others. Ossification of the interspinous ligaments is seen.*

Neuropathic spine and the role of instability

Grosser changes of end-plate irregularity, sclerosis, fragmentation and discal narrowing may be seen in patients with a neuropathy (Figure 8.48) and also following major trauma to the spine with instability, e.g. after a car crash.

Patients with ankylosing spondylitis have a rigid osteoporotic spine. Should they trip and fall, spinal fractures may occur. These can be cervical, thoracic or lumbar, with resulting neural deficit.

Fractures occur (1) through the ossified disc and (2) adjacent to the end-plate. The fracture line continues across the canal into the posterior elements. A

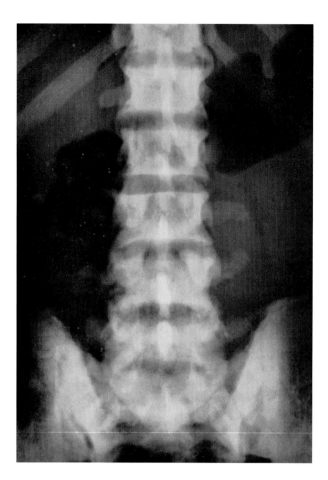

Figure 8.46 *This patient has X-linked hypophosphataemic osteomalacia with paradiscal syndesmophyte formation. The sacroiliac and spinal changes resemble those seen in ankylosing spondylitis, but the bones are dense and there is bowing of the long bones. Such bowing is not present in fluorosis.*

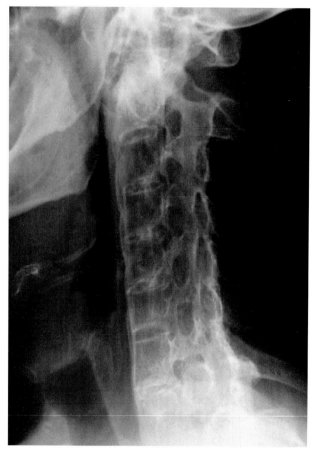

Figure 8.47 *Ankylosing spondylitis. There is loss of normal curvature in the cervical region with squaring of vertebral bodies and ossification of the anterior longitudinal ligament. Discal calcification occurs in areas of vertebral fusion.*

pseudarthrosis with instability results and a neuropathic pattern emerges, with all the features mentioned above (Figure 8.49). Lateral views taken in flexion and extension show the instability and the fracture line opens up upon extension.

DIFFUSE IDIOPATHIC SKELETAL HYPEROSTOSIS (DISH; FORESTIER'S DISEASE)

Diffuse idiopathic skeletal hyperostosis (DISH) is more common in older men who generally have well-preserved bone density. Ossification of musculo-tendinous insertions is a general feature, so that there is dense, prominent new bone formation, for example at iliac crests, ischia, iliac spines and trochanters (Table 8.2, page 360).

In the spine, the new bone is particularly dense and prolific, seeming to flow in continuity over four or more vertebral bodies with relative or total preservation of the underlying discs. Indeed, the extradiscal new bone probably prevents discal narrowing. New bone formation is much more profuse than in degenerative disc disease and, of course, in the latter, discal narrowing accompanies the osteophytes.

In the cervical spine, the change occurs especially from C4 down (Figure 8.50). The accretion of new bone is such that it may equal the sagittal diameter of the underlying vertebral bodies. Local pseudarthroses

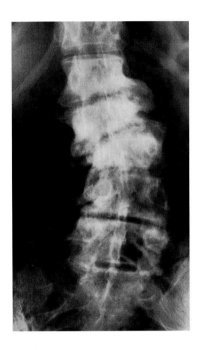 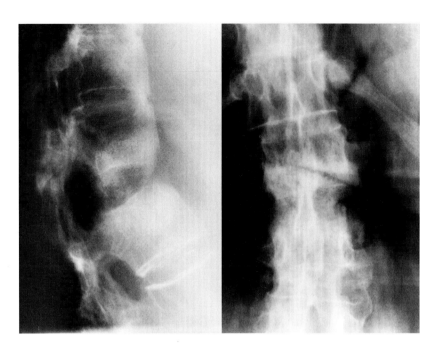

Figure 8.48 *Charcot spine with instability, discal narrowing, vertebral body resorption and sclerosis in this patient with neurosyphilis.*

Figure 8.49 *Ankylosing spondylitis—Romanus lesions and trauma. The lateral view of the lumbar spine demonstrates marked squaring of the vertebral bodies, and superior and inferior erosion of the anterior vertebral margins, accompanied by local sclerosis. A fracture has occurred through an affected disc space, which is therefore widened with posterior facetal dislocation. This is a relatively uncommon complication of ankylosing spondylitis and follows a fall. Patients may end up paraplegic. Hypermobility and instability occur at the level of the fracture and result in end-plate irregularity visible on the AP view.*

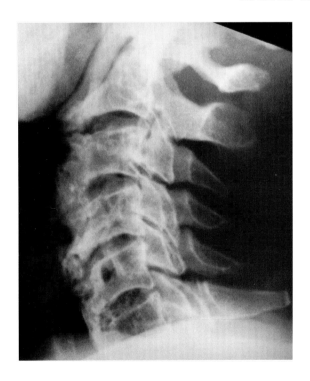

Figure 8.50 *Diffuse idiopathic skeletal hyperostosis (DISH). Marked new bone formation is demonstrated anterior to the vertebral bodies from C2 down. In places the new bone is continuous but pseudarthroses are seen.*

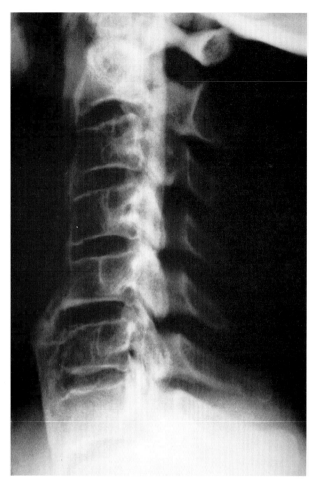

a

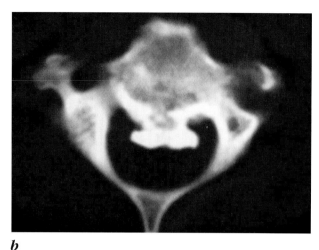

b

Figure 8.51 *DISH and ossification of the posterior longitudinal ligament (OPLL). (**a**) The lateral view shows quite marked skeletal hyperostosis from C5 down. The bone is smooth and continuous. The disc spaces are well preserved. Lesser changes are seen from C2 down. OPLL is demonstrated posteriorly from C2 to C5. (**b**) The CT scan shows new bone formation anteriorly on the vertebral body and posteriorly in OPLL. The canal is substantially narrowed at the level.*

and clefts may be seen in the new bone. Severe dysphagia may result from oesophageal impression.

An association occurs with *ossification of the posterior longitudinal ligament* (OPLL). This may occur as an isolated phenomenon and is more common in Japanese. It can result in cord compression (Figure 8.51).

DISH is most commonly present in the mid and lower thoracic spine and is often seen on the chest radiographs of middle-aged and elderly patients as prominent, anterolaterally directed, continuous spurs of bone, mainly on the right side (not usually on the left side because of the pulsation of the descending aorta, unless a right-sided descending aorta is present). DISH is also commonly seen on CT scans of the thorax or abdomen. Sometimes the aorta sits between two spurs; stress trabeculae extend into them (Figure 8.52). Peridiscal ankylosis may result in nuclear calcification, as in ankylosing spondylitis.

In the lumbar spine, the changes are most prominent superiorly, that is from L1 to L3. Disc spaces are relatively less likely to be narrowed in DISH (Figure 8.53). New bone formation in degenerative disc disease is more prominent in the lower lumbar spine.

Besides the changes in the pelvis mentioned above, that is, of new bone formation at musculotendinous insertions (Figure 8.54), ossification of ileosacral ligaments also occurs and generally at musculotendinous insertions from the neck to the tarsus (Figure 8.55). This new bone formation is less commonly seen in elderly females, who are more osteoporotic, outside of the thoracic spine. Laboratory findings are normal.

Bone changes in ankylosing spondylitis start earlier and are inevitably associated with true sacroiliac joint fusion. New bone and syndesmophyte formation is generally rather more delicate and not so florid in ankylosing spondylitis.

REITER'S SYNDROME AND PSORIASIS

Syndesmophyte formation here may be nonmarginal or 'floating', that is, not attached to a vertebral body at all (Figure 8.56).

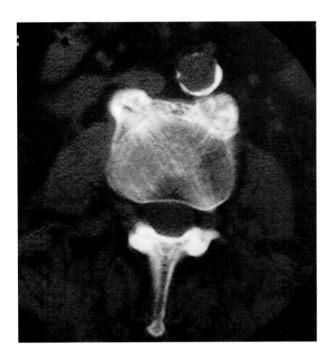

Figure 8.52 *CT of the lumbar spine in a patient with DISH. Note the stress lines leading to the new bone.*

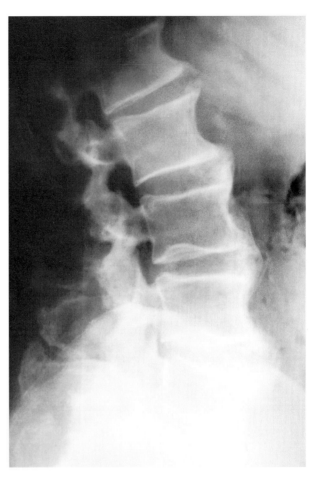

Figure 8.53 *DISH of the lumbar spine. There is new bone around the discs in association with well preserved disc spaces.*

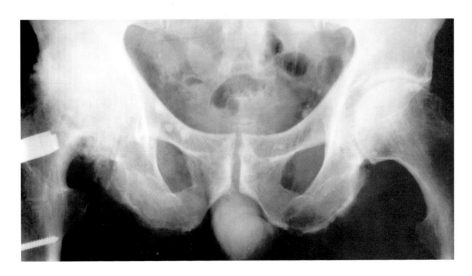

Figure 8.54 *This patient with DISH has osteoarthritis of the right hip and preserved bone density. There is whiskering at the ischia, but the sacroiliac joints are patent.*

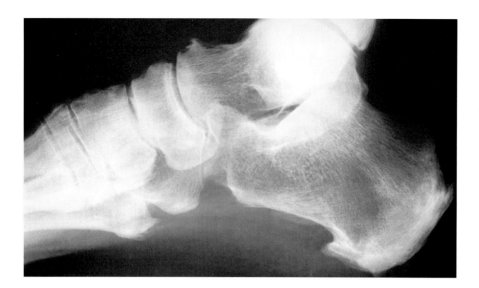

Figure 8.55 *DISH. A talar beak is present and new bone is also seen on the adjacent navicular. New bone formation is also present posteriorly and inferiorly on the calcaneus and on the base of the fifth metatarsal.*

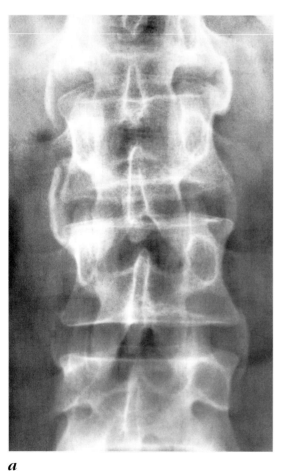

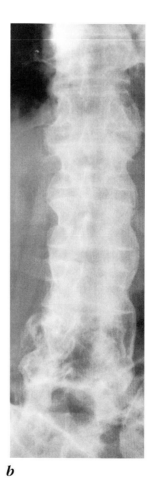

a

b

Figure 8.56 *(a) Psoriatic spondylitis. There are both bridging nonmarginal and floating syndesmophytes, more typical of psoriasis and Reiter's syndrome than of ankylosing spondylitis, though they may also be seen in the latter (by courtesy of Dr JT Patton). (b) Reiter's disease. Paraspinal new bone can be seen around the discs, but is not attached to the vertebral margin. A floating or nonmarginal syndesmophyte is more typical of Reiter's disease.*

CHANGES AT SACROILIAC JOINTS

In ankylosing spondylitis erosions occur initially on the lateral margins of the sacroiliac joints at the mid or lowest portions. The upper parts of the sacroiliac joints are not synovial, but bound only by ligaments. Erosions make the articular cortices indistinct. Ankylosing spondylitis almost inevitably proceeds to symmetrical involvement of the sacroiliac joints; in Reiter's syndrome and psoriasis, however, the sacroiliac joints may remain unilaterally involved (Figure 8.57).

Eventually, in ankylosing spondylitis, the medial cortices of the sacroiliac joints erode, reactive sclerosis is seen behind and between erosions, and the joints fuse. Confirmation of fusion may often be obtained by oblique views, or prone views, supine 30° shoot-up views, all at plain radiography (Figure 8.58) or, best of all, CT scanning (Figure 8.59). The inferior margin of the joint at the pelvic brim shows bony continuity, confirming fusion. Isotope bone scans may be positive even before plain film changes occur, but fused sacroiliac joints may be normal if the disease is quiescent. Radionuclide bone scanning gives a ratio of sacroiliac to sacral uptake of more than 1.4:1 in ankylosing spondylitis, but this examination is little used (Figure 8.60).

Bilateral erosions followed by fusion are the pathognomonic findings in ankylosing spondylitis. Changes in these joints are difficult to assess in children as their sacroiliac joints appear wider and more poorly corticated than in the adult, and are often apparently hotter on the bone scan. Changes at the sacroiliac joints are unusual, however, in juvenile ankylosing spondylitis below the age of 18 years.

In DISH, sacroiliac joint fusion may be found on an AP radiograph of the pelvis (Figure 8.61), but CT scans usually show anterior or posterior ankylosis. Only infrequently is the joint space itself obliterated.

Erosions are more likely to be unilateral in infection (Figure 8.62), psoriasis (Figure 8.63) and Reiter's syndrome (Figure 8.57).

Erosions occur elsewhere at characteristic sites in ankylosing spondylitis and the seronegative spondylarthritides. The ischia and pubic bones (Figure 8.64), femoral trochanters, calcaneal bones (Figure 8.65) and iliac blades are eroded and heal with the formation of new bone extending perpendicularly into the soft tissues, a phenomenon which has been described as 'whiskering' (Figure 8.64).

Lateral sclerosis of some depth occurs on the iliac sides of the sacroiliac joints as a stress phenomenon,

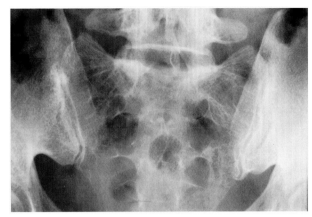

a

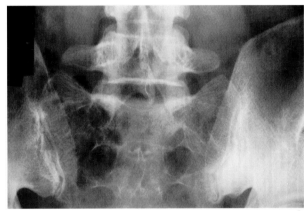

b

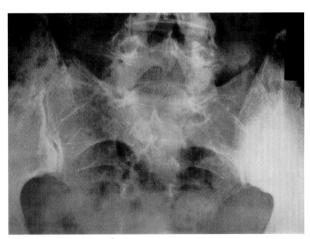

c

Figure 8.57 *Reiter's syndrome. The three radiographs taken over a 12-year period demonstrate the progression of a unilateral sacroiliitis.*

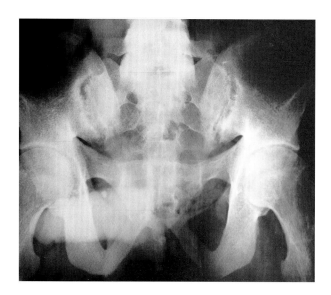

Figure 8.58 *As ankylosing spondylitis progresses, erosive change is evident on both sides of the sacroiliac joints, symmetrically and bilaterally. In this patient the changes of an erosive arthritis are also present at the hips, and appear more severe on the left side, where the joint space is reduced and the articular surfaces are irregular. There is little reactive sclerosis. 'Whiskering' is seen at the ischia (shoot-up view).*

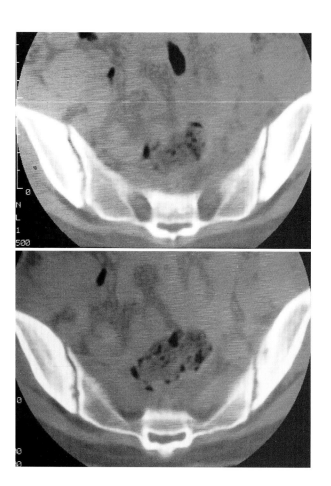

Figure 8.59 *Early ankylosing spondylitis. The CT scans show sclerosis and erosions on the lateral sides of the joints.*

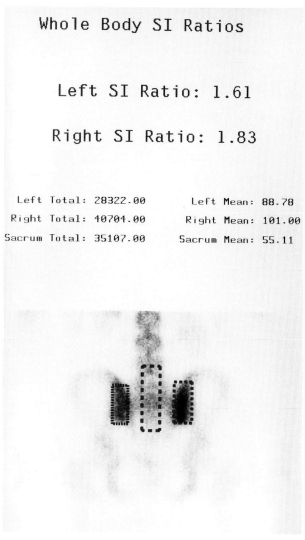

Figure 8.60 *Ankylosing spondylitis. Posterior radio-isotope bone scan to show the sacroiliac joint/sacral uptake ratios. There is greater uptake in the right sacroiliac joint than on the left. The mean uptake on both sides is given, together with the mean uptake in the sacrum (by courtesy of Dr A Hilson).*

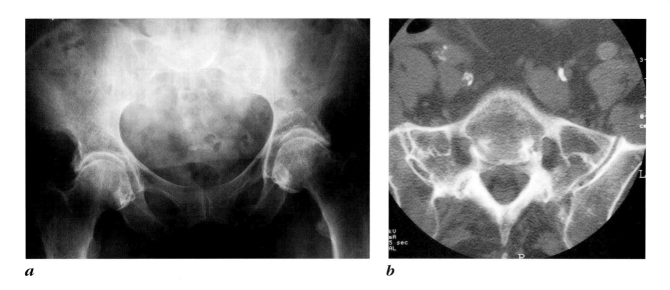

a *b*

Figure 8.61 *DISH. (**a**) The plain film shows right sacroiliac joint fusion. There is also new bone formation in the region of the anterior inferior iliac spines. (**b**) A CT scan demonstrates new bone on the anterior aspect of the first sacral vertebra together with sacroiliac joint fusion on the right.*

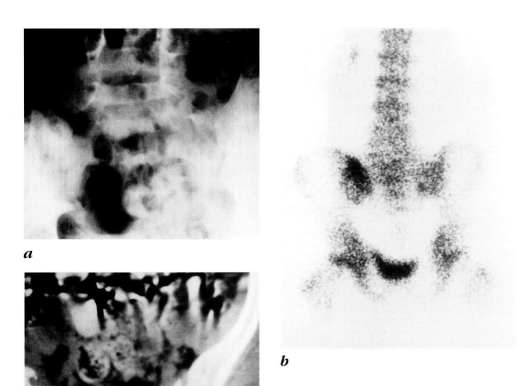

a

b

c

Figure 8.62 *Infective sacroiliitis. (**a**) The plain film shows widening of the right sacroiliac joint. Detail is obscured by bowel. The left sacroiliac joint appears normal. (**b**) The radioisotope bone scan shows local increase in uptake. (**c**) The CT scan shows the abnormal sacroiliac joint and local soft tissue thickening (by courtesy of Professor H Carty).*

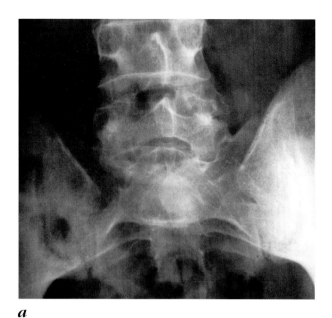

a

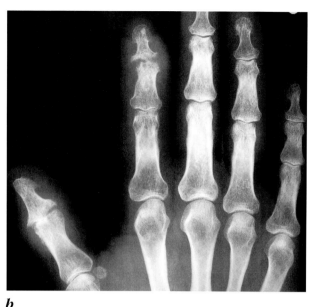

b

Figure 8.63 *Psoriasis. (**a**) A unilateral sacroiliitis is demonstrated. (**b**) Gull's wing appearances are shown at the bases of the distal phalanges of the thumb and index finger. Overlying soft tissue swelling is prominent.*

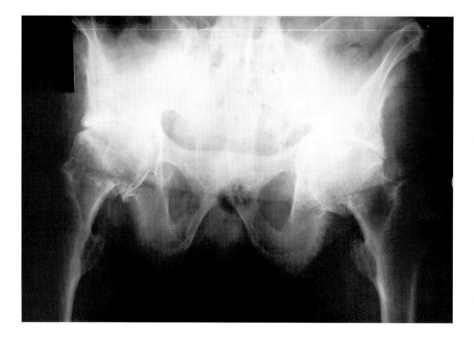

Figure 8.64 *Ankylosing spondylitis. The sacroiliac joints are fused, with little or no reactive sclerosis; the disease is quiescent. Both hip joints are narrowed. The femoral heads have a fringe of new bone around them—another feature of ankylosing spondylitis. Much irregular new bone is laid down upon the ischia, the original contours of which can still be seen. Similar fringing occurs at all the muscle attachments. The symphysis pubis is also fused and there is ossification of the interspinous ligaments.*

for example with a scoliosis, or in osteitis condensans ilii, in the absence of erosions (Figure 8.66).

Fusion is the end-stage of sacroiliitis in ankylosing spondylitis (Figure 8.45) but is also seen in other conditions (Figures 8.61 and 8.67).

FLUOROSIS

Fluorosis is usually associated with drinking water containing more than 8 parts/million of fluorine and occurs in endemic areas. The bones are increased in

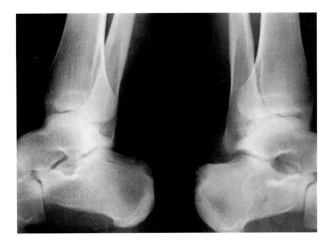

a

Figure 8.65 *Ankylosing spondylitis. (**a**) Erosions can be seen on the posterior aspects of the calcaneal bones. In this patient these are at the insertion of the Achilles tendons and also superiorly in the region of the retrocalcaneal bursa. (**b**, **c**) Sagittal T₂-weighted MR sequences show posterior calcaneal erosions, Achilles tendinitis and retrocalcaneal bursitis (arrow).*

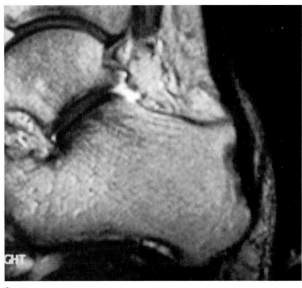

b

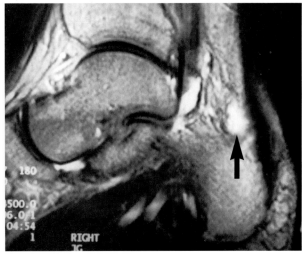

c

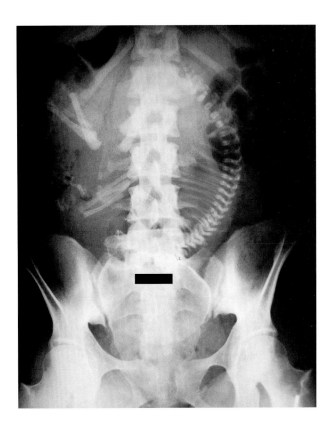

Figure 8.66 *Osteitis condensans ilii in pregnancy. These changes usually follow multiple pregnancies. Note the separation of the symphysis pubis.*

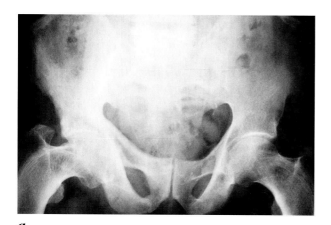

a

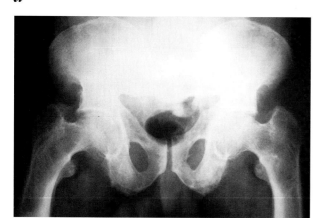

b

Figure 8.67 *Apparent sacroiliac fusion. This is seen in diseases other than the seronegative spondylarthropathies. (**a**) Paget's disease. (**b**) X-linked hypophosphataemic rickets. It also occurs in DISH (see Figure 8.61) and in thalassaemia.*

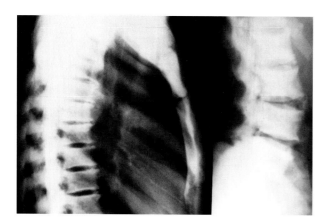

Figure 8.68 *Fluorosis. An increase in bony density is associated with paradiscal ossification.*

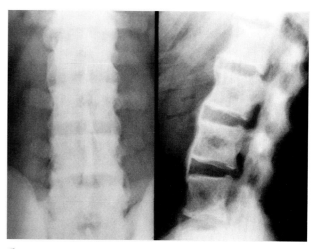

a

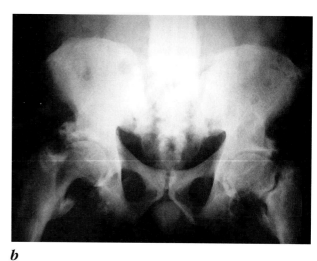

b

Figure 8.69 *X-linked hypophosphataemic osteomalacia. (**a**) The lumbar spine shows increase in bony density and marked new bone formation around the annulus at multiple levels. The facet joints are poorly visualized. (**b**) In the pelvis an increase in bony density is associated with marked new bone formation at the musculotendinous insertions throughout the pelvis and proximal femora. In addition, a Looser's zone through the left femoral neck has extended to cross the entire bone. The fracture is wavy rather than straight. Looser's zones need not be straight, but may be serpiginous. The sacroiliac joints appear fused but the film is underpenetrated for this region.*

density and new bone extends into soft tissues beneath the ribs, around the pelvis and at other insertions (Figures 2.54 and 8.68). These changes should not be confused with the increase in bony density and cortical thickening seen in osteopetrosis, where the bones are diffusely expanded (see Chapter 2, pages 95–97).

X-LINKED HYPOPHOSPHATAEMIC OSTEOMALACIA

The bones become thickened with increase in density; bowing of long bones is a characteristic feature. Looser's zones are seen, and whiskering occurs at musculotendinous insertions, as well as paraspinal ossification (Figures 8.46, 8.67b and 8.69).

SPINAL INFECTION

Simple infection, usually due to *Staph. aureus*, *E. coli* or *Salmonella*, enters the vertebral body:

(1) by haematogenous spread. This may be via the arteries entering at the posterior aspect of the vertebral body through the posterior foramen or via penetrating arteries entering the cortex from the surrounding soft tissues;

(2) via Batson's valveless vertebral venous plexus. This system allows malignant disease to metastasize from the pelvis to the spine and, similarly, pelvic infections, especially from the bladder, to infect the vertebrae;

(3) by direct inoculation at discography or percutaneous discectomy (Figure 8.22);

(4) by contiguous spread from a site already involved. An infection spreads via the disc to adjacent vertebrae or beneath the anterior longitudinal ligament to the vertebral body above or below (Figure 8.70). Local soft tissue infections can spread to the underlying bone. *Grisel's syndrome* of cervical vertebral instability follows a retropharyngeal abscess or a foreign body in the precervical soft tissues; infection results in ligamentous laxity and subluxation (Figure 8.71).

Types of spread (Figure 8.72)

(1) Infection starts beneath the vertebral end-plate in the subend-plate vascular cysterns, spreads through the end-plate into the adjacent disc and subsequently into the vertebral body above or below. The elderly are especially affected, often those with chronic urinary tract infections. Pain, spasms and fever are found, together with haematological features of infection—raised erythrocyte sedimentation rate, c-reactive protein and white cell count.

While the radiographs may be normal initially, the radionuclide bone scan will be abnormal early on in the disease. The plain film appearances lag behind changes demonstrated at radionuclide bone scanning (Figure 8.73) and MRI. Local loss of bone density is followed by cortical destruction (Figure 8.22), especially well seen by comparison with normal end-plates elsewhere. Disc destruction follows and disc height is lost. In malignant disease, loss of disc height follows herniation into the diseased body without actual loss of discal mass.

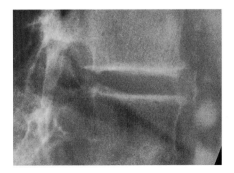

a

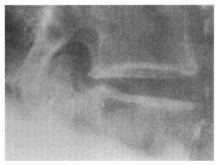

b

Figure 8.70 *Infective spondylodiscitis. (**a**) This radiograph shows disc space narrowing and some loss of definition of adjacent end-plates. (**b**) After 3 weeks there is further destruction of the surrounding vertebral bodies by infection.*

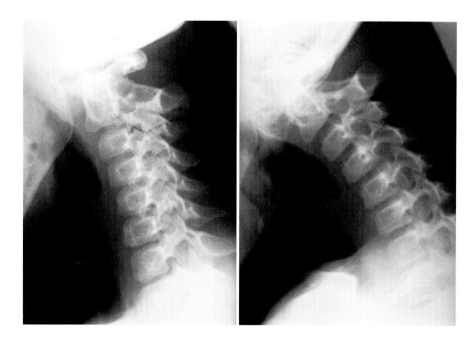

Figure 8.71 *Grisel's syndrome. Soft tissue swelling is demonstrated anterior to C1 and C2 and there is instability in flexion, as shown by forward slip of C1 on C2.*

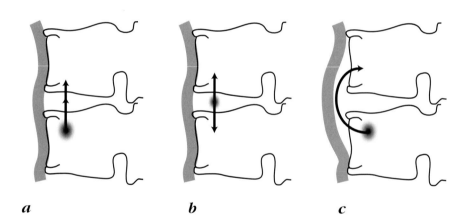

a   *b*   *c*

Figure 8.72 *Types of spread from a septic focus in bone and disc: (**a**) originating in the subend-plate region of bone, (**b**) in the disc and (**c**) subligamentous spread.*

Similarly, end-plate depressions in Scheuermann's disease also result in loss of disc height, but the end-plates are sclerotic, even if irregular.

Subsequent extension into the adjacent vertebral bodies causes further bone destruction, involving first the cortex, then the medulla. These changes may be obscured by overlying gut gas. Linear tomography shows the lesions more clearly and gives a more accurate estimation of the area of destruction, often showing it to be larger than the area seen on the plain film.

CT scanning with sagittal and coronal reconstruction is of similar value in assessing cortical, medullary and disc destruction. Soft tissue masses around infected vertebrae are also clearly seen on axial scans.

MRI demonstrates both anatomic change and local features of inflammation. Trabecular and end-plate destruction, and marrow and discal inflammatory changes are seen. If marrow is mainly red, inflammatory changes are best seen as an increase in signal on T_2-weighted sequences or as an area of signal loss in fat on T_1-weighted images (Figure 8.74). Gadolinium results in an increase in signal on T_1-weighted sequences.

(2) Infection may arise directly in the disc, especially in adolescents, as blood vessels still penetrate the end-plates to enter the discs. Subsequently, the disease spreads to adjacent end-plates and vertebral bodies.

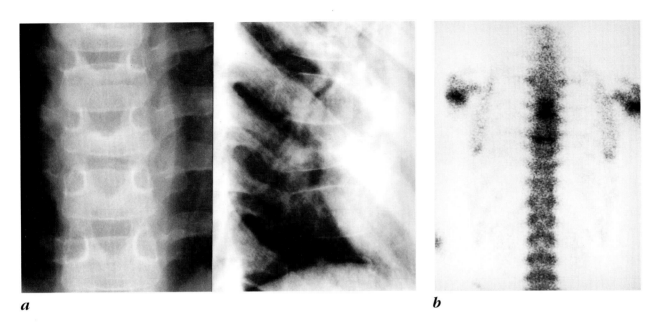

a   *b*

Figure 8.73 *Spinal osteomyelitis at T8.* (***a***) *On the plain radiographs destruction of the upper surface of the vertebral body of T8 is associated with a paraspinal soft tissue mass, which is widest at the point of vertebral body destruction. The lower end-plate of T7 is intact.* (***b***) *The radionuclide bone scan shows increase in uptake at T8 but also at T5, which is radiologically normal.*

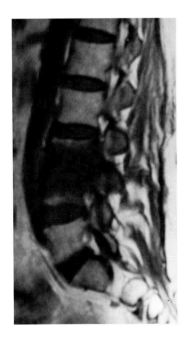

Figure 8.74 *Spinal osteomyelitis. Loss of signal affects the disc and adjacent vertebral bodies. The inflammatory process replaces fat in this sagittal T$_1$-weighted MR image.*

In all cases, posterior extension into the spinal canal is demonstrated at CT and MR imaging.

The presence of a vacuum phenomenon indicates an absence of inflammatory change; when a vacuum phenomenon vanishes and adjacent end-plates lose density or clarity, infection in the elderly patient is quite likely (Figure 8.75).

TUBERCULOUS SPONDYLITIS

This disease is rarely seen in the UK, but occurs (1) in immigrants from Asia and Africa, (2) in those who are immune-compromised and (3) in those living in poor or crowded environments such as hostels, or in vagrants. Fifty per cent of patients have evidence of tuberculosis on a chest radiograph.

Some 50% or more of cases of skeletal tuberculosis occur in the spine (Figure 8.76), often at the cervicothoracic, thoraco-lumbar or lumbosacral junctions. The anterior aspects of the vertebral bodies are often involved and large soft tissue masses result (Figure 2.34). Paraspinal abscesses are formed, clearly seen on plain films due to displacement of the overlying psoas fat stripe or lung (Figure 8.77).

(3) Subligamentous spread beneath the anterior longitudinal ligament causes anterior erosions of adjacent vertebral bodies. Here, soft tissue masses are especially prominent and enhance with gadolinium.

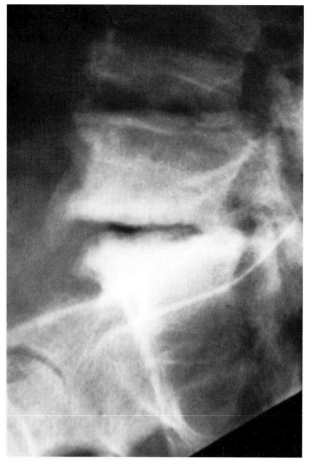

a

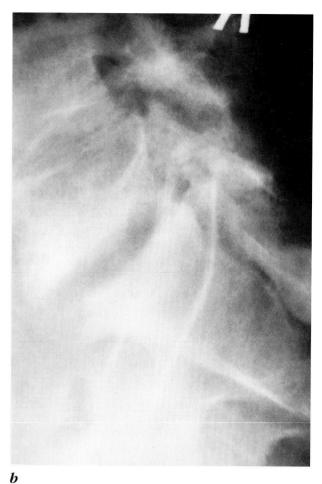

b

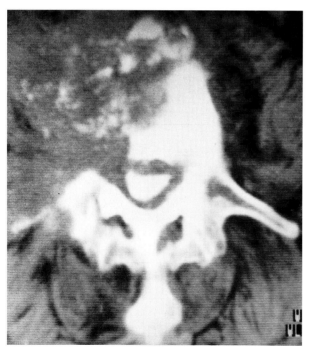

c

Figure 8.75 *Spinal osteomyelitis. (**a**) There is forward slip of L5 on S1 with obliteration of the disc space. A vacuum phenomenon is demonstrated. There is new bone formation anteriorly and reactive sclerosis at the end-plates. (**b**) A subsequent radiograph shows loss of the vacuum phenomenon and, if anything, an increase in the height of the disc space, presumably due to the infective process. (**c**) A CT scan taken at the time of the last radiograph shows a massive destructive process involving the right side of the vertebral body with a large soft tissue mass in which ossific fragments are demonstrated. The theca is impressed upon.*

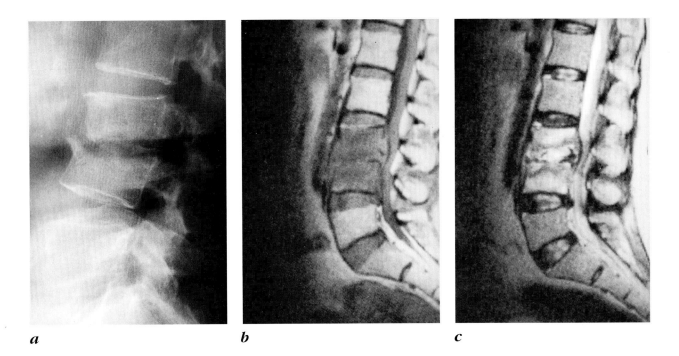

a   b   c

Figure 8.76 *Tuberculous spondylitis. (**a**) End-plate and discal destruction with the beginnings of a kyphos are seen. (**b**, **c**) The sagittal T$_1$- (left) and T$_2$-weighted (right) MR sequences show extensive vertebrodiscal destruction with oedema in the underlying bone. The spinal canal is encroached upon by a soft tissue inflammatory mass.*

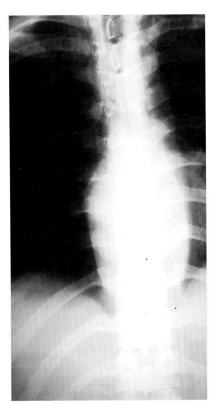

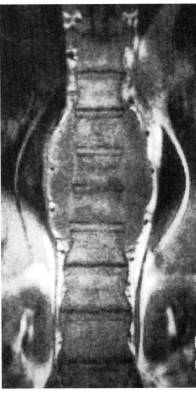

a   b

Figure 8.77 *Spinal tuberculosis. (**a**) Extensive paraspinal soft tissue swelling extending from T6 to T10 is shown on the plain radiograph. The disc spaces between T6 and T8 are poorly visualized. (**b**) The coronal T$_1$-weighted MR image demonstrates discal and end-plate destruction and large soft tissue masses on either side of the spine.*

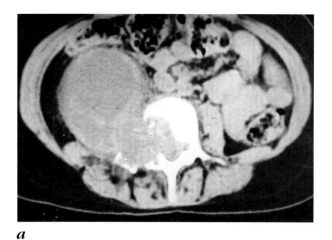

a

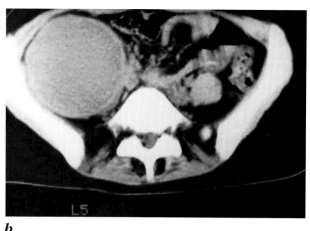

b

Figure 8.78 *Psoas abscess demonstrated at CT scanning. (**a**) A proximal scan of the lumbar spine shows destruction of a vertebral body and a large mass in the psoas which, anteriorly, is of relatively low attenuation, compatible with fluid. The process enters the spinal canal. (**b**) In the pelvis the abscess occupies much of the pelvic cavity. It is well defined and homogeneous, replacing psoas.*

Linear tomography shows the combination of disco-vertebral destruction and a soft tissue mass. Large psoas abscesses extend to the groin.

Psoas abscesses are demonstrated on CT scans in the presence of cortical and medullary bone destruction (Figure 8.78). The lytic lesions in bone are often surprisingly well defined. Multiple vertebral bodies and discs are involved, unlike the situation usually

seen with simple pyogenic disease, where only one to two vertebral bodies may be involved.

The soft tissue abscesses may show areas of differing attenuation at CT scanning with a thick wall surrounding a necrotic centre (Figure 8.78). At MRI, too, communication of the destructive vertebral lesion with the overlying abscess is seen (Figure 8.79), and the extent of the disease can be fully

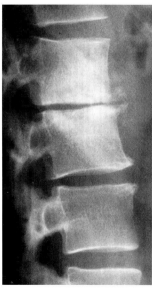

a

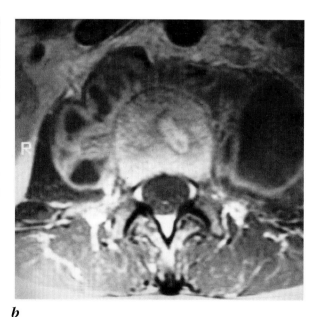

b

Figure 8.79 *Tuberculous spondylitis. (**a**) The plain radiograph shows vertebrodiscal destruction; a soft tissue mass can be seen anterior to the involved segment. (**b**) The axial T$_1$-weighted post-contrast MR image shows vertebral destruction centrally together with large abscesses in both psoas muscles. On the left there is a relatively smooth-walled cavity, while on the right there is a more multilocular thick-walled cavity.*

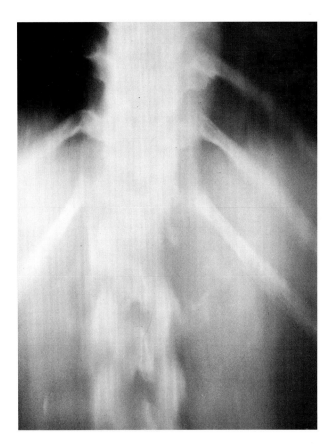

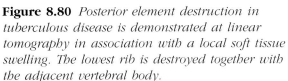

Figure 8.80 *Posterior element destruction in tuberculous disease is demonstrated at linear tomography in association with a local soft tissue swelling. The lowest rib is destroyed together with the adjacent vertebral body.*

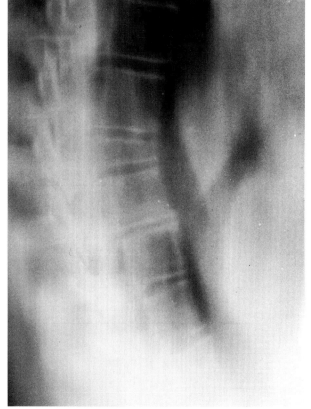

Figure 8.81 *Tuberculous spondylitis in this non-Caucasian patient results in vertebra plana with preservation of discs and end-plates.*

appreciated on sagittal and coronal scans. The abscess itself may be of mixed signal due to the presence of fluid, soft tissue and necrotic tissue. Increased signal on T_2-weighting and fat suppression sequences indicates fluid and inflammation. Vascular granulation tissue shows increased signal on T_1-weighted images after gadolinium.

While anterior subligamentous spread is common and causes anterior vertebral destruction on several adjacent vertebral bodies, a significant proportion (up to 20%) have involvement of the posterior elements. The lateral vertebral margins, transverse processes and laminae must be inspected on plain films (Figure 8.80). Instead of the usual kyphos due to anterior vertebral destruction, posterior collapse results. Ribs or transverse processes become crowded posteriorly. Posterior changes are easily recognized at axial imaging. Cord compression may result.

Vertebra plana with preserved discs and end-plates is occasionally seen, usually in immigrants into the UK (Figure 8.81).

Healing is by bone fusion and soft tissue calcification. Psoas abscesses may show extensive egg-shell, peripheral or central calcification extending to the groin (Figure 8.82). Sedimentation of calcium may be seen in the abscess. Calcification may also be seen within destroyed or fused areas of bone. Reactive bone sclerosis was said to be more common in tuberculosis than in simple infection.

BRUCELLOSIS

This infection, acquired from milk, is prevalent around the Mediterranean and in Saudi Arabia. It should be considered in a patient from these areas presenting with a spondylitis involving a long segment which shows disc destruction and fusion associated with proliferation of sclerotic and irregular bone laid down on affected vertebral bodies. The sclerosis is often more extensive, proliferative and irregular than in other infective lesions (Figures 8.83 and 8.84).

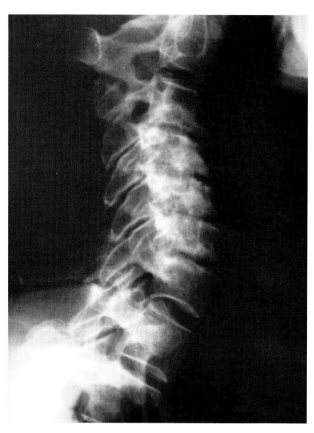

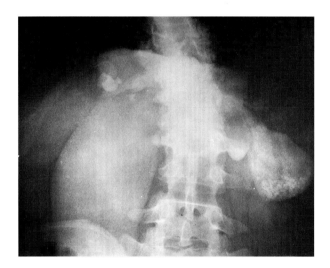

Figure 8.82 *Healed tuberculous disease with large psoas abscesses which are partially calcified. There is spinal destruction and fusion.*

Figure 8.83 *Brucellosis. There is widespread end-plate destruction with subsequent fusion and reactive new bone formation. The sclerosis and irregularity over a wide area of the cervical spine is a feature of brucellosis.*

Figure 8.84 *Brucellosis. (a) In an earlier stage of the disease there are typical changes of infective spondylitis with disc and end-plate destruction, a large soft tissue mass anteriorly and the beginnings of new bone formation. (b) A subsequent radiograph demonstrates reactive sclerosis and further proliferative new bone formation.*

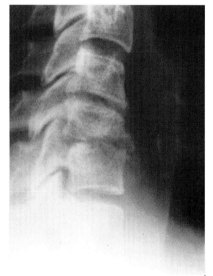

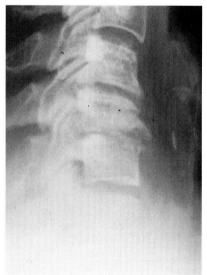

a

b

TUMOURS OF THE SPINE (Table 8.5)

BENIGN TUMOURS

Haemangiomas

These lesions have been found in 11% of anatomic specimens. The lesions are more common in females (M:F = 1:1.5) and occur in an older age group, often over 60 years of age.

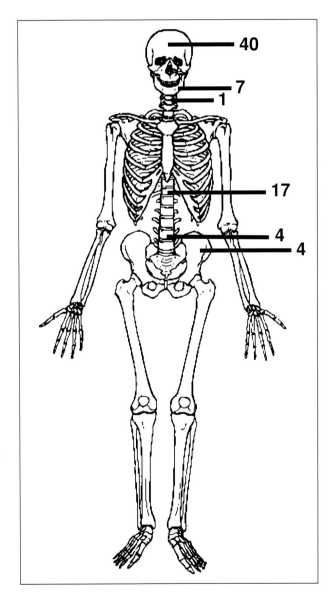

Figure 8.85 *Haemangioma. Sites of percentage distribution at major sites only. (After Unni, 1996, with permission.)*

Table 8.5 Lesions occurring in the spine (after Unni, 1996).

	Spine (%)	Sacrum (%)	Posterior elements (P) Body (A)
Osteochondroma	2.5	0.4	P
Chondroma	1.7	—(<1)	—
Osteoid osteoma	9.0	2.1	P
Osteoblastoma	34.0	9.1	P
Giant-cell tumour	5.5	9.2	A
Haemangioma	25.9	—	A
Fibrous dysplasia	0.71	0.53	A or P
Benign total*	**6.2**	**3.3**	
Myeloma	28.8	4.3	A
Lymphoma	11.8	4.8	P
Chondrosarcoma	6.0	2.6	
Osteosarcoma	2.2	1.1	A
Fibrosarcoma	3.5	7.0	?
Chordoma	14.3	47.4	A>P
Ewing's sarcoma	3.1	6.2	A

*Does not include aneurysmal bone cyst or simple bone cyst.

As only larger lesions are seen on plain films, their incidence is lower. They are rare in the cervical spine and commoner in the thoracic and lumbar spine (Figure 8.85). Smaller lesions are seen at MRI.

Multiple lesions are seen in at least 30% of patients and are of two types: (1) multiple primary lesions or (2) diffuse cystic angiomatosis without periositis.

Plain film changes are those of residual vertical trabeculation or honeycomb-like spaces en face (Figure 8.86). The cortex is thinned but vertebral expansion is absent. They are diagnosed on CT scanning as a low attenuation area within sparse but thickened trabeculae (Figure 8.87).

At MRI the lesions are bright on T_1-weighted images because they are high in fat, which contributes the bulk of signal from these tumours (Figures 8.88 and 8.89). On T_2-weighted sequences the lesions can also be of high signal intensity. Subarticular haemangiomas may resemble Modic Type II changes, i.e. bright on T_1- and T_2-weighted sequences (see page 362). It seems that a high amount of fat in a haemangioma indicates benignity, while a low level of fat at MRI indicates a more aggressive lesion.

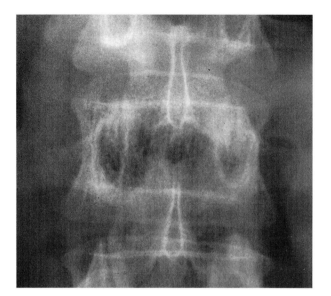

a

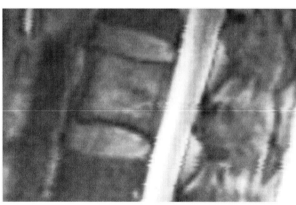

c

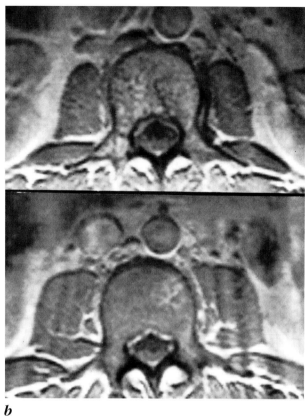

b

Figure 8.86 *Haemangioma of the spine. (**a**) On the plain radiograph the lumbar vertebral body is not expanded. The cortices are present but thinned. Residual vertical trabeculation is shown. (**b**) Axial T$_1$-weighted MR sequences show areas of increased signal compatible with fatty change in a haemangioma. (**c**) The sagittal T$_2$-weighted MR image shows a rather more diffuse increase in signal, not as bright as the fluid in the adjacent CSF space.*

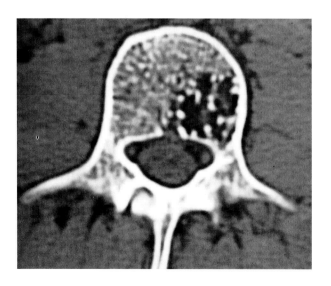

Figure 8.87 *Haemangioma at CT scanning. Residual vertical trabeculae remain in an area of low attenuation.*

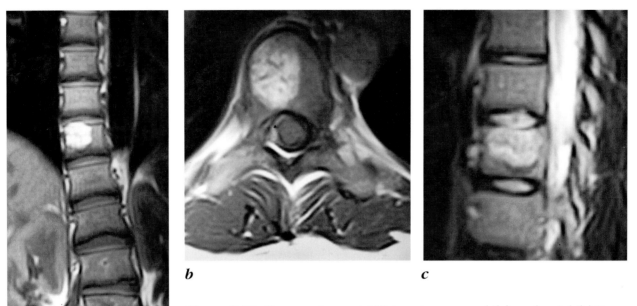

Figure 8.88 *Haemangioma at MR imaging: coronal (**a**) and axial (**b**) T$_1$-weighted and (**c**) sagittal T$_2$-weighted sequences. The low signal material in the lesion in (**b**) is presumably related to residual bone trabeculation.*

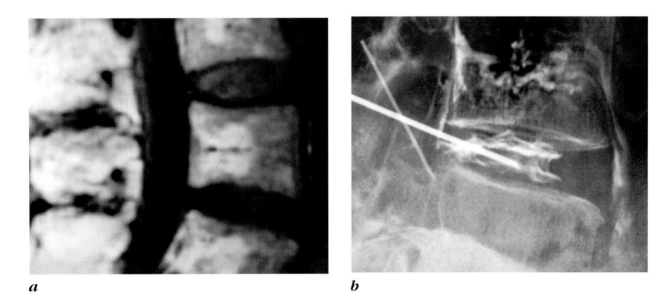

Figure 8.89 *Haemangioma. (**a**) The T$_1$-weighted MR image shows signal change in many lumbar vertebral bodies compatible with haemangiomata. (**b**) At discography the haemangioma in the adjacent superior vertebral body opacifies with contrast. Prominent vessels are shown in and around the vertebral body and in the haemangioma.*

Fibrous dysplasia

Involvement of the spine is uncommon in polyostotic disease and even less common as a monostotic phenomenon. The body or appendage is enlarged. The cortex may be thinned. Changes of lysis, sclerosis, ground-glass or a mixed pattern are found (Figure 8.90).

Extensive involvement of the body may result in vertebral collapse, with cord compression. Extradural soft tissue fibrous masses may be found.

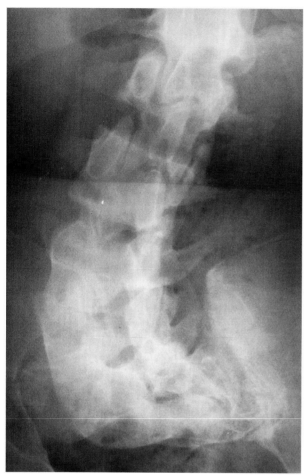

a

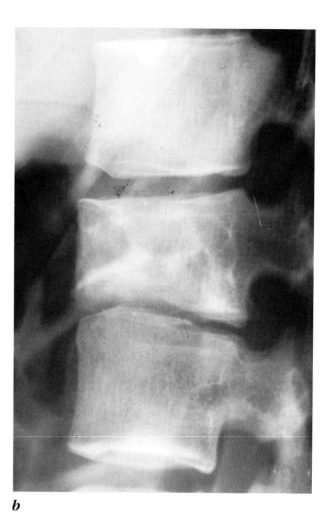

b

Figure 8.90 *Fibrous dysplasia of the spine. (**a***) Polyostotic disease. There is a scoliosis with bone expansion, cortical thinning and a generalised ground-glass texture. (**b***) Fibrous dysplasia with vertebral deformity and collapse. There is a mixture of sclerosis and lysis. The adjacent discs are preserved.*

Neurofibromatosis

See Chapter 7, pages 349–50.

Giant-cell tumour
(see also Chapter 3, pages 154–62)

The spine is not usually involved. Lesions most commonly arise in the sacrum (Figure 8.91). Unlike the aneurysmal bone cyst, which is found in the posterior elements, changes predominate in the vertebral bodies, with an expansile osteolytic lesion (see Figure 3.90), allowing the posterior elements to be shown with remarkable clarity on the antero-posterior film due to lack of overlying bone.

Osteochondromatosis

Spinal involvement is unusual, but can have serious consequences as the enlarging tumour compresses the cord. Tumours arise especially in the cervical spine on the posterior elements. Enlargement of the cartilage cap and malignant transformation result in the early compression of the spinal cord (Figure 8.92).

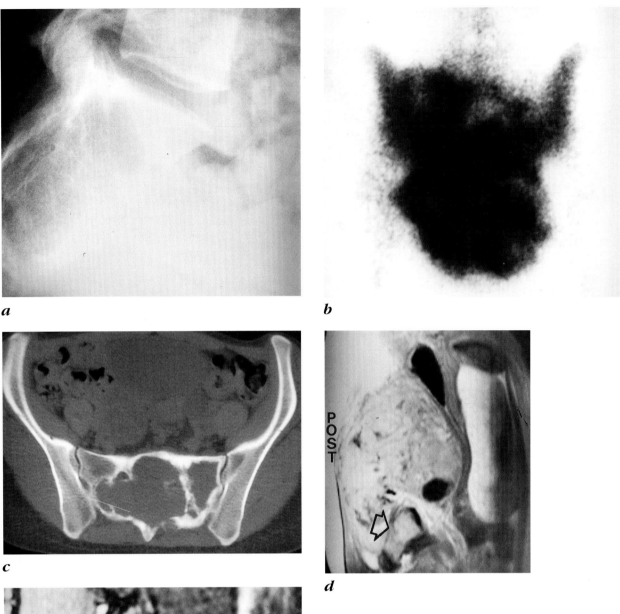

Figure 8.91 *Giant-cell tumour of the sacrum. (**a**) There is an expansile osteolytic lesion of the sacrum, seen on the lateral radiograph. (**b**) The radionuclide bone scan shows substantial increase in uptake in the sacrum, especially inferiorly, associated with expansion of the bone. (**c**) The CT scan demonstrates a large osteolytic expansile lesion which is well defined and does not cross the sacroiliac joint. (**d**) The sagittal post-gadolinium T_1-weighted MR sequence shows a highly vascular and expansile lesion, indenting rectum and bladder. The coccyx is inferior (arrowed). (**e**) The sagittal T_2-weighted MR image through the same area shows a largely soft tissue mass lesion.*

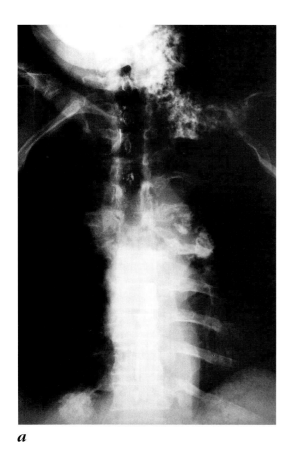

a

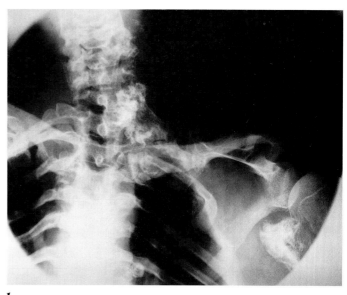

b

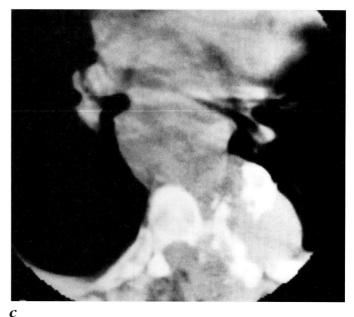

c

Figure 8.92 *Diaphyseal aclasia. (a, b) Exostoses are seen associated with the spine in this patient who developed paraplegia. (c) CT scan showing intrathoracic and spinal masses.*

PRIMARY MALIGNANT TUMOURS OF THE SPINE

Chordoma

Incidence: 4% of primary malignant tumours.
Sex: Male predilection, especially in the sacrum.
Age: Those in the occiput occur at an earlier age than those in the sacrum. Peak incidence is around the fourth and fifth decades.

Sites: see Figure 8.93.
Fifty per cent of lesions arise in the sacrum, 40% around the clivus and otherwise at C2. Lesions are classically in the midline, resulting from their notochordal origin. They are usually anterior, related to vertebral bodies, but may be posterior.

Because of the limited space available in the neck, clival and cervical lesions present much earlier than sacral, which, in turn, present as large masses with pathological fractures, pain or even rectal obstruction.

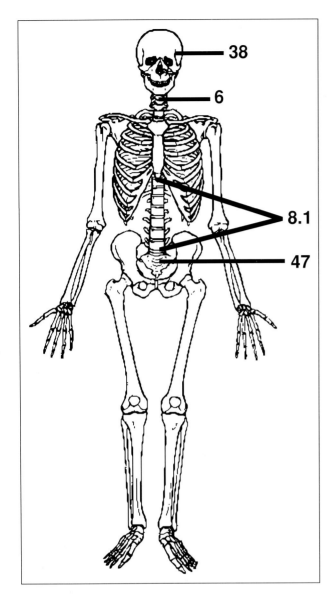

Figure 8.93 *Chordoma. Sites of percentage distribution at major sites. (After Unni, 1996, with permission.)*

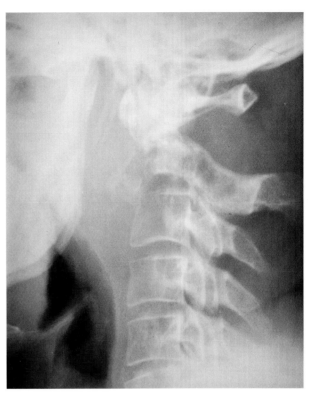

Figure 8.94 *Chordoma of C2. A pathological fracture has occurred through an osteolytic lesion affecting the vertebral body. The cortex is thinned and there is a large associated soft tissue mass.*

In the cervical spine, a pathological fracture of the affected body, normally C2, is associated with an anterior soft tissue mass. There is usually little mineralization, perhaps a few residual trabeculae remain (Figure 8.94). The lesions metastasize.

CT and MR scanning are of great value in showing the extent of tumour at the clivus and of C2. Sacral lesions, of whatever type, are difficult to visualize because of overlying gas and faeces. The sacrum also is a relatively blind area on an AP view of the pelvis because it is a flat bone parallel to the plane of the film, as are the iliac blades. Little cortex is visible and overlying soft tissue swelling is poorly visualized in the absence of axial images, unless gross. Special attention must be paid to the integrity of the sacral foramina as their loss is an early sign of anterior or posterior cortical destruction (Figure 8.95).

At MR scanning, chordomas are of soft tissue intensity on T_1-weighted images and bright on T_2-weighting. CT scanning demonstrates bone destruction, cortical thinning and soft tissue extension, as well as occasional mineralization in spinal lesions.

Other causes of sacral destructive lesions are given in Table 3.8, page 117.

Osteogenic sarcoma

Spinal disease accounts for only 3% of all osteosarcomas and around 5% of all primary spinal tumours.

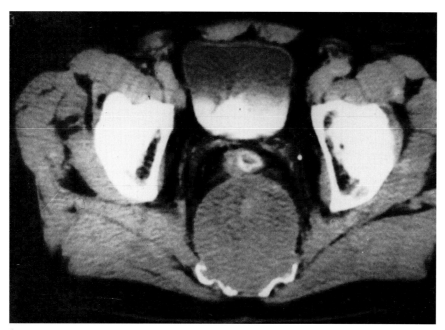

a

Figure 8.95 *Chordoma. (**a**) The lower part of the sacrum and coccyx are not visualized on the radiograph, being overlain by a large soft tissue mass. This has the appearance of the bladder but represents the rounded sacral tumour. (**b**) The post-contrast CT scan shows a large osteolytic, expansile, soft tissue lesion extending forward from the sacrum displacing the rectum. (**c**) A sagittal T$_1$-weighted MR image shows a largely homogeneous mass of soft tissue signal arising from the lower sacrum and extending into the pelvis, displacing the rectum anteriorly.*

b

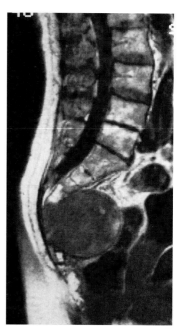

c

There is no difference in incidence between the sexes and patients tend to be much older than usual, with a mean age of 38 years. At this later age of presentation, Hodgkin's disease may be suggested.

Radiologically, in the spine a larger number of tumours (50%) are lytic than elsewhere in the skeleton (see Figure 2.35). Change is most common in the lumbosacral region (see Figure 2.36), least common in the neck (see Figure 2.35). Cord compression and extraspinal extension are seen at CT (Figure 8.96), myelography and especially well at MRI.

Ewing's sarcoma of the spine (see below) occurs in younger patients.

Ewing's sarcoma

Spinal involvement is unusual, but is most often seen in the sacrum. Vertebral body infiltration, destruction and collapse are associated with soft tissue masses and cord compression (Figure 8.97). The disease may spread to posterior elements.

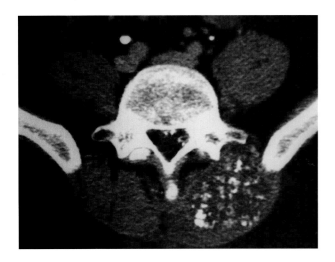

Figure 8.96 *Osteogenic sarcoma. The CT scan demonstrates a large ossifying soft tissue mass posterior to the spine. The soft tissues show mixed attenuation in the area of ossification. There is metastatic ossification within the spinal canal.*

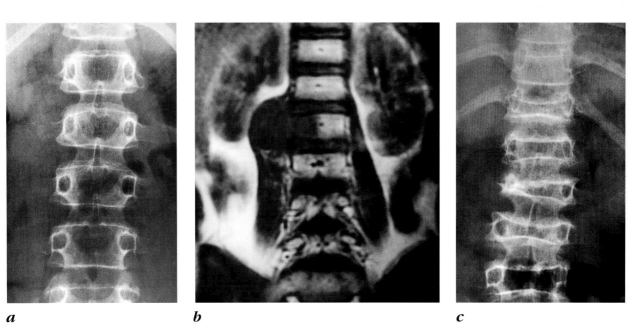

a   *b*   *c*

Figure 8.97 *Ewing's sarcoma of the spine. (**a**) The initial radiograph is minimally abnormal. There is some loss of clarity of the right pedicle of L2 together with early collapse of the upper surface of L2 on the right. The psoas shadow is displaced. (**b**) The coronal T$_1$-weighted MR sequence shows a large mass of soft tissue signal occupying the right lateral half of the body of L2 with extension into the psoas muscle. (**c**) After chemotherapy and radiotherapy, vertebral collapse is shown on the plain film throughout the lumbar spine and at T12. The body of L2 is now well defined, as is the right pedicle.*

Metastatic disease

Over 40% of skeletal metastases occur in the spine. This is the result of the local presence of red marrow in the adult and also because Batson's vertebral venous plexus connects, for instance, both pelvic organs and breasts with the spine. Primary breast and prostate lesions especially, but also kidney, thyroid and lung cancers, metastasize to the spine. Trabecular compression by tumour causes resorption of trabeculae. Sclerosis in prostatic deposits results from reactive new bone formation. The cells themselves may also stimulate osteoclastic and osteoblastic activity.

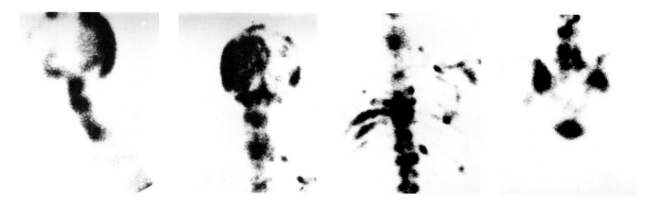

Figure 8.98 *Metastatic disease. The radionuclide bone scan demonstrates widespread areas of increase in uptake, the distribution of which is completely random.*

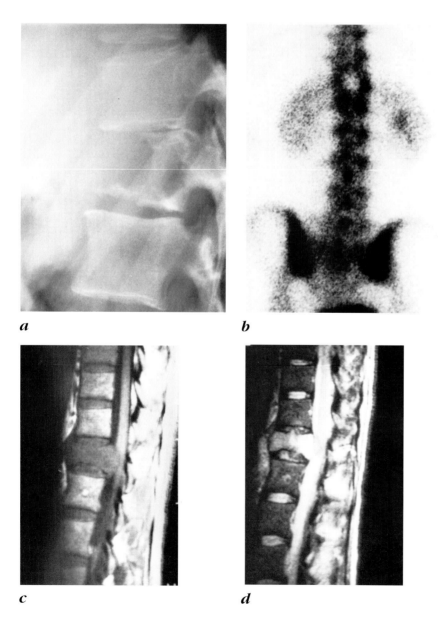

a

b

c

d

Figure 8.99 *Metastatic disease. (**a**) There is a large osteolytic metastasis in the body of T12. The anterior and superior cortices of this body are no longer to be seen. (**b**) The radioisotope bone scan shows a generalized increase in uptake locally with a photopenic area centrally. Presumably this region is avascular. (**c**) Sagittal T$_1$-weighted MR image showing a soft tissue mass with posterior protrusion into the canal compressing the cord. (**d**) On this T$_2$-weighted MR sequence the posterior part of the lesion protrudes into the canal.*

Radionuclide bone scanning demonstrates the presence of multiple skeletal metastases and is more sensitive in detecting early bone loss than plain radiography (Figure 8.98). CT scanning confirms vertebral medullary and cortical bone destruction, and cord compression in the presence of soft tissue masses.

Radiculography is used together with CT to assess the status of the canal, cord and roots, and to demonstrate the presence of intrathecal and intramedullary metastases. It may not be possible to induce contrast medium past a block and cervical puncture may be needed. Lesions away from the canal are of course not seen. Radiculography may result in a deterioration of neurological symptoms.

MRI demonstrates changes in the vertebral body, canal, thecal space, cord and also in the surrounding soft tissues (Figure 8.99). Sagittal scans show long lengths of canal, demonstrating both the upper and lower levels of block as well as soft tissue changes

outside the spine. MRI is also more sensitive in detecting spinal metastases than is radionuclide bone scanning. Myeloma presents similarly but is said to spare the pedicles, unlike secondary metastatic disease (Figure 8.100).

Diffuse metastatic disease may present with generalized demineralization on a plain film and a 'superscan' on radionuclide bone scanning with widespread increase in uptake. At MRI, T_1-weighted sequences following intravenous gadolinium will show marked increase in signal in the presence of diffuse metastatic disease compared with the pre-enhancement T_1-weighted images, unlike normal marrow where enhancement is absent. Fat suppression scans are also abnormal with focal or general osteolytic malignancy.

Sclerotic metastases replace fat and haemopoietic marrow, resulting in low signal change in affected vertebrae.

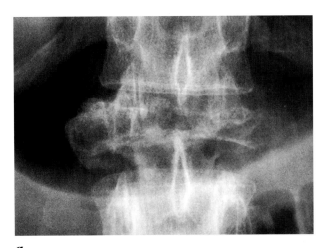

a

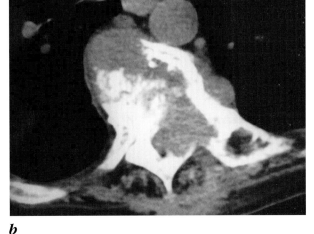

b

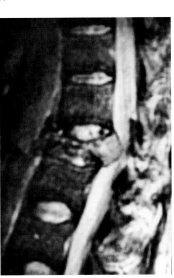

c

Figure 8.100 *Myeloma presents similar appearances to metastatic disease in the elderly. (**a**) The plain film shows vertebra plana. The pedicles are not clearly seen. (**b**) The CT scan shows widespread vertebral body destruction with an anterior soft tissue mass. The spinal canal is invaded posteriorly. (**c**) The sagittal* T_2-*weighted MR image shows vertebral collapse, marrow replacement by tumour and canal stenosis at the level of the flattened and expanded vertebral body.*

SCOLIOSIS

This term describes a lateral curvature of the spine. Usually, but not always, there is a primary curve, with a compensatory curve above and below. If the primary curve lies in the lumbar spine, a curve cannot exist below it as there can be no mobility at or below the lumbosacral junction. Clinically, the compensatory curves straighten out in forward flexion of the spine; the primary curve is *structural*.

Curves may be classified thus (after Cobb, 1948):

1. Idiopathic
2. Osteogenic
   (a) congenital, e.g. hemivertebra, or acquired, e.g. in Scheuermann's disease, ankylosing spondylitis, tumour, infection with vertebral destruction and following irradiation
   (b) skeletal dysplasias, including neurofibromatosis (Table 8.6)
   (c) irritable, e.g. with osteoid osteoma, pneumonia, renal colic
3. Neuropathic, e.g. polio, syringomyelia
4. Myopathic, e.g. muscular dystrophy
5. Thoracogenic, e.g. post-thoracoplasty

IDIOPATHIC SCOLIOSIS

This is the most commonly seen form and is further divided into the following groups:
- Infantile—age of onset 0–3 years (Figure 8.101)
- Juvenile—age of onset 4–9 years
- Adolescent—age of onset 10 years, to the cessation of growth (Figure 8.102). It is much more common in girls (M:F = 1:8).

Idiopathic scoliosis is so-called because no aetiology is recognized; the diagnosis is made by exclusion. Most are seen on routine chest radiographs, existing unknown to the patient. They are often discovered on routine medical examination, or when the child bends over and rib protrusion is made prominent. Skeletal maturity may be retarded.

Idiopathic curves are associated with spinal rotation.

AP and lateral whole spine films are obtained. Prior to surgery, lateral bending films are obtained to see whether the compensatory curves are flexible. It would be wrong to straighten the main or primary curve if the curves above and below are inflexible and would persist after straightening of the primary curve.

Table 8.6 Scoliosis associated with syndromes.

Arthrogryposis multiplex congenita
Chondrodysplasia punctata
Diastrophic dysplasia
Down's syndrome
Ehlers–Danlos syndrome
Larsen's syndrome
Laurence–Moon–Biedl syndrome
Marfan syndrome
Mucopolysaccharidoses
Neurofibromatosis
Prader–Willi syndrome
Spondyloepiphyseal dysplasia congenita
Spondylometaphyseal dysplasia

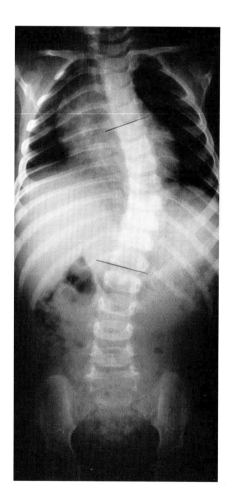

Figure 8.101 *Infantile idiopathic scoliosis concave to the right in the lower thoracic region. A degree of spinal rotation is also shown.*

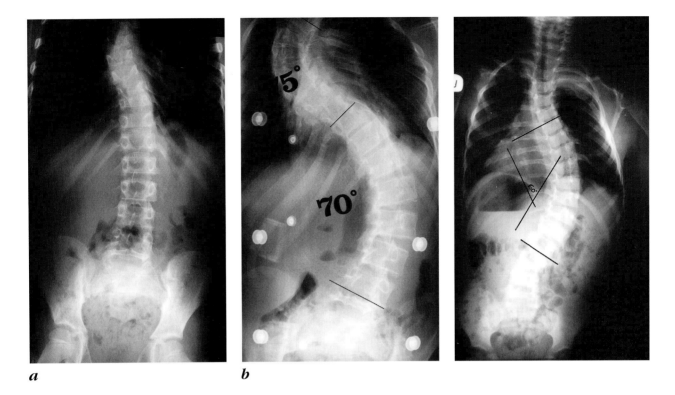

a   b

Figure 8.102 *Adolescent idiopathic scoliosis. (**a**) The initial radiograph shows a moderate thoracic scoliosis with compensation inferiorly. (**b**) Four years later the curves have increased in the coronal plane, as well as the degree of spinal rotation. This is especially apparent in the lumbar region.*

Figure 8.103 *Measurement of the curve by the method of Cobb. Perpendiculars are drawn to lines at the uppermost and lowest endplates of the curve. The angle at which the perpendiculars meet is the angle of the curve.*

Structural curves are not flexible. Deformity may be permanent and associated with compression of vertebral bodies on the side of the concavity. Rotation is present in idiopathic scoliosis and the spinous processes deviate to the site of the concavity. Rotation is greatest at the apex of the curve. In keeping with the general rotation of the spine, the pedicles move towards the concavity, and that at the apex of the concavity has a flattened or hypoplastic appearance.

The curve is measured by the method described by Cobb (1948). Lines are drawn on the upper surface of the highest vertebra in the curve and on the lower surface of the lowest vertebra; these are the highest and the lowest vertebral bodies with the greatest endplate angulation from the horizontal (Figure 8.101). As the angle subtended between these two lines usually cannot be read on the film, perpendiculars are drawn to these lines; the angles at which they meet is the *angle of the curve* (Figure 8.103). Severe curves are 100° or more, mild curves less than 69°, and moderate in between.

The earlier the onset of disease, the more marked the curve at the time of spinal skeletal maturity, after which little further deterioration is to be expected (Figure 8.102). Disc degeneration at the concavity, however, allows subsequent further deformity, together with the formation of buttressing osteophytes on the concavity. Spinal skeletal maturity is reached when the apophysis for the iliac crest turns down towards and reaches that for the anterior superior iliac spine and, for this reason, films of the iliac crests are routinely obtained.

It is likely that multiple radiographs will be obtained and even more if surgery is undertaken. Radiation to thyroid, breasts and gonads is substantial and should be kept to a minimum.

Cord stretching and tethering

Prior to surgery, or should neurological symptoms supervene, the status of the spinal cord should be assessed. It is stretched over the concavity. A normal situation of the conus (T12–L1) excludes cord tethering.

OSTEOGENIC SCOLIOSIS

This may be localized, for example a hemivertebra (Figure 8.104), or more extensive. There may be multiple vertebral anomalies, diastematomyelia (Figure 8.105) and rib abnormalities. Associated soft tissue anomalies may be present in the heart, gut or renal tract. If spinal anomalies exist, in an osteogenic scoliosis, Arnold–Chiari or other cord anomalies such as a tethered cord with a low conus may be present (Figure 8.106). Previously examined with intrathecal contrast medium, MRI is now used routinely to exclude cord abnormality.

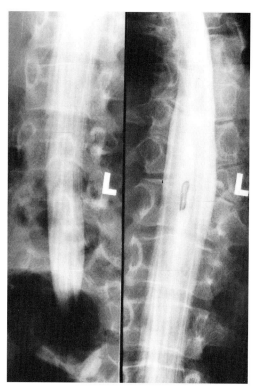

a

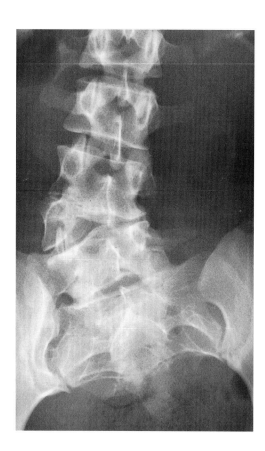

Figure 8.104 *Osteogenic scoliosis with a hemivertebra. The concavity is on the side that is deficient.*

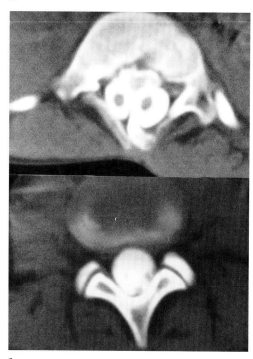

b

Figure 8.105 *Diastematomyelia. (**a**) At radiculography a bony spur is seen dividing the cord into two. (**b**) The subsequent CT radiculogram confirms these changes.*

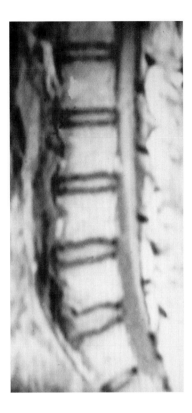

Figure 8.106
Cord tethering demonstrated at MRI. The thinned cord is demonstrated as far as the sacrum.

Unilateral radiation

Used, for example, for Wilm's tumours in infancy, this causes cessation of growth and a resulting mainly non-rotatory curve (Figure 8.107).

Dysplasia

Many dysplasias feature spinal abnormalities, including scoliosis (Table 8.6). Spondyloepiphyseal dysplasia (Figure 8.108a), mucopolysaccharidoses (Figure 8.108b) and pseudoachondroplasia (Figure 8.108c) which may all be associated with scoliosis.

In neurofibromatosis an acute kyphoscoliosis may be seen in the absence of a local tumour, or in the presence of one (Figure 8.109). MRI demonstrates local tumours, as well as other spinal manifestations of the disease, such as dural ectasia and vertebral scalloping, as does radiculography (see Chapter 7, page 351).

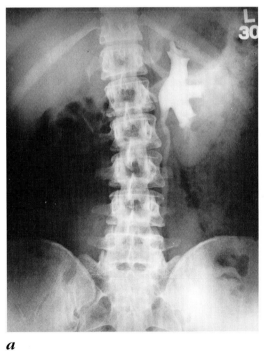

a

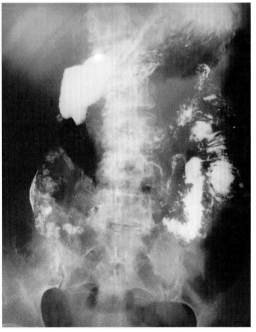

b

Figure 8.107 *Scoliosis following irradiation.* (**a**) *The patient had a Wilm's tumour excised and irradiated as a child. The subsequent radiograph demonstrates a scoliosis concave to the side of irradiation with contralateral renal hypertrophy. Scoliosis results from local vertebral hypoplasia after irradiation and presumably also from fibrosis in the adjacent soft tissues.* (**b**) *Subsequently the patient developed radiation necrosis of the gut.*

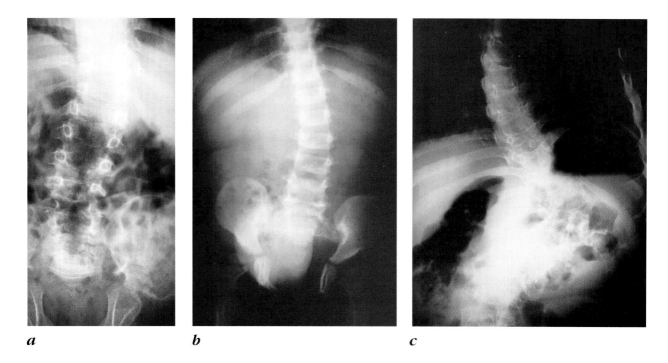

a *b* *c*

Figure 8.108 *Scoliosis.* **(a)** *Spondyloepiphyseal dysplasia.* **(b)** *Myopathic Hurler's syndrome (MPS I-H). There is vertebral deformity, probably related to muscle weakness and imbalance. Note the large anterior hernia, the dysplastic pelvis and hips and the paddle-shaped ribs.* **(c)** *Pseudoachondroplasia.*

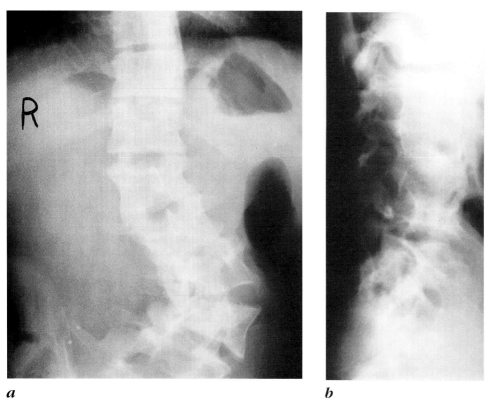

a *b*

Figure 8.109
Scoliosis in neurofibromatosis. **(a)** *There is a very acute curve in the lumbar spine with marked rotation.* **(b)** *Dural ectasia is seen on the lateral view.*

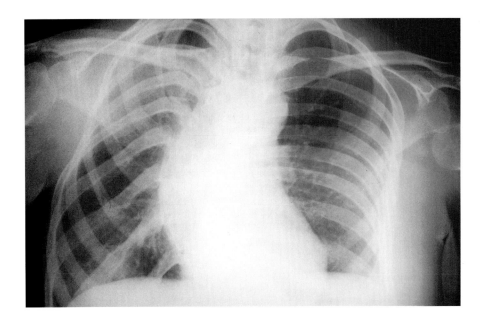

Figure 8.110 *Scoliosis in anterior poliomyelitis. Muscle wasting of the right thoracic wall is seen. The scoliosis is concave to the side of muscle activity.*

Irritable or painful scoliosis

Pneumonia, renal colic, appendicitis and spinal tumours, for example osteoid osteoma, all cause painful scoliosis, usually but not inevitably concave to the side of the lesion, due to guarding and spasm. *There is no rotation* (see Figure 3.8)

If a chronic painful scoliosis is present for which no cause is seen on the radiograph, a radionuclide bone scan should be performed. Generally, idiopathic scoliosis is pain-free and associated with vertebral rotation.

NEUROGENIC SCOLIOSIS

These are smooth and long. The curve may be related to muscle imbalance, as in polio (Figure 8.110). The pelvis may be tilted, bones and soft tissues hypoplastic and hips subluxed or dislocated.

POST-THORACOPLASTY

This operation is no longer performed, but patients with the deformity are still occasionally seen (Figure 8.111)

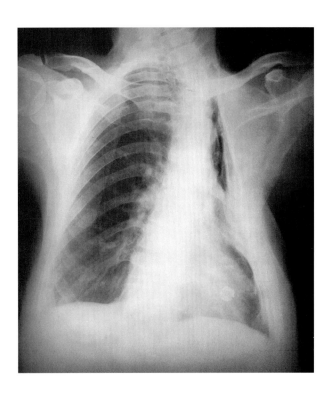

Figure 8.111 *Scoliosis following thoracoplasty. There is a left thoracoplasty with a scoliosis. The concavity is to the right, presumably due to muscle pull.*

INEQUALITY OF LIMB LENGTH

This may result in pelvic tilt and a secondary scoliosis.

DEGENERATIVE DISEASE

A scoliosis is often seen in the elderly in association with degenerative change. A scoliosis may have been present since childhood and the discs subsequently become degenerate, but disc degeneration and facet slip result in an acquired curvature secondary to degeneration. This will often deteriorate under observation in late adult life, and other features of idiopathic scoliosis, rotation and vertebral compression may be absent (Figure 8.11).

BIBLIOGRAPHY

Aisen AM, Martel W, Ellis JH, McCune WJ (1987) Cervical spine involvement in rheumatoid arthritis. MR imaging. *Radiology* **165**: 159–63.

Andersson O (1937) Röntgenbilden vid spondylarthritis ankylopoetica. *Nordisk Medicin* **14**: 2000.

Birney TJ, White JJ Jr, Berens D, Kuhn G (1990) Lumbar discography followed by computed tomography. *Spine* **15**: 690.

Birney TJ, White JJ Jr, Berens D, Kuhn G (1992) Comparison of MRI and discography in the diagnosis of lumbar degenerative disc disease. *J Spinal Disord* **5**: 417–23.

Cobb JR (1948) Outline for the study of scoliosis. *Instructional Course Lectures, American Academy of Orthopaedic Surgeons* **5**: 248. Ann Arbor: Edwards.

Collins CD, Stack JP, O'Connell DJ et al (1990) The role of discography in lumbar disc disease. Comparative study of magnetic resonance imaging and discography. *Clin Radiol* **42**: 252–7.

Cowan NC, Bush K, Katz DE, Gishen P (1992) The natural history of sciatica: a prospective radiological study. *Clin Radiol* **46**: 7–12.

Dequeker J, Goddeeris T, Walravens M, De Roo M (1978) Evaluation of sacroiliitis. Comparison of radiological and radionuclide techniques. *Radiology* **128**: 687–9.

Einig M, Higger HP, Meairs S et al (1990) Magnetic resonance of the craniocervical junction in rheumatoid arthritis: value, limitations, indications. *Skeletal Radiol* **19**: 341–6.

Farfan HF (1973) *Mechanical Disorders of the Low Back.* Philadelphia: Lea & Febiger.

Forrester DM (1990) Imaging of sacro-iliac joints. *Radiol Clin North Am* **28**: 1055–72.

Griffiths HJ (1991) *Imaging of the Lumbar Spine.* Aspen: Gaithersburg.

Jones MD, Pais MJ, Omiya B (1988) Bony overgrowths and abnormal calcifications about the spine. *Radiol Clin North Am* **26**: 1213–34.

Karlin CA, Brower AC (1977) Multiple primary hemangiomas of bone. *Am J Roentgenol* **129**: 162–4.

Modic MT, Steinberg PM, Ross JS et al (1988) Degenerative disk disease: assessment of changes in vertebral body marrow with MR imaging. *Radiology* **166**: 193–9.

O'Brien JP (1984) Mechanisms of spinal pain. In: *Textbook of Pain* (eds PD Wall and R Melzack), pp 2–13. Edinburgh: Churchill Livingstone.

Osti OL, Fraser RD (1992) MRI and discography of annular tears and intervertebral disc degeneration. A prospective clinical comparison. *J Bone Joint Surg* **74B**: 431–5.

Resnick D (1995) *Diagnosis of Bone and Joint Disorders*, 3rd edn. Philadelphia: WB Saunders.

Resnick D, Guerra J Jr, Robinson CA, Vint VC (1978) Association of diffuse idiopathic skeletal hyperostosis and calcification and ossification of the posterior longitudinal ligament. *Am J Roentgenol* **131**: 1049–53.

Romanus R, Yden S (1955) *Pelvo-spondylitis Ossificans*, p 104. Copenhagen: Munksgaard.

Ross JS, Masaryk TJ, Modic MT et al (1987) Vertebral hemangiomas: MR imaging. *Radiology* **165**: 165–9.

Sanjay BK, Sim FH, Unni KK et al (1993) Giant-cell tumors of the spine. *J Bone Joint Surg* **75B**: 148–54.

Unni KK (1996) *Dahlin's Bone Tumors*, 5th edn. Philadelphia: Lippincott-Raven.

Wiltse LL, Newman PH, Macnab F (1976) Classification of spondylolysis and spondylolisthesis. *Clin Orthop* **117**: 23–9.

Zucherman J, Derby R, Hsu K et al (1988) Normal magnetic resonance imaging with abnormal discography. *Spine* **13**: 1355–9

Chapter 9 **Imaging of soft tissues**

Soft tissues should always be satisfactorily imaged and carefully assessed. This should take place prior to inspection of the underlying bone and joint and, if possible, two views usually at right-angles should be assessed. As a generalization, abnormal soft tissues may be related to underlying bone or joint disease, while normal soft tissues may well exclude underlying bony change.

Besides plain films, soft tissues can be examined with ultrasound, radionuclide scanning, CT and MRI.

Plain film changes include:

- Soft tissue swelling
- Fat plane displacement
- Fat plane loss
- Soft tissue ossification
- Soft tissue calcification
- Soft tissue atrophy

Soft tissue swelling is seen as an increase in both thickness and density as a result of local pathology or subjacent bone or joint disease. Thus, for example, if soft tissue swelling is seen over the ulnar styloid, the involved tissues will also appear denser. The underlying bone is then less well seen because of local X-ray filtration. If a swelling is central, fat planes may be displaced and the muscle appears denser. This may be as a result of trauma or tumour. With infection, oedema may result in loss of the fat planes.

SPECIFIC AREAS OF PLAIN FILM SOFT TISSUE CHANGE

Skin

Following trauma, infection, ulceration (Figure 9.1) or at the site of foreign bodies (Figure 9.2).

Cervical spine

On the lateral view in the adult, soft tissues are closely (2–3 mm) applied to the anterior aspects of the bodies of C1–4. Below C4 (that is, from the larynx down), the soft tissues are around 1 cm in thickness.

Air may be seen in the oesophagus and, occasionally, a precervical fat stripe may be present. In children, the adenoids may protrude into the nasopharynx, but should involute in adolescence. Recurrence of local soft tissue swelling may occur with malignancy or may reflect local trauma or infection (see Figure 8.71).

Displacement of the pharyngeal gas shadow occurs with local infection (Figure 9.3), trauma or tumour in the underlying spine or soft tissues.

Thoracic spine

Here, the paraspinal soft tissue lines are seen between the underlying vertebral density and overlying lung lucency and are well seen on an adequately penetrated AP film. Displacement of these planes follows tumour, trauma or infection (Figures 8.77 and 9.4), and also osteophyte formation. The soft tissue mass is usually widest at the site of maximal spinal disease.

Lumbar spine

The lumbar spine is surrounded by soft tissues and these may be displaced and distorted (Figures 2.34 and 8.82). The margin of psoas is represented by its overlying fat plane, which is displaced, for example, in tuberculosis, on an AP film. On the lateral view, gut shadows may be displaced away from the spine (see Figure 8.79). Lesions of the sacrum displace the overlying rectum.

Shoulder

Deltoid thickening or atrophy may be seen, as well as axillary recess distension, with a local increase in density and fat plane displacement (Figures 4.22 and 9.5).

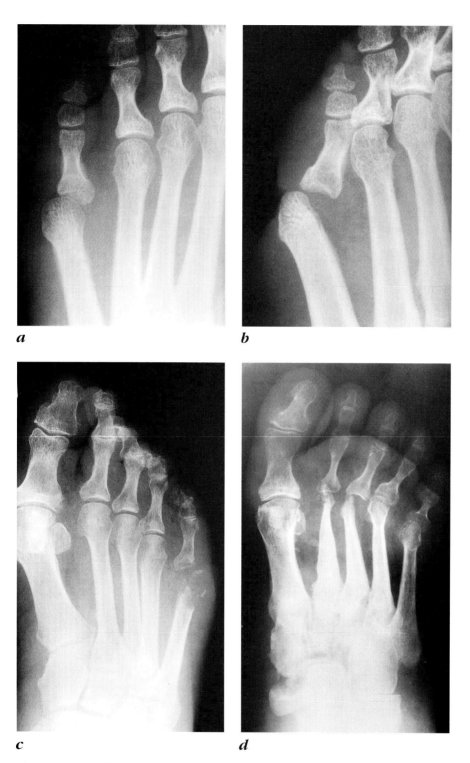

a

b

c

d

Figure 9.1 *Diabetic ulcer. (**a**) There is marked soft tissue swelling over the fifth metatarsophalangeal joint associated with demineralization, and subluxation of the proximal phalanx. The local joint space is narrowed. A periostitis is demonstrated on the proximal phalangeal shaft. (**b**) The oblique view demonstrates a penetrating ulcer in this patient with a diabetic neuropathy. (**c**) A different patient showing subsequent osteomyelitic destruction of the fifth metatarsal head in this condition with subluxation of the joint. (**d**) In another patient following treatment and healing, the remaining bone becomes dense and well defined. A pointed tubular bone results.*

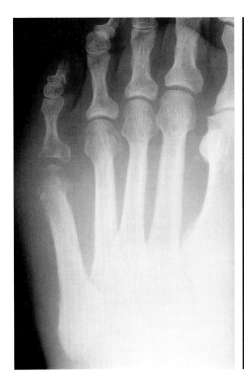
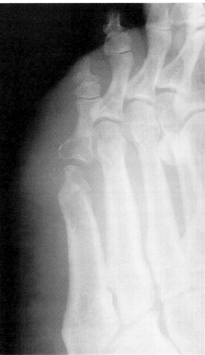

Figure 9.2 *A penetrating injury as an occupational hazard. The patient was a dustman who trod on a rusty nail. There is soft tissue swelling, bone destruction and widening of the joint space. The infection was progressive because of antibiotic resistance.*

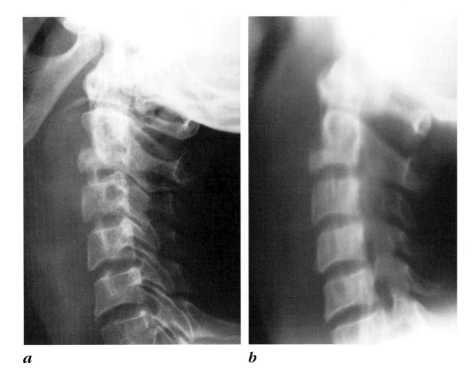

a   *b*

Figure 9.3 *(a) Plain film, (b) linear tomogram. Tuberculosis of C2 associated with substantial enlargement of the precervical soft tissues. Anterior vertebral destruction is seen.*

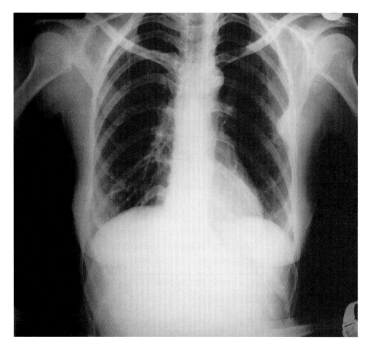

a

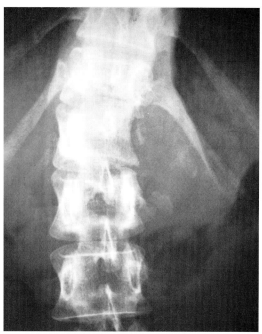

b

Figure 9.4 *Paraspinal soft tissue swelling in thoraco-lumbar tuberculosis. (**a**) The chest radiograph of this patient from the Indian subcontinent shows a scoliosis at the thoraco-lumbar junction concave to the left, together with a soft tissue mass on the concavity overlying the lowest rib. (**b**) The penetrated view of the thoraco-lumbar junction confirms the presence of a soft tissue mass associated with destruction of bone, including the posterior elements (see Chapter 8, page 397), and disc. There is enlargement of the paraspinal soft tissues extending into the upper lumbar region.*

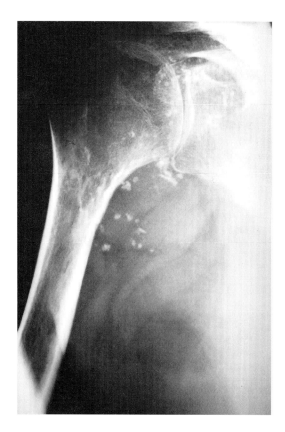

Figure 9.5 *Synovial osteochondromatosis. There is a soft tissue mass in the axilla associated with irregular calcification and bone erosion.*

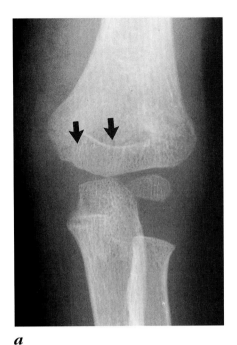

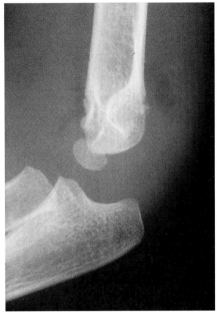

a   *b*

Figure 9.6 (**a**, **b**) *Anterior and posterior fat pad displacement following a supracondylar fracture. The supracondylar fracture is difficult to visualise on the AP view (**a**) (arrowed) and should not be confused with the growth plate at the distal humerus.*

Elbow

Displacement of the anterior and posterior fat pads result from joint effusion, giving the 'sail' sign (Figure 9.6). The fat pads lie superficial to the synovium, but beneath the fibrous capsule. Because the lateral view of the elbow is taken in flexion, with triceps pressing down on the back of the joint, the presence of a posterior sail sign indicates a larger amount of fluid; following trauma, this almost inevitably denotes an underlying fracture.

Wrist

Numerous tendons, tendon sheaths and bursae exist around the wrist in association with a complex series of joints—radio-ulnar, radio-carpal, mid-carpal and carpometacarpal (Figure 9.7).

Bursal and tendon sheath pathology may be seen in rheumatoid arthritis. Trauma to bone also results in local soft tissue swelling. The navicular or scaphoid fat pad lies beneath abductor pollicis longus tendon (Figure 9.8); it is displaced or blurred by trauma to the scaphoid or radial styloid. On the lateral view of the wrist, filling in of the normal dorsal soft tissue concavity behind the wrist and displacement of the fat plane anteriorly over the pronator quadratus are shown with wrist trauma (Figure 9.9).

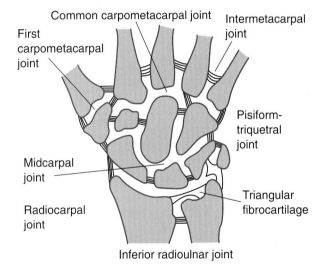

Figure 9.7 *Diagram of synovial compartments of wrist (after Resnick, 1995).*

Pelvis

A line of fat is seen over obturator internus, roughly parallel to the ilio-pectineal line. Trauma to the acetabulum or local malignancy, as well as infection, displace this fat line (Figure 9.10).

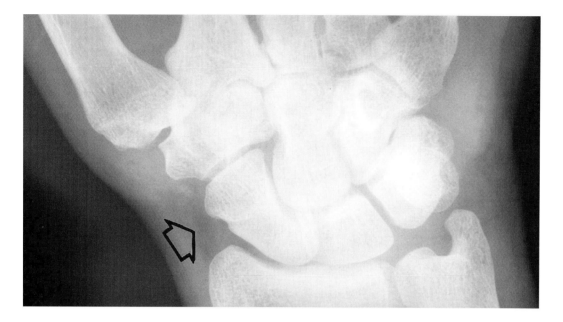

Figure 9.8 *Normal AP radiograph of wrist. There is a fat plane in the angle between the distal scaphoid and the radial styloid beneath the abductor pollicis longus tendon (arrow).*

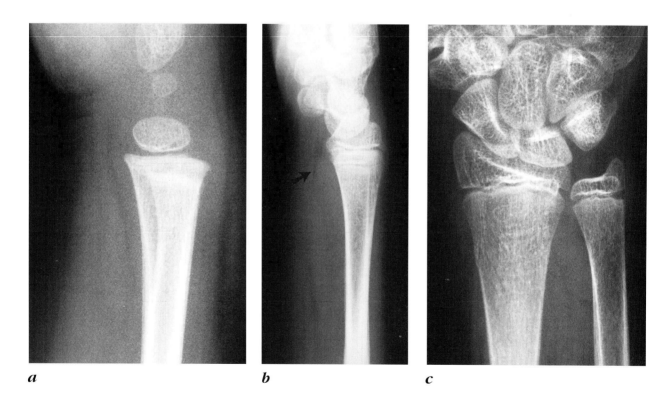

a   *b*   *c*

Figure 9.9 *(a) Lateral radiograph of wrist. The fat line over pronator quadratus is normally straight or parallel to the distal radius. (b, c) Following trauma, there is displacement of the fat plane over pronator quadratus (arrowed). The child, who has a mild form of osteogenesis imperfecta, as does her father, slipped whilst ice-skating. A very minor greenstick fracture is demonstrated.*

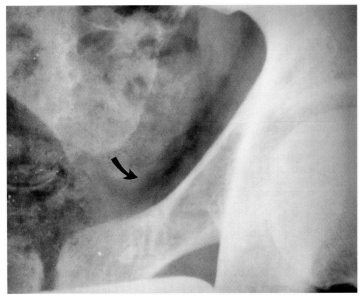

a

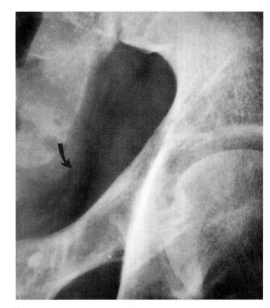

b

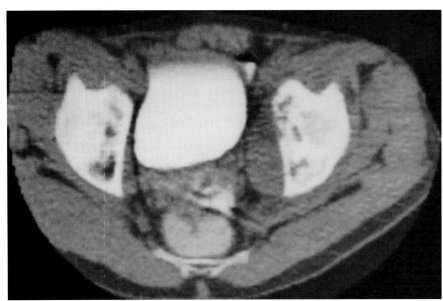

c

Figure 9.10 *Displacement of the fat line over obturator internus due to tumour. (**a**) The patient has a malignant lymphoma of bone which is difficult to visualize on the initial radiograph, but the displaced fat plane is clearly evident (arrow). (**b**) The subsequent radiograph shows the development of the tumour and further displacement of soft tissue planes. (**c**) This change is clearly seen at CT scanning.*

Assessment of hip joint stiffness should include the fat lines around the femoral neck (Figure 9.11). Controversy exists as to whether hip joint effusions do displace these fat lines, but if apparent distension is seen on a plain film, it can be confirmed at ultrasound, which is the examination of choice (see Figure 4.59).

Knee

An effusion in the joint is associated with progressive distension of the suprapatellar pouch, seen on the lateral view as a lenticulate structure of soft tissue density surrounded by fat, rising from between the upper pole of patella and adjacent femur (see Figure 4.141).

The lateral view also shows the ligamentum patellae down to its insertion into the tibial tuberosity, where soft tissue thickening and apophyseal fragmentation occur in Osgood–Schlatter's disease (Figure 4.104). MRI occasionally shows a bursa at the insertion. Similar changes can occasionally be seen around the upper (Hoffa's disease) and lower (Sinding–Larsen disease) patellar poles. A Baker's

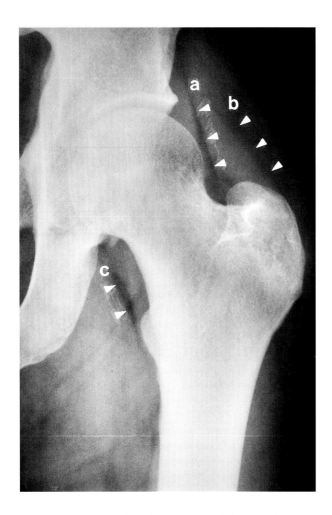

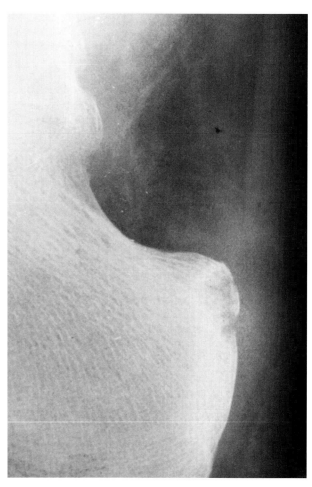

Figure 9.11 *The fat planes around the hip (a: capsular; b: gluteus; c: iliopsoas).*

Figure 9.12 *Retrocalcaneal bursa in rheumatoid arthritis. The tendo-Achillis is thickened and an erosion is seen at its insertion.*

cyst can also be seen on the lateral view as a lobulated, soft tissue density as the surrounding popliteal fossa is largely fat-filled. Densities may be seen in this bursa, usually due to loose bodies, less often to synovial osteochondromatosis (Figure 4.23).

On the AP view of the knee, progressive distension of the joint capsule displaces the fat planes which normally lie against the bone, away from the distal femur. This pattern of distension can be appreciated on coronal MRI sequences (see Figure 4.142).

Ankle

On the lateral view, distension of the capsule can be seen anterior to the ankle joint and especially posteriorly, against the fatty triangle which lies between the

ankle and the Achilles tendon—Kager's triangle (Figure 9.12). Similarly, the Achilles tendon is normally clearly seen because of fat around it. Trauma, inflammation and necrosis thicken the Achilles tendon, which then loses definition on conventional lateral images (Figure 4.168). Similarly, enlargement of the retrocalcaneal bursa displaces fat and thickens the tendon at its insertion into the back of the calcaneum, often in the presence of local erosions (Figure 9.12).

The plantar fascia origin should be sharply defined against overlying fat and this, too, may become poorly defined with plantar fasciitis.

On the AP view, soft tissues are closely applied to, and are parallel with, the malleoli. Trauma to malleoli elevates the soft tissues over them, while injury to the ligaments distal to the malleoli causes swelling distal to the bone.

Foot

Changes may mirror those seen in the hand, for example with trauma, over the base of the fifth metatarsal, and with rheumatoid disease, especially over the fifth metatarsal head. Flexion of the toes makes visualization of bone and soft tissues over the phalanges difficult.

SOFT TISSUE TUMOURS—GENERAL PRINCIPLES

Soft tissue masses are much more likely to be benign than malignant. Soft tissue sarcomas are rare, comprising less than 1% of all malignancies, and they occur in an older age group than primary malignant tumours of bone, often in the fifth decade or later. Some tumours can be positively diagnosed as benign, for example lipoma, and others have features strongly suggestive of malignancy. Many cannot be easily diagnosed radiologically and biopsy may then be necessary.

Plain films demonstrate the presence of soft tissue masses, their margins and, to some extent, the density changes within soft tissue tumours. There may be diminished density, as in lipomas (see below), or increased density in mineralizing tumours or in areas of soft tissue necrosis.

Phleboliths in veins and linear arterial calcification are seen in vascular malformations (see Chapter 7, page 346).

Ultrasound permits localization and biopsy of soft tissue lesions and demonstrates their tissue characteristics; it can also differentiate solid from cystic masses.

Computed tomography for soft tissue tumours has largely been superseded by MRI, though CT and plain films demonstrate calcification in and around soft tissue lesions better than MRI, where low signal change may reflect calcification, arterial flow, gas in the soft tissues or tissue necrosis or fibrosis.

Magnetic resonance imaging permits accurate localization and, to some extent, characterization of soft tissue masses and demonstrates their relationship to muscle, the neurovascular bundle and bone.

Angiography is performed as a precursor to tumour embolization (see Figure 3.99).

MAGNETIC RESONANCE IMAGING OF SOFT TISSUE TUMOURS

At MR imaging, certain features lead to the diagnosis of benignity or malignancy.

Homogeneity

Benign lesions tend to homogeneity. A lipoma, haematoma, cyst or bursa may be totally homogeneous and have features that are totally diagnostic at MRI. Malignant lesions are heterogeneous because of pathological vascularity, cystic change, necrosis, mineralization and the signal from the basic stroma (see Table 3.11).

Benign lesions, however, may also be heterogeneous. Septation, mineralization, necrosis and vascular hypertrophy may be found in benign lesions, such as haemangioma, and the MR appearances vary accordingly.

Size

Smaller lesions tend to be benign and larger lesions malignant. This alone cannot be used as a criterion; some small (<5 cm) lesions turn out to be malignant. However, a small homogeneous lesion is probably, but not inevitably, benign.

Tumour margination

A narrow zone of transition generally distinguishes a benign from a malignant lesion at plain radiography. What is evident, however, is that this is not necessarily the case at MRI. Peripheral oedema often surrounds malignant lesions, but this may represent a stress phenomenon in the surrounding tissues rather than a direct feature of malignancy.

Septation is also seen at MRI in malignant lesions of soft tissue.

COMMON BENIGN SOFT TISSUE LESIONS

Lipoma

This is diagnosed as a lucent lesion on plain films (Figure 9.13) and, because of low attenuation, on CT

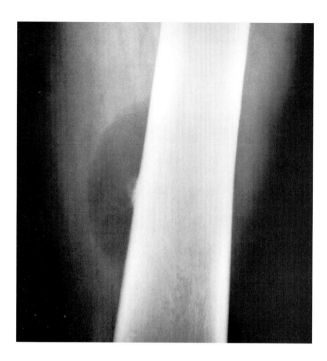

Figure 9.13 *Lipoma. A well demarcated hypertranslucent soft tissue mass which excites a small periosteal reaction.*

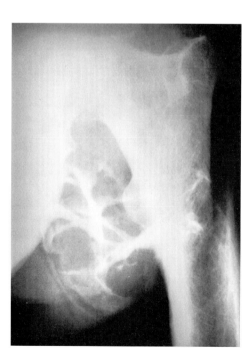

Figure 9.14 *Parosteal lipoma. There is a little evidence of fat within the tumour, but some loss of density is demonstrated between the aborescent (tree-like) strands of bone.*

with a negative value on the Hounsfield scale (see Chapter 3, page 146). With liposarcomatous change, less mature fat cells are present and fibrous change occurs. Features of a fatty tumour may then not be seen. Bizarre calcification or ossification may be seen in lipomatous tumours (Figure 9.14).

Lipoma is the most common soft tissue tumour seen at MRI scanning. They are often larger than many benign lesions and may lie in muscle (Figures 9.15 and 9.16) or actually in subcutaneous fat (Figure 9.17). Generally smoothly marginated, they may infiltrate between adjacent muscle fibres, giving a serrated edge (Figure 9.18).

Septation may be seen but generally the lesion is homogeneous, characteristically bright on T_1-weighted

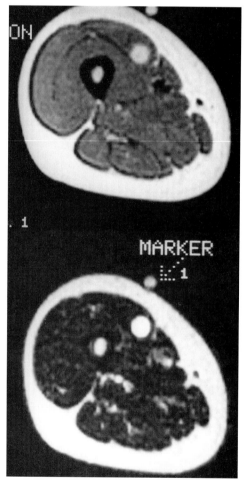

Figure 9.15 *Lipoma. Axial T$_1$- (top) and T$_2$-weighted (bottom) MR images. A well demarcated soft tissue mass lies within rectus femoris. This has the same signal strength as the surrounding subcutaneous fat.*

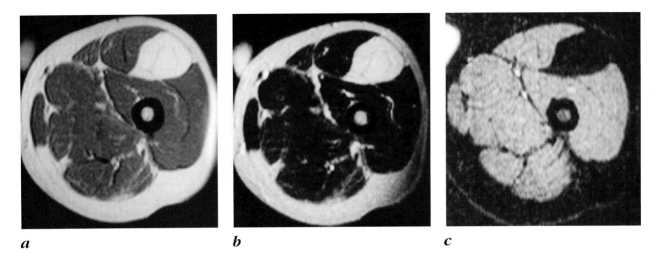

Figure 9.16 *Septal lipoma. Here, a lipoma is seen on* T$_1$- *(a) and* T$_2$-*weighted (b) as well as fat suppression (c) MR sequences. It lies in the fascial plane between rectus femoris and vastus lateralis. The lesion is totally suppressed in the fat suppression image.*

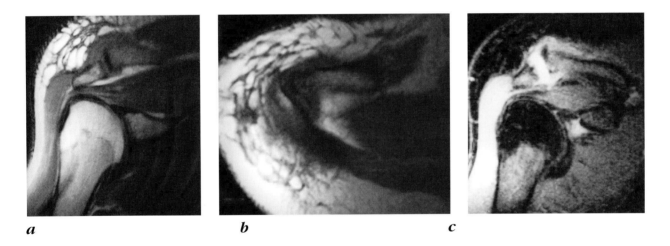

Figure 9.17 *Lipoma in subcutaneous fat. (a) Coronal, (b) axial* T$_1$-*weighted and (c) fat suppression MR sequences. The mass lesion has a different signal and texture to the fat elsewhere. It is brighter and shows numerous septations, but suppresses well.*

images and totally suppressed on fat suppression sequences.

A rare entity, *lipoma aborescens*, fills a whole joint, usually the knee, with fat.

Fluid-containing lesions—cysts

These are generally smoothly marginated. Fluid is of intermediate signal on T_1-weighting, bright on T_2-

weighting and not suppressed on fat suppression sequences (see Figure 4.27).

Haemangioma

This is a benign tumour seen as a heterogeneous mass on MRI scanning. Arteries have rapid flow, giving a signal void; veins are brighter on T_2-weighting because of slow flow, as are blood pools. Fibrous

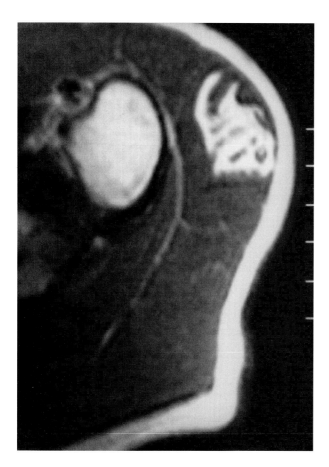

Figure 9.18 *Lipoma—axial* T$_1$*-weighted MR image. Serration of the margins is demonstrated in this intramuscular lesion (by courtesy of Mr Richard Browne FRCS).*

tissue gives a low signal and fat is bright on T_1-weighted images. Signal void may also be due to phleboliths, best seen with plain radiography (see Figure 7.25).

Neurofibromatosis

Tumours are aligned along the course of a nerve. The lesions are lobulated, septate and of an intermediate signal on T_1-weighting, higher on T_2-weighting (see Figure 7.36b, c).

Haematoma

An acute collection of blood in soft tissues may be well defined and cystic. Haematomas often occur in

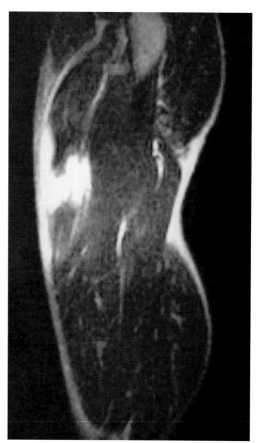

a

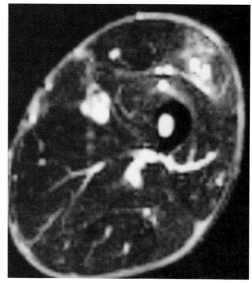

b

Figure 9.19 *Haematoma.* **(a)** *The sagittal* T$_1$*- and* **(b)** *axial* T$_2$*-weighted MR images show a haematoma surrounded by more diffuse infiltration of blood in the surrounding muscle.*

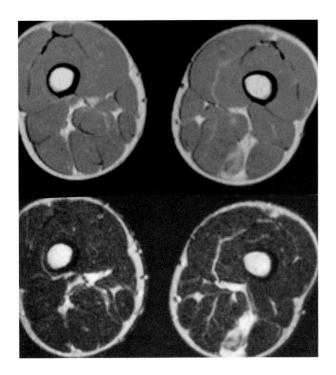

Figure 9.20 *Haematoma. Axial T₁- (top) and T₂-weighted (bottom) MR images showing reduction in size and progressive signal loss in an old organizing haematoma.*

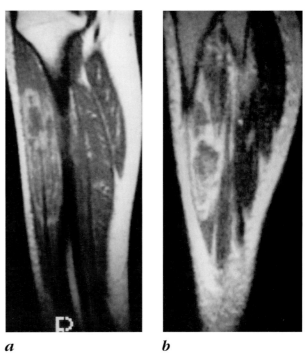

a   *b*

the lower limbs due to sporting injuries. Initially they are bright on *T₂*-weighted images and are not suppressed on fat suppression sequences.

Haematomas are best seen on axial slices, where their location is easily assessed. They may lie in muscles or in intramuscular septae, often tracking vertically for a considerable distance. The surrounding muscle may be entirely clear of change, but may be the site of diffuse infiltration by blood (Figure 9.19).

Fluid collections persist longer than the clinical signs, gradually shrinking (Figure 9.20) and losing bright signal. Finally, a low signal scar replaces the haemorrhagic collection.

OTHER BENIGN MUSCLE LESIONS

Anterior compartment syndrome

Raised pressure in a tightly contained compartment leads to vascular compression, oedema and muscle necrosis. The MRI changes reflect these features (Figure 9.21).

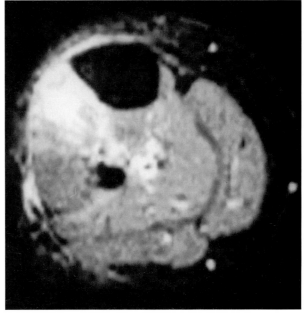

c

Figure 9.21 *Anterior compartment syndrome. The sagittal T₁- (**a**) and coronal T₂-weighted (**b**) MR sequences show change in tibialis anterior. Fluid surrounds islands of muscle which themselves show local increase in signal. Presumably they are oedematous and necrotic. (**c**) The axial fat suppression MR image demonstrates fluid in the abnormal muscle.*

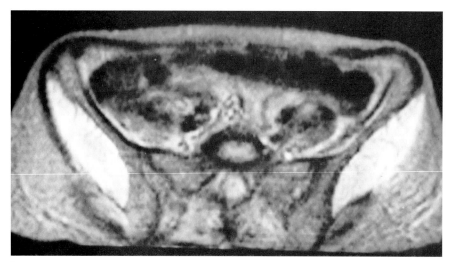

a

b

Figure 9.22 *Polymyositis— (**a**, **b**) axial and (**c**) coronal fat suppression MR images, (**d**) coronal T$_1$-weighted MR sequence. There is muscle atrophy with diffuse infiltration and increase in signal in the muscles. This is not fatty, as shown on the fat suppression sequences, but inflammatory. The signal from muscle is brighter than that from fat in the fat suppression sequences.*

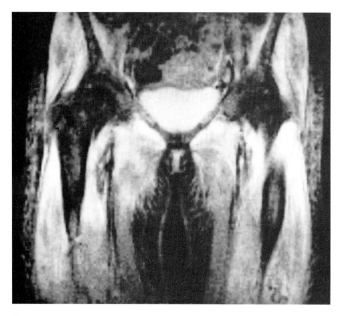

c

d

Polymyositis

This results in generalized muscle atrophy and increased signal with oedema (Figure 9.22). Remission after therapy can be assessed at MRI scanning.

MALIGNANT LESIONS OF SOFT TISSUE

Liposarcoma

Liposarcomas vary in their degree of differentiation. On plain films, malignancy is associated with varying degrees of loss of the normal radiolucency associated with fatty tumours (Figures 9.23 and 9.24). Progressive fibrosis, haemorrhage and necrosis result in a pattern of inhomogeneity at MRI with total or partial loss of the normal signal from fat (Figure 9.25).

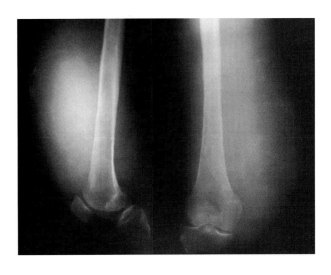

Figure 9.23 *Liposarcoma. The plain film demonstrates a large soft tissue mass with only a few areas of lucency. There is rim calcification.*

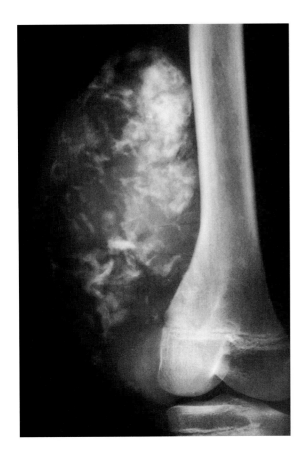

Figure 9.24 *Liposarcoma. A separate case showing bizarre mineralization in the tumour which still displays some areas of translucency, suggesting mature fat.*

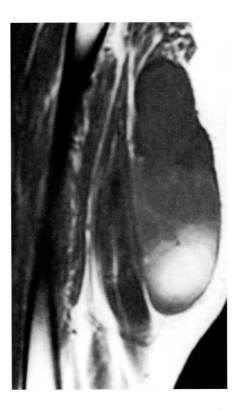

Figure 9.25 *Myxoid liposarcoma. The sagittal T₁-weighted MR sequence shows increased signal in the lower part of the tumour due to focal haemorrhage. More proximally there is dishomogeneity of signal, which resembles muscle. The lesion also shows septation. There is little to suggest the fatty origin of the tumour.*

Myosarcoma

This presents as a large mass lesion with a heterogeneous pattern of intermediate mixed signal on T_1-weighted images which, with intravenous gadolinium, enhances centrally and peripherally. Areas of vascularity and necrosis may be present (Figures 9.26 and 9.27).

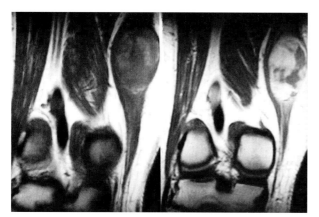

a

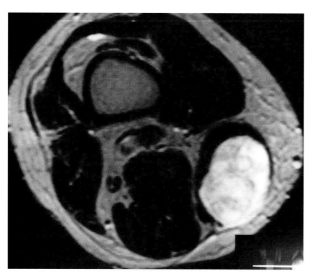

b

Figure 9.26 *Rhabdomyosarcoma. Two examples showing well demarcated tumours despite malignancy, but which also show inhomogeneity of signal.* **(a)** *Coronal T$_1$-weighted MR images, pre-(left) and post-gadolinium (right). The tumour arises in vastus medialis. The lesion is highly vascular.* **(b)** *The axial fat suppression MR sequence shows the lesion to be very well defined despite its malignant nature.*

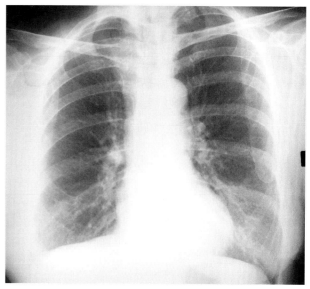

a

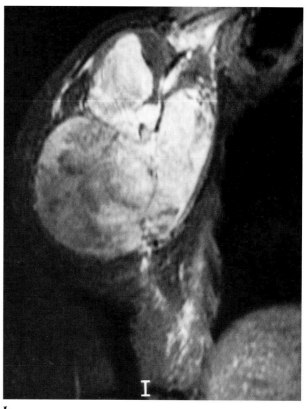

b

Figure 9.27 *Soft tissue sarcoma.* **(a)** *The chest radiograph shows a large soft tissue mass arising in the right axilla.* **(b)** *Coronal fat suppression MR image showing septation in this oedematous tumour. Although there is inhomogeneity of signal, it remains relatively well demarcated at MRI.*

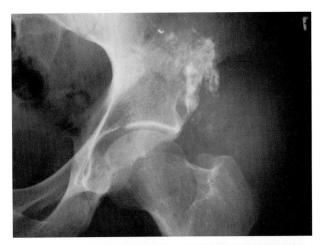

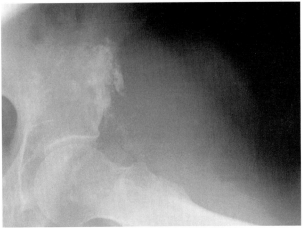

Figure 9.28 *Soft tissue osteosarcoma. A large soft tissue mass is mineralizing. The mineralization is irregular. The lesion does not arise from the underlying bone.*

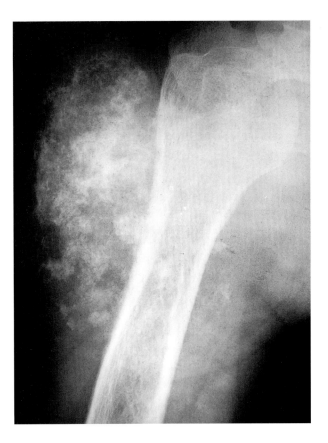

Figure 9.29 *Soft tissue chondrosarcoma. A large irregularly mineralizing soft tissue mass is demonstrated which causes saucerization or scalloping of the underlying proximal humerus.*

MALIGNANT BONE-FORMING TUMOURS IN SOFT TISSUE

Soft tissue osteosarcoma (Figure 9.28), *chondrosarcoma* (Figure 9.29) and *fibrosarcoma* (Figure 9.30) may all be found. Irregular mineralization is seen in the soft tissues. The diagnosis is made by biopsy. The features are those of a mineralizing, irregular malignant soft tissue mass.

Recurrence of malignancy should also be assessed on the plain film. The presence of a metal prosthesis may make interpretation by CT or MR imaging difficult because of artefact, but the recurrence of the tumour in the soft tissues may be ossified (Figure 9.31).

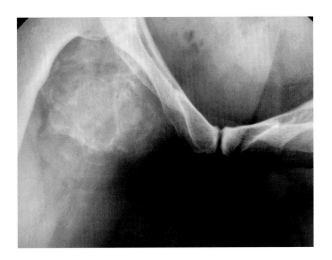

Figure 9.30 *Soft tissue fibrosarcoma. Another irregularly ossifying mass with no specific diagnostic features is demonstrated in the thigh, perhaps resembling an ossifying haematoma.*

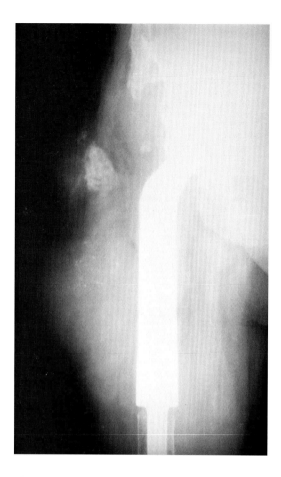

Figure 9.31 *Recurrence of chondrosarcoma in the soft tissues. The patient had had a chondrosarcoma of the proximal femur resected. A massive replacement was performed. Recurrence is shown by the appearance of a large ossifying soft tissue mass.*

SOFT TISSUE CALCIFICATION (Table 9.1)

Calcification in and around tendons occurs most commonly in the shoulder and less commonly at the hip.

Shoulder

Deposition of hydroxyapatite crystals around the tendons of the rotator cuff is seen in around 3% of adults and is a common cause of shoulder pain. Supraspinatus is most often affected (Figure 9.32). Calcific masses of varying sizes may be seen proximal

Table 9.1 Sites of soft tissue calcification.

Situation	Disease
Peri- and intra-articular	Osteoarthritis
	Tumoural calcinosis
	CPPD and other crystal deposition diseases
	Ageing
	Hyperparathyroidism and renal osteodystrophy
	Familial hypercalcaemia
	Haemochromatosis
	Haemosiderosis
Vascular	
Arterial:	Old age
	media—pipestem
	interna—plaque
	Diabetes
	Hyperparathyroidism and renal osteodystrophy
	Tumours
Venous:	Phleboliths
	Haemangioma
Nervous	Leprosy
Subcutaneous	Scleroderma
	Dermatomyositis
	Mixed connective tissue disease
Deep calcification	Compartment syndrome
	Injection site calcification
Discal calcification	Immobilization
	Ankylosing spondylitis
	Post-infective
	DISH
	Idiopathic (in cervical spine in children)
	Degeneration
	Ochronosis
Parasitic calcification	Loa-loa
	Guinea worm
	Cysticercosis
	Armiliffer armilatus

to the tendinous insertion (Figure 9.33a,b). These may be hidden on internal rotation views and are better visualized in external rotation. Calcifications are seen at ultrasound and as areas of low signal around an abnormal tendon on MR (Figure 9.33c). At one time

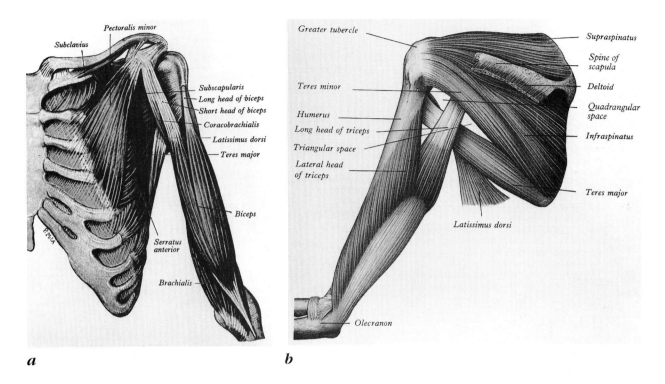

Figure 9.32 *Diagram showing insertion of shoulder tendons.* (**a**) *Anterior view;* (**b**) *posterior view. (Reproduced from* Gray's Anatomy, *38th edition, by kind permission of Churchill Livingstone, Edinburgh.)*

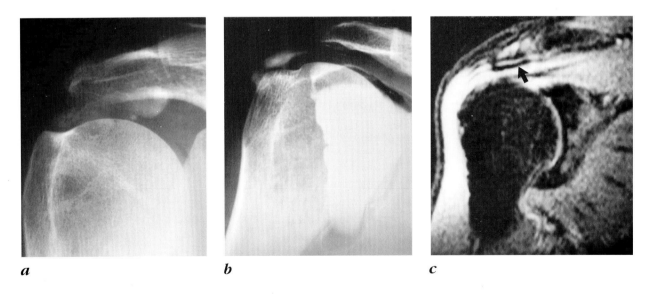

Figure 9.33 (**a**) *Calcific tendinitis in the supraspinatus insertion. Extensive calcification is shown proximal to the greater tuberosity.* (**b**) *Calcific tendinitis. In another patient the rotator cuff is still intact, as demonstrated by the arthrogram.* (**c**) *Rotator cuff calcification seen at MRI. On the fat suppression sequence a transverse band of low signal is situated immediately beneath the acromion (arrow).*

it was thought that the presence of calcification on the tendon implied that the tendon was intact and that when the tendon ruptured, the calcification dispersed and the pain vanished. It is now realized that the calcification commonly occurs in the presence of partial or total rotator cuff tears.

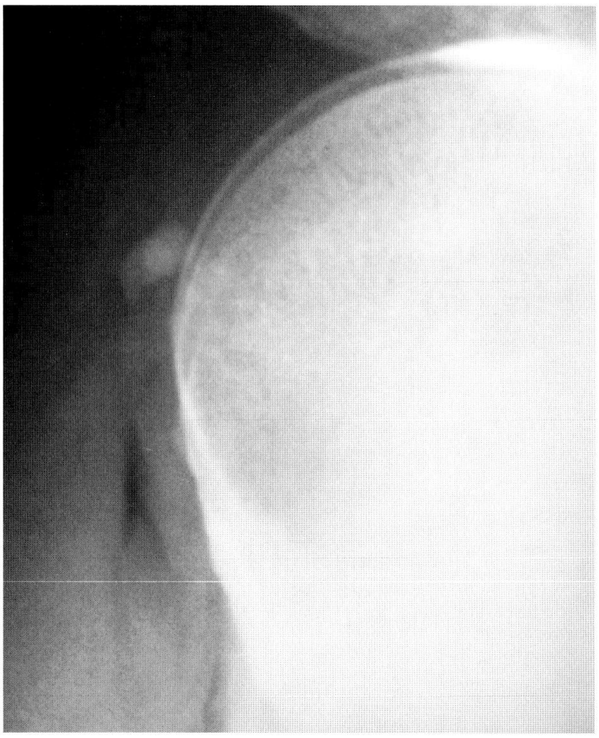

Calcification in infraspinatus is projected below that for supraspinatus, as befits the lower insertion of the tendon (Figure 9.34). Calcification may be extensive (Figure 9.35).

Bicipital tendon calcification may arise proximally along the line of the tendon for the long head and, more commonly, distally in the bicipital groove. Subscapularis calcification is also seen, anteriorly, related to its insertion into the lesser tuberosity (Figure 9.36).

Hip

Just as calcifications are seen in the tendons inserting into the greater tuberosity of the shoulder, so too are they seen at the tendons around the hip (Figure 9.37), especially at the greater trochanter. Gluteus medius may be affected. Rectus femoris may be affected at the anterior inferior iliac spine (Figure 9.38).

Figure 9.34 *Infraspinatus calcification projected beneath the summit of the humeral head.*

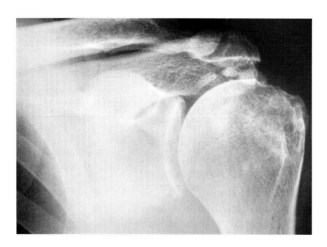

Figure 9.35 *Widespread dystrophic calcification in the rotator cuff.*

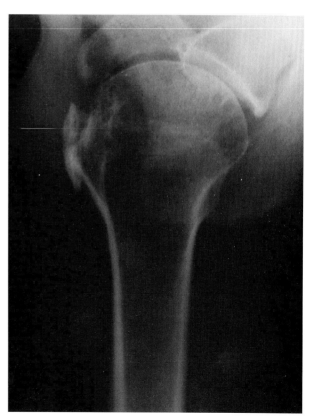

Figure 9.36 *Calcification in the subscapularis tendon. This is anteriorly situated.*

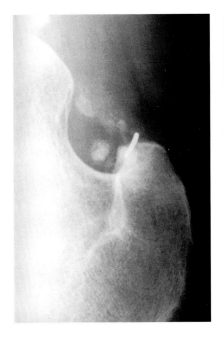

Figure 9.37 *Calcification at the greater trochanter prior to attempted aspiration.*

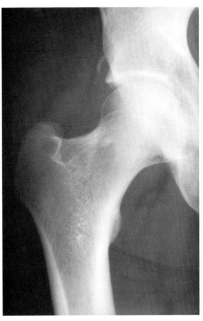

Figure 9.38 *Calcification in rectus femoris origin.*

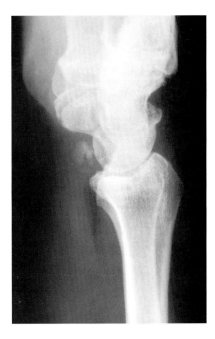

Figure 9.40 *Calcification in flexor carpi ulnaris tendon.*

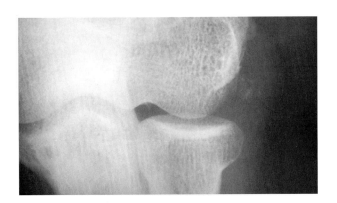

Figure 9.39 *Irregular calcification is seen at the common extensor origin.*

Table 9.2 Causes of cartilage calcification.

Old age
Hyperparathyroidism
Gout
Pseudogout
Ochronosis
Wilson's disease
Haemochromatosis
CPPD crystal deposition disease
Repeated intra-articular steroid injections
Chondrodysplasia punctata

Elbow

Dystrophic calcification is seen in both the common extensor (Figure 9.39) and flexor origins.

Hand and wrist

The commonest site for calcific tendinitis in the hand is in flexor carpi ulnaris, related to repetitive strain injury. Calcification may be seen on a lateral view anterior and proximal to the pisiform (Figure 9.40).

CHONDROCALCINOSIS (Table 9.2)

Visualization of calcification in cartilage is usually related to calcium pyrophosphate dihydrate (CPPD) crystal deposition. Calcification in patients with CPPD

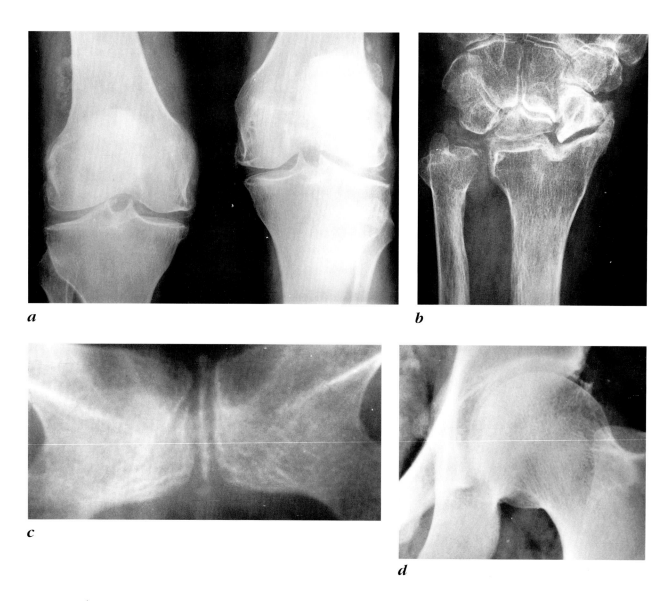

Figure 9.41 (*a*) *Chondrocalcinosis in the meniscal and articular cartilages, as well as synovium, of the knee.* (*b*) *Chondrocalcinosis in the triangular fibrocartilage at the wrist, together with calcium pyrophosphate dihydrate crystal deposition in the distal radio-ulnar joint. The patient, in addition, had probably suffered a waist of scaphoid fracture and the proximal pole of the scaphoid has been resorbed. A prominent spur on the proximal pole of the distal portion erodes the adjacent radius. Overall, the bones show severe demineralization.* (*c*) *Chondrocalcinosis in the symphysis pubis and* (*d*) *in articular cartilage at the hip.*

crystal deposition disease is commonest at the knee, then at the wrists, hands, ankles and hips.

According to Resnick (1995), up to 30% of patients with cartilage calcification are asymptomatic. Twenty per cent have a clinical pattern of pseudogout characterized by acute attacks of arthritis, especially at the knee, hip, shoulder and other major joints. A more chronic form of the disease also occurs in large joints in association with degenerative joint disease.

In gout, up to 30% of patients have chondrocalcinosis involving fibrocartilage, again usually at the knee, but also at the wrist, hip and symphysis pubis.

Patients with hyperparathyroidism will have an elevated serum calcium and, while hyperparathyroidism is a rare cause, chondrocalcinosis is seen in 30% of patients with hyperparathyroidism. This occurs especially at the knee, in those with longstanding disease, and at an earlier age (sixth

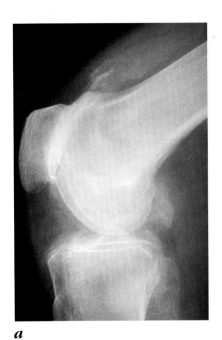

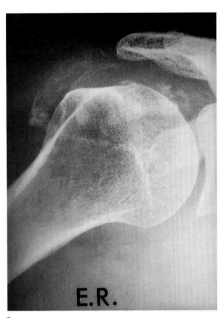

a　　　　　*b*

Figure 9.42 *(a) Synovial calcification at the knee is associated with degenerative change. This is seen in the suprapatellar pouch and also in the posterior joint capsule on the lateral view. (b) Calcific bursitis around the shoulder (film obtained in external rotation). The subacromial bursa is enlarged and lined with calcium.*

decade) than in 'senile' chondrocalcinosis (seventh to eighth decades).

Deposits occur both in fibrocartilage—the menisci of the knee (Figure 9.41a), the triangular fibrocartilage at the wrist (Figure 9.41b), the labra and the symphysis pubis (Figure 9.41c), as well as in hyaline or articular cartilage, especially at wrists, knees and hips (Figure 9.41d), as thin layers of calcification parallel to the adjacent articular cortex.

Synovial calcification also occurs, especially at the knee (Figure 9.42a) and wrist, as well as in the shoulder (Figure 9.42b).

HAEMOCHROMATOSIS

In this condition haemosiderin is deposited in the soft tissues, either in a genetic form or, in an older patient, as a complication of iron overload. Males are affected more commonly than females, and changes are usually seen in middle age. Iron deposition occurs in the liver and pancreas, causing failure of these organs, as well as in the gonads.

An arthropathy is associated with haemochromatosis which resembles the changes seen in rheumatoid arthritis. There is joint swelling, pain and stiffness. An acute arthritis also occurs relating to CPPD crystal deposition, which occurs in addition to the deposition of iron in the synovial tissues (Figure 9.43a, b).

Chondrocalcinosis occurs in patients with haemochromatosis at the knee, wrist and symphysis pubis.

Radiologically, osteoporosis and articular calcification are seen. Subsequently an arthritis resembling that of osteoarthritis occurs, especially at the metacarpophalangeal joints in the hand, with joint space narrowing and subarticular cyst formation with articular collapse (Figure 9.43c). The appearances therefore are those of degenerative joint disease at the metacarpophalangeal joints—an unusual site for degeneration—in association with chrondrocalcinosis, especially at the wrist.

PHLEBOLITHS

Phleboliths are 2–5 mm round densities, often with a central lucency. Usually multiple, they form in varicosities, around the urinary bladder, in the scrotum and in varicose veins in the lower limbs.

Multiple phleboliths in soft tissues may be seen in haemangiomas and Maffucci's syndrome in association with multiple enchondromas. There is a high incidence of chondrosarcomatous degeneration in the latter condition (see Chapter 7, page 345).

In the Ehlers–Danlos syndrome, rounded areas of subcutaneous calcification (spheroids) are related to fat necrosis. Calcifications are often subcutaneous (Figure 9.44).

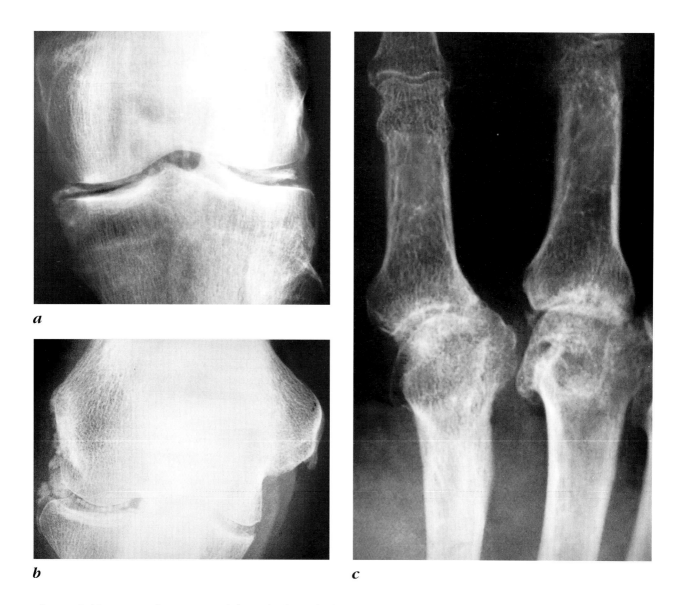

Figure 9.43 *Haemochromatosis. (**a**) At the knee both articular and meniscal cartilages are involved. (**b**) At the elbow articular and soft tissue calcification is seen at the flexor and extensor origins. (**c**) Osteoarthritic change with a rheumatoid arthritis distribution in the hand.*

VARICOSE VEINS

Varicose veins can be seen on plain films as sinusoidal tortuous soft tissue densities in subcutaneous fat. Local oedema results in thickening of soft tissues and blurring of the muscle–fat–skin interfaces. An underlying periostitis may result (see Chapter 6, page 319). Ulceration is also seen in the soft tissues which, if chronic, may undergo granulomatous (Figure 9.45) or malignant degeneration (Marjolin's ulcer), with subsequent erosion of underlying bone.

ARTERIAL CALCIFICATION

Arterial calcification is of two basic types. Intimal plaques of degenerative calcification, discontinuous and irregular, occlude the lumen. Medial calcification

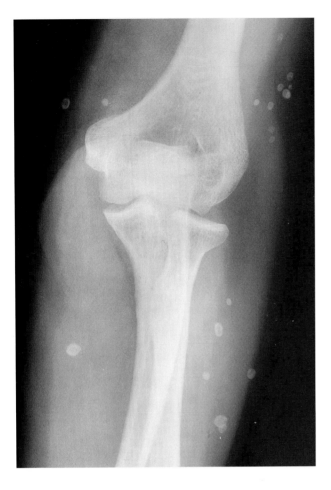

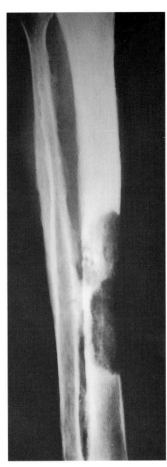

Figure 9.45 *Varicose ulceration with granulomatous erosion of the underlying bone. The patient was 81 years of age and had had varicose veins for 20 years. A large ulcer was present which was associated with bone destruction. This suggested malignant transformation of the ulcer, but the histology showed there to be granulomatous change only.*

Figure 9.44 *Subcutaneous calcification in Ehlers–Danlos syndrome. Rounded calcific densities with a lucent centre are shown.*

is continuous, better defined and ring-like in continuity along the line of major blood vessels. This is seen in diabetes and Buerger's disease.

NEURAL CALCIFICATION

This is rare, but is described in leprosy (Figure 9.46).

PARASITIC CALCIFICATION

Cysticercosis

Calcified cysts of *Taenia solium* lie in the muscles arranged along the plane of the fibres. They are 2–3 mm in length, may number in their hundreds and are clearly seen on a plain film (Figure 9.47).

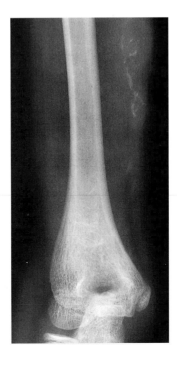

Figure 9.46 *Calcification in the nerves in leprosy. This is rare.*

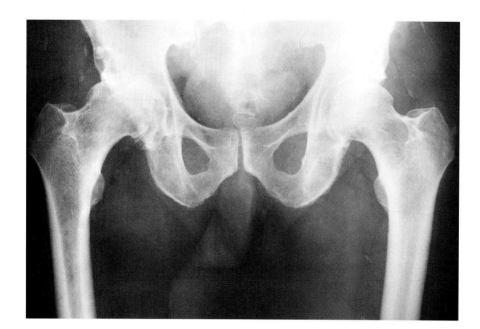

Figure 9.47 *Cysticercosis— 3 mm calcific densities are arranged along the plane of the muscular fibres. Note fat lines around the hip joints.*

Loa-loa

Small, thin, calcified, coiled densities can best be seen in the relatively sparse soft tissues of the hand (Figure 9.48) and are associated with polyarthritis. The parasite is found in Nigeria, central Africa and Angola.

Guinea worm

The parasite is found in Arabia, Iran, the Sudan and in West Africa. This larger, denser, calcified, dead worm—*Dracunulus medinensis*—is seen in bulkier muscles—thigh and calf. It may be associated with septic arthritis (Figure 9.49).

CORAL FRAGMENTS

Plantar densities in the soft tissues of the feet result from walking barefoot in the sea (Figure 9.50).

CALCIFIED INJECTIONS

Bilateral round calcified opacities, often with a denser rim, are found in the buttocks. They may be up to 2 cm in diameter. Dystrophic calcification follows fat necrosis (Figure 9.51).

Heavy metal injections tend to have a denser, linear track.

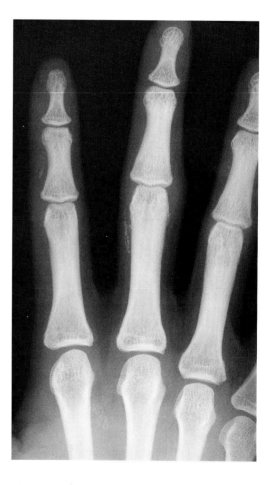

Figure 9.48 *Loa-loa: small, curled-up, calcified, dead parasites are shown in the relatively sparse soft tissues of the hand.*

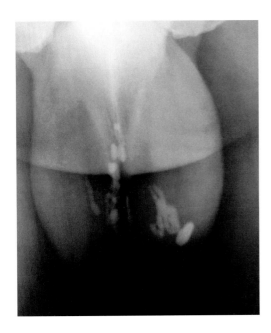

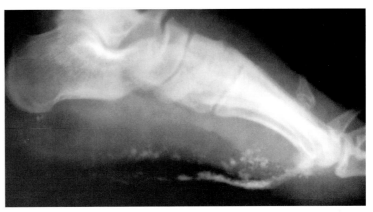

Figure 9.50 *Coral fragments in the sole of the foot. Bizarre calcifications are demonstrated in the soft tissues of the sole in a native of the Fiji Islands (by courtesy of Professor HG Jacobson).*

Figure 9.49 *Guinea worm, in this instance, in the scrotum. Phleboliths occur here more commonly.*

Figure 9.51 *Calcified injection remnant. The patient had been previously treated with injections in both buttocks for a tropical illness. The appearance is of peripheral calcification around the soft tissue mass and is typical for quinine injection. At histology the lesion consisted of necrotic fat and calcification of the capsule.*

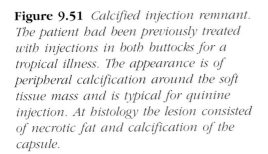

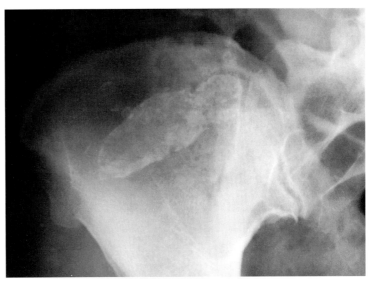

SCLERODERMA

Scleroderma is a cause of acro-osteolysis (see Figure 4.21) in association with pulp atrophy, as well as of a similar soft tissue contraction and bone resorption at the mandible (Figure 9.52). Bone resorption also occurs at the clavicle, cervical spinous processes and ribs as in rheumatoid arthritis (Table 1.10).

This resorption of bone and soft tissue in the hand may be associated with calcification in the pulp around the tuft (Figure 9.53). Calcifications resembling those seen in tumoural calcinosis (see below) also occur around major joints—hip (Figure 9.54), knee, elbow and wrist—and around small joints in the hand or foot, in soft tissues, tendons, capsule or in the joint space.

DERMATOMYOSITIS

Muscle weakness, fatigue and pain are associated with skin rashes, often facial. Raynaud's phenomenon and acro-osteolysis occur. Arthritis, which does not usually have erosive features is present, although occasionally in patients who are seropositive, changes resembling rheumatoid arthritis may be

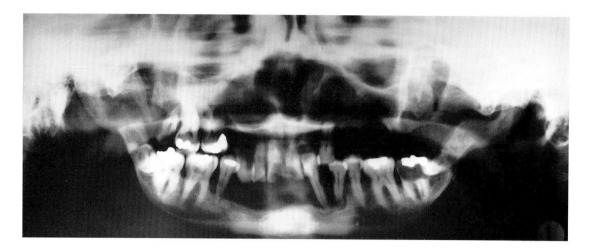

Figure 9.52 *Mandibular atrophy in scleroderma. Clinically, the patient had a pointed chin and the radiograph demonstrates almost total resorption of the mandible, leaving only the supporting bone at the sockets.*

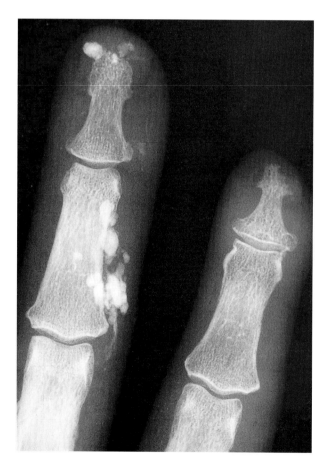

Figure 9.53 *Scleroderma. Pulp atrophy, acro-osteolysis and soft tissue calcification.*

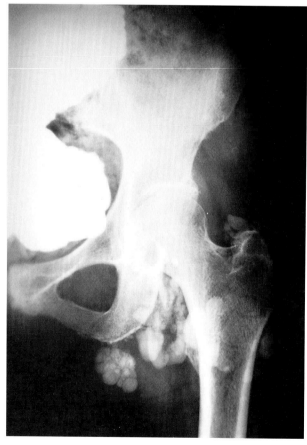

Figure 9.54 *Scleroderma. Calcific deposits around the hip joint resembling those seen in tumoural calcinosis.*

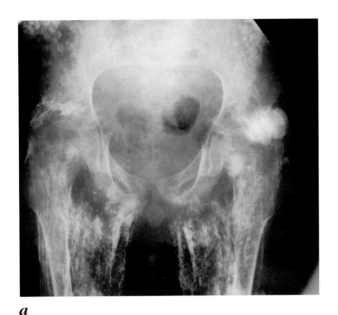

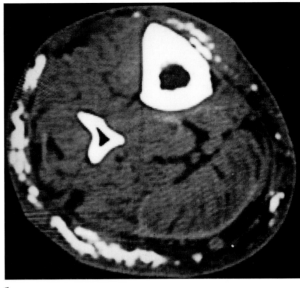

a *b*

Figure 9.55 *Dermatomyositis. (**a**) Sheet-like plaques of calcification are shown wrapped around the thigh in association with periarticular calcification similar to that seen in scleroderma. (**b**) CT scan showing plaque-like calcification in the subcutaneous fat.*

seen, so that an overlap syndrome may be present. Older patients may have an underlying neoplasm.

Calcification typically occurs in intermuscular fascial planes and especially in sheets in the subcutaneous fat (Figure 9.55). Calcification also occurs in tendons and in soft tissues over distal phalanges associated with resorption of bone, as in scleroderma.

HYPERPARATHYROIDISM

Soft tissue calcification is more commonly seen in patients with renal osteodystrophy than in those with primary hyperparathyroidism (Figure 9.56). Calcification may occur in non-visceral (periarticular and subcutaneous) and visceral (heart, lung and muscle) sites (see Figure 2.66). The calcific material in the latter contains a greater amount of magnesium.

Large lobulated calcific masses around major joints resemble changes seen in tumoural calcinosis, but the latter is an essentially idiopathic phenomenon without the major biochemical and radiological bone changes seen in secondary hyperparathyroidism.

Calcific deposits are also seen in periarticular situations around swollen joints in association with the other changes of renal osteodystrophy. The

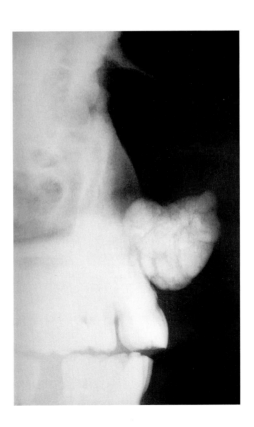

Figure 9.56 *Soft tissue calcification in renal osteodystrophy.*

calcification may regress in patients with renal osteodystrophy on haemodialysis.

TUMOURAL CALCINOSIS

Large well-defined or lobulated calcific masses are seen, often symmetrically, in the soft tissues around large joints, usually on the extensor aspect, but also in the vicinity of small joints in the hand. Men are more often affected than women. The lesions are common in Africa and may be related to chronic trauma. The mass lesions are not uniformly dense, but are rather patchily calcified (Figure 9.57) and, in larger lesions, sedimentation may occur, with a less dense supernatant layered on a rather denser lower calcification. Occasionally, the lesions ulcerate through the skin and discharge their contents. They may be solitary or multiple and are usually seen in the second and third decades of life.

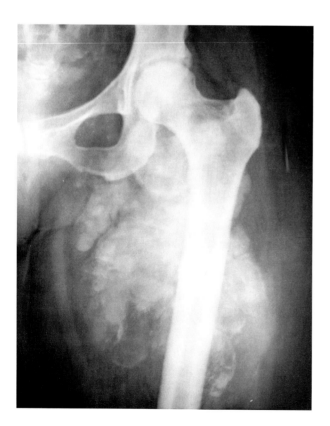

Figure 9.57 *Tumoural calcinosis. A very large, lobulated, calcific soft tissue mass is demonstrated below the hip extending into the upper thigh.*

Table 9.3 Ossification in soft tissues.
Neurologic around bones and joints
In decubitus ulcers
Primary tumours in soft tissue or secondary to a primary in the underlying bone
Pseudomalignant tumour of soft tissues
Trauma
Fibrodysplasia ossificans progressiva
Melorheostosis
Post-operative

OSSIFICATION IN THE SOFT TISSUES (Table 9.3)

AVULSION INJURIES

Muscle traction on apophyses prior to growth plate fusion results in displacement of the apophysis with subjacent haemorrhage and new bone formation. This typically appears around the pelvis (Figure 9.58a).

A large bony mass, initially irregular, then well defined, forms at these sites. Both radiologically and histologically in a susceptible age group a malignant tumour of bone might be considered (Figure 9.58b, c), but the site and history should avoid even the need for biopsy.

Similar lesions arise with pathologically soft bone, for example in Paget's disease. Here, 'pull off' lesions also arise at sites of musculotendinous insertions and may resemble exostoses (see Figure 2.10).

NEUROGENIC HETEROTOPIC NEW BONE FORMATION (Table 9.3)

New bone formation around major joints occurs following head injury or with paraplegia secondary to spinal cord injury, especially in those with spastic paralysis (Figure 9.59). It may be that over-vigorous physiotherapy ruptures muscles, and soft tissue ossification results around joints. Ankylosis may follow.

Patients with sensory loss develop decubitus ulcers, which on penetration allow infective destruction of underlying bone. This is subsequently associated with irregular local new bone formation (Figure 9.60).

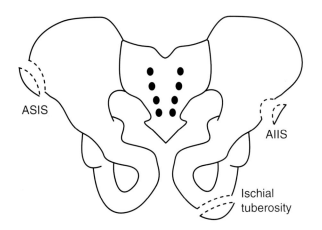

a

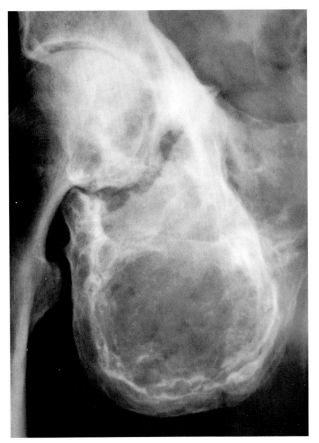

c

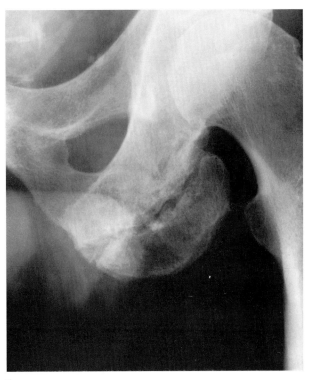

b

Figure 9.58 (*a*) *Diagram to shows sites of avulsion at apophyses around the pelvic ring. ASIS: anterior superior iliac spine; AIIS: anterior inferior iliac spine.* (*b*, *c*) *Avulsion at the ischial apophysis results in new bone forming between the distracted apophysis and the underlying metaphysis.*

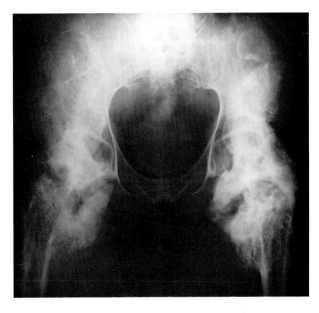

Figure 9.59 *Paraplegic myositis ossificans. The cord had been severed at T7, following a mining accident 3 years before. There is extensive new bone formation around both hips.*

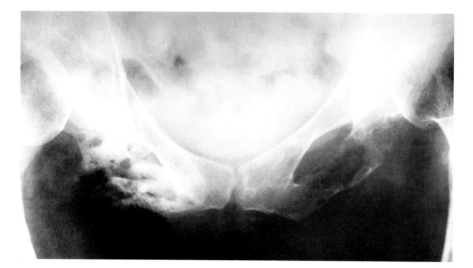

Figure 9.60 *New bone formation at a decubitus ulcer. The patient was paraplegic. Gas is seen in the soft tissues, indicating ulceration. The ischium is in part destroyed, but there is local irregular new bone formation on the right. On the left, the ischial changes are mainly destructive.*

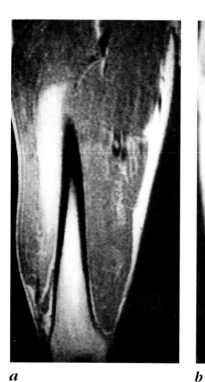

a

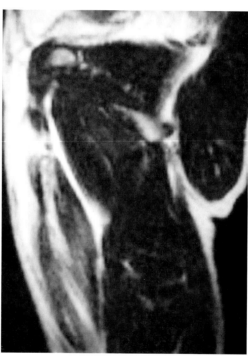

b

Figure 9.61 *Intramuscular haematoma demonstrated at MRI. (**a**) A coronal T₁-weighted MR sequence shows a haematoma and disruption of muscle. (**b**) In another patient a sagittal T₂-weighted image demonstrates diffuse intramuscular haemorrhage.*

MYOSITIS OSSIFICANS TRAUMATICA

CT, ultrasound and especially MRI (Figures 9.61, 9.62 and 9.63) are much more sensitive than the plain film in the diagnosis of post-traumatic muscle haemorrhage and in the follow-up of progression and healing of the haematoma but, in previous years, the plain film was used to confirm the presence of ossification in muscles—a late sequel of trauma, occurring at 4–6 weeks after the traumatic episode (Figure 9.64). On the plain film, a central more lucent area is surrounded by a denser shell of mineralization. A transradiant zone is said to be present between the cortex of the underlying bone and the lesion itself (Figure 9.65a). This lucent zone may be lacking with a parosteal sarcoma, in which part of the tumour is attached to bone, but the margin need not be (Figure 9.65). As the traumatic lesion may also be attached,

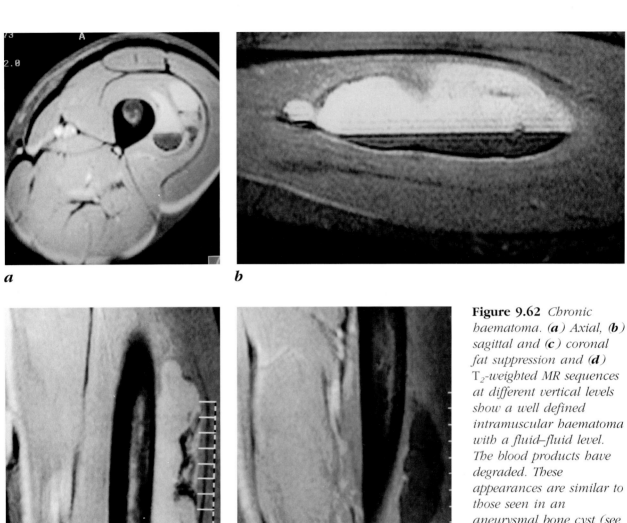

a

b

c

d

Figure 9.62 *Chronic haematoma. (**a**) Axial, (**b**) sagittal and (**c**) coronal fat suppression and (**d**) T$_2$-weighted MR sequences at different vertical levels show a well defined intramuscular haematoma with a fluid–fluid level. The blood products have degraded. These appearances are similar to those seen in an aneurysmal bone cyst (see Figure 3.93).*

this is not always a helpful differentiating feature. Subsequently the mineralized lesion matures, becomes more dense, smaller and may incorporate onto the underlying cortex (Figure 9.66). The lesion may then resemble a sessile osteochondroma and will be dense, smooth and corticated.

PSEUDOMALIGNANT OSSEOUS TUMOUR OF SOFT TISSUE

Pain and soft tissue swelling, usually without antecedent trauma, affects the upper or lower limbs in adolescents and young adults. The history may

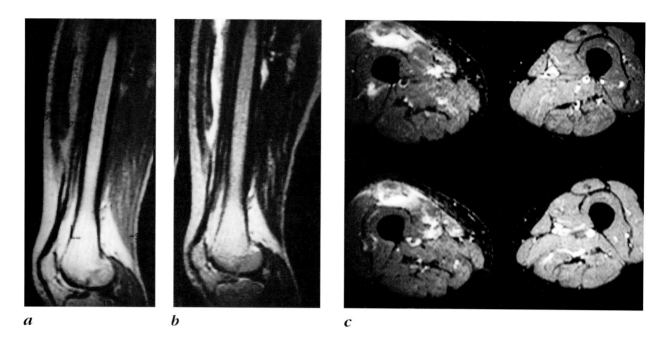

a   *b*   *c*

Figure 9.63 *Haematoma.* (*a*) *Sagittal proton density weighted,* (*b*) T$_2$-*weighted and* (*c*) *axial fat suppression MR images show extensive disruption of the anterior musculature of the thigh. The change affects rectus femoris on the right.*

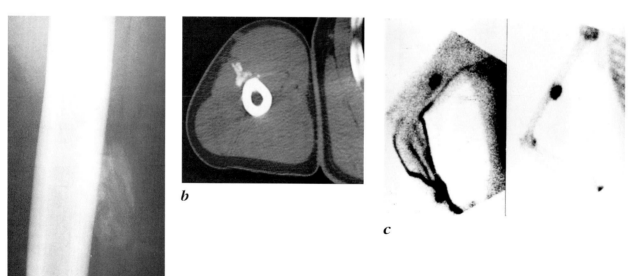

b

c

a

Figure 9.64 *Ossifying haematoma.* (*a*) *The plain radiograph shows an irregular ossifying mass situated adjacent to the mid-shaft of the humerus, not clearly separate from the underlying cortex. The periphery is slightly more dense than the centre of the ossifying mass.* (*b*) *The CT scan confirms the appearance seen on the plain film and shows the plane of cleavage between the lesion and the underlying bone.* (*c*) *The radioisotope bone scan shows increased uptake locally;* (left) *vascular phase,* (right) *delayed scan.*

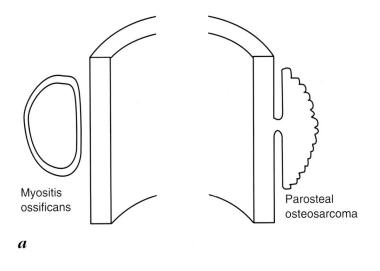

Myositis
ossificans

Parosteal
osteosarcoma

a

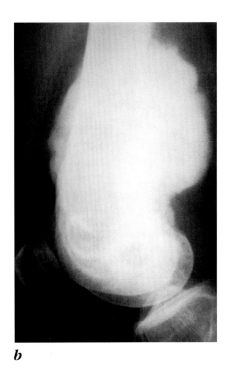

b

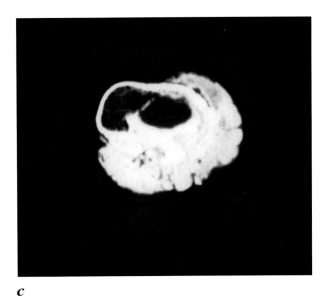

c

Figure 9.65 *(a) Line drawing representing the theoretical difference between myositis ossificans and a parosteal osteosarcoma. In fact, the distinction is not easily made on this basis alone (after Resnick, 1995). (b, c) Parosteal osteosarcoma. The initial radiograph shows the ossifying mass situated around the distal femoral shaft with an anterior plane of cleavage between the tumour and the cortex, but none posteriorly. (c) The CT scan shows the extensive nature of the lesion and a plane of cleavage anteriorly but not posteriorly.*

thus mimic that found with osteogenic sarcoma. Absence of trauma should rule out myositis ossificans traumatica.

The history precedes radiographic change by 2–3 weeks. Radiologically, a well defined mineralizing mass with a denser periphery than centre is seen (Figure 9.67). Histology shows a core of central fibrous with peripheral cartilaginous and bone metaplasia. The peripheral bony density may help distinguish this process from osteogenic sarcoma of soft tissue radiologically and the natural history also differs, the benign condition usually being self-remitting.

FIBRODYSPLASIA OSSIFICANS PROGRESSIVA (MYOSITIS OSSIFICANS PROGRESSIVA; MUNCHMEYER'S SYNDROME)

This is a true congenital dysplasia of bone associated with soft tissue ossification. Skeletal anomalies involve the great toe (Figure 9.68) and thumb and are seen at birth (Figure 9.68). Fusion of cervical vertebral bodies with a widened cervical canal are seen (Figure 9.69). The vertebral bodies elsewhere tend to be tall. Femoral and mandibular condylar necks are broad.

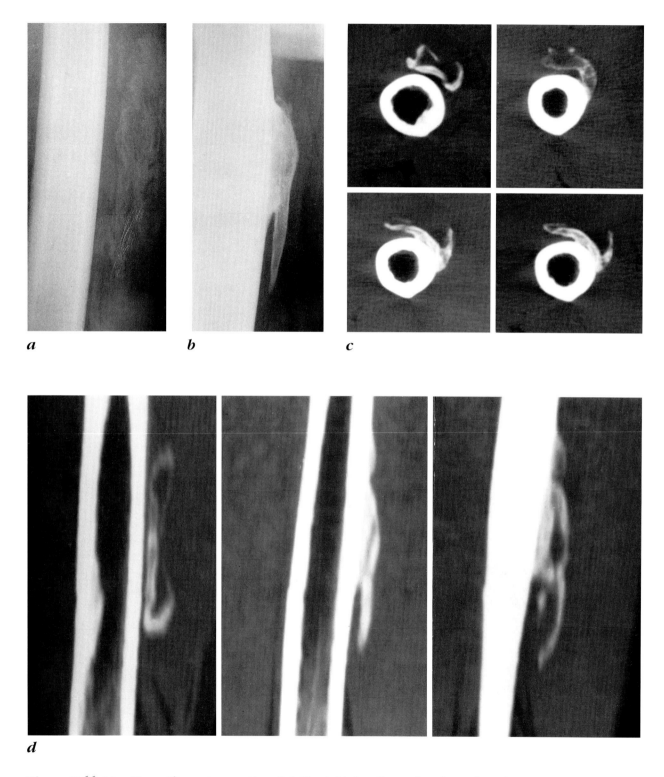

a   *b*   *c*

d

Figure 9.66 *Myositis ossificans traumatica. (**a**) The initial radiograph, taken when the patient was a young rugby player, shows soft tissue ossification. (**b**) A subsequent radiograph obtained 17 years later shows incorporation of a well defined exostosis onto the underlying bone (by courtesy of Dr RO Murray). (**c**) Axial images obtained at CT scanning in another patient who fell off his bicycle 4 months previously. The lesion is undoubtedly cortically based in the main but, due to the effect of partial voluming, in places it will appear separate from the underlying bone. (**d**) This tendency is reinforced on the sagittal reconstruction images.*

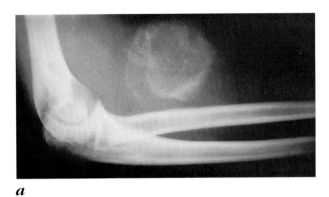

a

Figure 9.67 *Pseudomalignant tumour of soft tissue. (**a**) The radiograph shows a rounded, well defined and highly mineralized lesion, denser at the margin. (**b**) The CT scan confirms these features.*

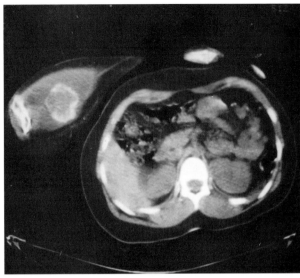

b

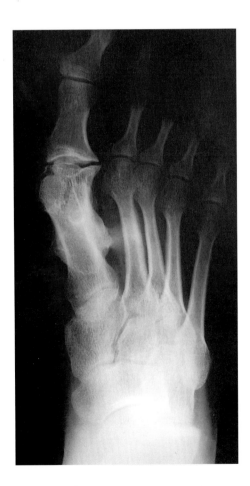

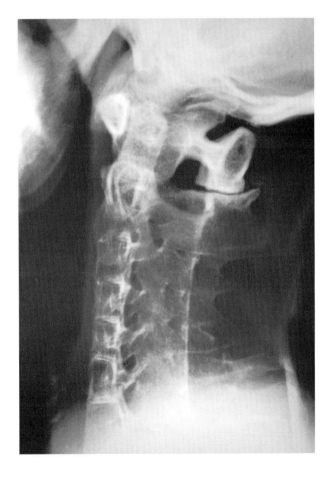

Figure 9.68 *Fibrodysplasia ossificans progressiva. A grossly dysplastic great toe is demonstrated. It is enlarged. The metatarsophalangeal joint is irregular and exostoses are shown.*

Figure 9.69 *Fibrodysplasia ossificans progressiva. Fusion of cervical vertebral bodies results in vertebral hypoplasia. The laminae and spinous processes are also fused. The canal is wide.*

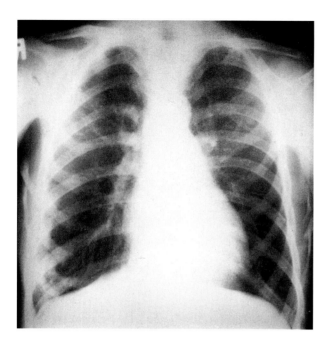

Figure 9.70 *Fibrodysplasia ossificans progressiva. Sheets of bone are demonstrated in the thoracic musculature.*

Ossification occurs in the fibrous tissue of muscle. Sheets of bone form in muscles, often attached to underlying bone, like exostoses (Figure 9.70). The changes occur proximally and only in voluntary muscle. Restriction of thoracic rib cage movement leads to pneumonia and death. Patterns of involvement of muscle may be identical in twins. Bleeding in soft tissues, even venepuncture, leads to ossification. Ankylosis occurs around joints.

BIBLIOGRAPHY

Bane BL, Evans HL, Ro JY et al (1990) Extraskeletal osteosarcoma. A clinicopathologic review of 26 cases. *Cancer* **65**: 2762–70.

Dias JJ, Finlay DBI, Brenkel JJ, Gregg PJ (1987) Radiographic assessment of soft tissue signs in clinically suspected scaphoid fractures: the incidence of false negative and false positive results. *J Orthop Trauma* **1**: 205–8.

Guerra J Jr, Armbuster TG, Resnick D et al (1978) The adult hip: an anatomic study. Part II. The soft-tissue landmarks. *Radiology* **128**: 11–20.

Lewis RJ, Ketcham AS (1973) Maffucci syndrome: functional and neoplastic significance. *J Bone Joint Surg* **55A**: 1465–79.

Pathria MN, Zlatkin M, Sartoris DJ et al (1988) Ultrasonography of the popliteal fossa and lower extremities. *Radiol Clin North Am* **26**: 77–85.

Sordillo PP, Hadju SI, Magill GB et al (1983) Extraosseous osteogenic sarcoma. A review of 48 patients. *Cancer* **51**: 727–34.

Resnick D (1995) *Diagnosis of Bone and Joint Disorders*, 3rd edn. Philadelphia: WB Saunders.

Wardle EN, Patton JT (1969) Bone and joint changes in haemochromatosis. *Ann Rheum Dis* **28**: 15–23.

Weatherall PT (ed) (1995) Musculoskeletal soft tissue imaging. *MR Imaging Clinics of North America* **3** (4).

Weekes RG, Berquist TH, McLeod RA et al (1985) Magnetic resonance imaging of soft-tissue tumors: comparison with computed tomography. *Magnetic Resonance Imaging* **3**: 345–52

Chapter 10 **Imaging techniques**

A brief résumé of imaging techniques used in diagnostic radiology is included here for the use of the clinician. The techniques currently available are listed in Table 10.1.

Table 10.1   Techniques used in musculoskeletal radiology.

Plain radiography
Linear tomography
Arthrography
Computed tomography (CT)
Radionuclide scanning, including DEXA (bone densitometry)
Ultrasonography
Magnetic resonance imaging

PLAIN FILM RADIOGRAPHY (Table 10.2)

This is usually the first radiological investigation undertaken. Films of bones and joints are often obtained in two planes at right-angles to each other, for example an AP and lateral view of the knee. The letters AP (anteroposterior) or PA (postero-anterior) indicate the direction of the beam from the X-ray tube through the patient and onto the film. The part

---

Table 10.2   Plain radiography.

Readily available
Cheap
Quickly processed
Easily read
Shows cortical bone especially well

---

to be examined should be nearest the film. The chest is examined PA, so that the heart is nearest the film, and thus not significantly magnified, while the thoracic spine is examined AP, so that it too is nearer the film.

A lateral view is not always helpful, for example at the hand or pelvis because of overlap and, under these circumstances, oblique views are used. These are often specific to the joints under investigation and may have a specific eponym, for example Judet views of the hip (45° oblique views). The use of eponyms is generally not helpful as they are not always recognized internationally. Short texts on orthopaedic radiography are available (see Appendix).

Digital imaging allows storage of images on disc and subsequent reconstruction (imaging) at outlying workstations. Irradiation levels are lower than with conventional plain film imaging.

Macroradiography is unobtainable outside specialist units. Generally, magnification of an imaged object results in loss of definition. For acceptable macro images, a very fine focal spot (< 15 µmd) is needed, as well as fine-grain film. The object is placed close to the X-ray tube and far from the film. 10 or 20 × magnification results and small objects around 25–50 µm can be seen. This technique has been of value in showing early erosions in rheumatoid arthritis and hyperparathyroidism.

TOMOGRAPHY

A single layer can be imaged when the tube and film rotate about the patient, the layer imaged being centred about the axis of rotation of tube and film. Multiple layers are imaged by moving the tube–film linkage up or down along the long axis of the patient. The thickness of plane imaged can be altered—the longer the arc of tube movement, the thinner the 'slice'. Linear, circular, elliptical or polycycloidal movements are available, the latter giving

Table 10.3 Uses of arthrography.

Site	Disease
Shoulder	Rotator cuff tear
	Frozen shoulder
	Biceps tendon integrity
	Loose bodies
	Labral integrity (combined with CT)
Elbow	Loose bodies
	Articular integrity
Wrist	Triangular cartilage integrity
	Midcarpal joint integrity
Hip	Labral integrity
	Articular integrity
	Loose bodies
	Diagnosing 'snapping' hips
	Determining the head-socket relationship, for example in congenital dislocation
	Perthes' disease and dysplasias
Knee	Loose bodies
	Meniscal and cruciate integrity
	Articular surface integrity
	Adventitious bursae and their complications
Ankle	Capsular and ligamentous integrity
	Articular integrity
Temporomandibular joint	TMJ malfunction syndrome
	Meniscal abnormalities
In general	To assess tumours, infections, prostheses

extremely fine detail. Since the advent of computerized axial tomography (CAT) scanning, conventional tomography is used less often.

Tomography has the major advantages over plain radiography in that a small lesion can be visualized in its entirety without the distraction of overlying structures, such as bowel gas, while larger objects are better defined. Radiation dosages are higher unless multiple films are loaded in a box cassette, when a single exposure suffices.

ARTHROGRAPHY (Table 10.3)

This facilitates visualization of the internal structure of a joint by negative (air) or positive (iodinated) contrast media, first used for the knee in 1904 and for the shoulder, using an oil-based medium, in 1939. Injection of contrast into a joint can be preceded by aspiration of joint contents for microbiologic or cytologic examination.

Arthrography has been used to demonstrate all the major joints, but minor joints, such as the metacarpophalangeal joints, can also be imaged. In the knee, arthrographic examination of the menisci is as accurate as arthroscopy, but the cruciate ligaments are better shown at arthroscopy.

Where magnetic resonance imaging (MRI) is available, routine arthrography is generally no longer performed. Dynamic studies, for example of the paediatric hip, may still currently be performed using fluoro-arthrography, although MRI will no doubt routinely be available for dynamic studies. Prosthetic loosening is still investigated by aspiration arthrography.

ULTRASONOGRAPHY (Table 10.4)

Diagnostic ultrasound uses sound frequencies higher than those audible to the human ear (>20 000 cycles per second). A hand-held probe contains arrayed piezo-electric crystals which generate sound pulses and receives them back in attenuated form after reflection from the target tissues. These are then processed by a computer and the images displayed.

The resulting images may vary because of:

(1) *ultrasound frequency*. The higher the frequency, the better the spatial resolution, but the poorer the depth of penetration of the tissues by the sound waves;
(2) *the nature of the underlying tissues*. Bone is totally refractory to sound waves (as is air). The deep soft tissues in joints therefore cannot be assessed. Ultrasound is thus of more limited use in the knee than in the shoulder, the internal structures of which are more accessible to the beam.

The speed of sound in tissues varies with the nature of the tissue: the greater the density, the greater the

Table 10.4 Uses of ultrasound in musculoskeletal disease (reproduced with kind permission of Dr S Burnett).

Site	Disease	Site	Disease
Shoulder	Rotator cuff, including subscapularis, for impingement, calcification and tears	Ankle and foot	Peroneal tendinitis or rupture
	Subacromial bursitis		Posterior tibialis tendinitis or rupture
	Biceps tendon integrity		Achilles tendinitis or rupture
	Labral defect		Ankle sprains
	Hill–Sachs defect		Morton's neuroma
Elbow	Triceps tendinitis		Plantar fasciitis
	Medial or lateral epicondylitis	Skin	Thickness of melanoma
	Distal biceps tendinitis or rupture		Epidermal or dermal lesions
Wrist	Tendinitis		Heel pad thickness
	Gamekeeper's thumb		Measurement of subcutaneous fat
	Triangular fibrocartilage complex tear	Miscellaneous	Muscle strain, partial or full thickness tear
	Carpal tunnel syndrome		Bursitis
Hip	Greater trochanter bursitis		Palpable mass
	Muscle strain—rectus femoris, sartorius, adductors, hamstrings		Vascularity of soft tissue tumours
	Prosthesis aspiration		Fracture healing, limb lengthening
Knee	Quadriceps rupture		Joint effusion
	Patellar dislocation, patellar tendinitis, evaluate retinaculum		Nonopaque foreign body
	Loose body		Aspiration—osteomyelitis/cyst/mass
	Tendinitis, bursitis, Baker's cyst		Biopsy guidance
	Collateral ligament injury		Tendon integrity in rheumatoid disease
	Posterior cruciate ligament		Synovial masses
	Osgood–Schlatter's disease		Subluxing tendons
	Sinding–Larsen syndrome		Ganglia
	Posterior and lateral meniscal tears and separations		Infective tenosynovitis—aspiration
		Paediatric	Tethered cord
			Hip dysplasia
			Transient synovitis
			Infantile skeletal trauma prior to bone mineralization

speed of the transmitted sound. Sound is reflected back at tissue interfaces, so that the returning pulses characterize the underlying tissues and tissue interfaces. Cystic lesions have a well defined margin and are echo-free with distal echo enhancement. Tumours of soft tissue are usually of altered echogeneity with altered texture, and have a more complex and irregular pattern than normal soft tissues.

COMPUTERIZED AXIAL TOMOGRAPHY (CAT SCANNING, CT SCANNING)
(Table 10.5)

A tomographic technique is used to give sequential axial slices of varying thicknesses. The X-ray source passes in an arc around the patient and the detectors lie opposite them in the arc. Because the information

Table 10.5   Computed tomography (CT).

Demonstrates bone well but has a significant
   radiation dose
Shows soft tissue also
Erosions seen
Permits reconstruction to any plane

Table 10.6   Radionuclide bone scanning.

More sensitive, but less specific
Gives accurate localization of disease
Significant radiation dose

obtained is stored in a computer, a much wider grey scale is reproduced compared with a conventional X-ray film–screen combination. Computer storage allows accurate assessment of tissue density, measured in Hounsfield units (after the inventor of the technique). Reconstructions can also be obtained in any plane, but the definition of these secondary images is not as good as the original. Three-dimensional CT reformatting is possible.

Vascular soft tissues can be enhanced by intravenous water-soluble contrast media, but soft tissues are better demonstrated at MRI.

CT is used especially to show bone, but also soft tissues in the axial or any other plane. In the spine, the state of the lateral recesses and facet joints can be accurately assessed. Conventional studies, such as arthrograms, radiculograms and discograms, are improved upon by subsequent axial imaging, where spatial relationships in the sagittal and coronal planes are demonstrated without the overlap seen on conventional imaging.

CT is better than MRI at assessing cortical bone, while MRI demonstrates soft tissues more clearly. CT is thus of particular value in the assessment of bone trauma and cortical changes with infection or tumour, as well as in the arthritides.

The radiation dose from CT scans may be high and it is estimated that 25% of the radiation dose to the public now comes from CT scans.

RADIONUCLIDE SCANNING (Table 10.6)

This minimally invasive technique is highly sensitive in detecting pathological change in bones and joints, but is of somewhat less specificity.

Abnormal areas of bone usually show increased perfusion in the early or vascular phase of the bone scan. Delayed scans demonstrate foci of increase in uptake at sites of increase in bone turnover due to isotope deposition on hydroxyapatite crystals.

While isotope scans demonstrate pathology, they do not indicate its nature, although often this too can be inferred by the distribution of the disease. Scans should be read together with radiographs, but often the scan is performed because the radiograph is perceived to be negative in the presence of clinical symptoms. It is well recognized that the radiograph may be normal for at least 7 days in osteomyelitis, while the isotope scan will rapidly reflect increased blood flow to the abnormal region. Similarly, children with a painful scoliosis should have a bone scan to exclude focal bony pathology, such as an osteoid osteoma.

Infections may also be located by the use of white blood cells labelled in vitro or in vivo.

Spatial discrimination has been improved by the use of SPECT (single photon emission computed tomography).

MAGNETIC RESONANCE IMAGING (MRI) (Table 10.7)

MRI scanning does not involve ionizing radiation but instead utilizes the different distribution of hydrogen ions or protons in the various structures of the body

Table 10.7   Magnetic resonance imaging (MRI).

Best imaging modality for soft tissues
Demonstrates anatomy and pathophysiology in any
   plane
Not as good for cortical bone as CT, but excellent
   for bone marrow
Very sensitive in the arthritides
Costly, time-consuming, not readily available

and their different behaviour when subjected to high-strength, externally applied magnetic fields. The field strength of the external magnets generally varies from 0.5 to 2.0 T (Tesla). Hydrogen nuclei gyrate at frequencies in the range of radio waves or radio frequency (RF) and, under the influence of the magnetic field, their random orientation is aligned along the central axis of the magnetic field. RF stimulation deflects spinning protons and brings them into phase with each other. When the RF pulse is turned off, the system returns to normal. A measure of the time taken for dephasing to occur is the T2 (transverse relaxation time), while the T1 (longitudinal relaxation time) is that taken for the protons to re-establish their orientation relative to the external magnetic field.

Structures which have the highest concentration of protons—fat, fluid and medullary bone—have the highest signal, while those structures most deficient in fluid have the lowest signal. Local increase in fluid due to oedema, haemorrhage or inflammation, or malignancy, therefore increases local signal, while infarction, cell death or soft tissue calcification decrease local signal.

Primary CT images are always in the plane of the scanning gantry. CT reformatting in other planes inevitably involves loss of definition and, because of the extra amount of information needed by the computer, often involves a greater amount of radiation. MR images are obtained in the plane of the operator's choice and are not subject to loss of definition. Vascular programmes and dynamic scans are also available. Joint function can be analysed.

Purpose-made coils are available for each body part, so that for instance the temporomandibular joints or a finger can be scanned with a high signal to noise ratio, while dedicated spinal coils are available to investigate scoliosis.

In most cases T_1- and T_2-weighted images are used (Table 10.8). T_1-weighted images show better anatomic detail. Fat is bright and fluid grey. With T_2-weighted sequences, fat is grey and fluid bright. In both, cortical bone, tendons, ligaments and menisci are black. Fat suppression sequences cause the bright fat signal to be suppressed in the marrow and in subcutaneous and muscle fat. Muscle then appears homogeneously dark grey and the marrow black. Fluid remains bright and so any pathology, with oedema, infection, haemorrhage or hypervascularity clearly stands out against the low signal from surrounding soft tissues. Intravenous paramagnetic contrast media enhance vascular lesions when compared with unenhanced T_1-weighted images.

To summarize, MRI is becoming the investigation of choice for the musculoskeletal system as both anatomy and pathophysiology are demonstrated in any plane. MRI is not only more specific than isotope scanning but is at least as sensitive.

MRI scanning may be stressful to the patient. Older scanners are rather confining, dark, noisy and claustrophobic, leading to a rejection rate of around 2%, while movement artefact causes image degradation. Sedation or anaesthesia may be needed, especially in children, but the patient then needs to be monitored. Nonferromagnetic anaesthetic equipment is needed. Modern scanners are less restricting or even open, allowing biopsies to be performed.

Patients with ferromagnetic implants cannot be scanned. Metal fragments in the eye (welders) may move—metal workers should have preliminary radiographs of the eyes—while surgical clips and some heart valves too may be displaced. Pacemaker function may be interfered with; heat induced in the leads may cause burns. Cochlear implants may be ferromagnetic. IUCDs are often made of copper; these may be safely scanned. It is often not possible to say whether bullets or shrapnel are ferromagnetic. Lists of forbidden implants are available. Orthopaedic implants cause a simple signal void if nonferromagnetic and this does not significantly impair image quality, but ferrous implants are associated with significant artefact.

BIBLIOGRAPHY

Berquist TH (1990) Technical considerations in magnetic resonance imaging. In: *Magnetic Resonance Imaging of the Musculoskeletal System* (ed TH Berquist), 2nd edn, pp 53–73. New York: Raven.

Berquist TH (1991) Magnetic resonance techniques in musculoskeletal disease. *Rheum Dis Clin North Am* **17**: 599–615.

Buckland-Wright JC (1984) Microfocal radiographic examination of erosions in the wrist and hand of patients with rheumatoid arthritis. *Ann Rheum Dis* **43**: 160–71.

Table 10.8 MR sequences in common use: signal intensities.

	T_1W	T_2W	*Fat suppression*
Fat	Bright	Less bright	Low
Fluid	Intermediate	Bright	Bright

Kreel L (ed) (1979) *Clark's Positioning in Radiography*, 10th edn. London: Heinemann.

Nixon JR (1987) Basic principles and terminology. In: *Magnetic Resonance Imaging of the Musculoskeletal System* (ed TH Berquist), pp 1–12. New York: Raven.

Shellock FG (1996) *Pocket Guide to MR Procedures and Metallic Objects*. Philadelphia: Raven.

Stripp WJ (1990) Special techniques in orthopaedic radiography. In: *The Radiology of Skeletal Disorders* (eds RO Murray, HG Jacobson, DJ Stoker), 3rd edn, pp 2045–105. Edinburgh: Churchill Livingstone.

Appendix

SUGGESTIONS FOR FURTHER READING

MAJOR TEXTBOOKS ON BONE DISORDERS

Greenfield GB (1990) *Radiology of Bone Diseases*, 5th edn. Philadelphia: Lippincott.

Marcove RC, Arlen M (1992) *Atlas of Bone Pathology*. Philadelphia: Lippincott.

Milgram JW (1990) *Radiologic and Histologic Pathology of Non-Tumorous Diseases of Bones and Joints*. Illinois: Lea & Febiger.

Murray RO, Jacobson HG, Stoker DJ (1990) *The Radiology of Skeletal Disorders*, 3rd edn. Edinburgh: Churchill Livingstone.

Reeder M, Bradley WG (1993) *Reeder & Felson's Gamuts in Radiology*, 3rd edn. Berlin: Springer.

Resnick D (1995) *Diagnosis of Bone and Joint Disorders*, 3rd edn. Philadelphia: WB Saunders.

Resnick D, Kang HS (1997) *Internal Derangements of Joints*. Philadelphia: WB Saunders.

GENERAL RADIOLOGICAL TEXTBOOKS WITH GOOD CHAPTERS ON ORTHOPAEDICS

Carty H, Shaw DG, Brunelle F, Kendall B (eds) (1994) *Imaging Children*. Edinburgh: Churchill Livingstone.

Grainger RG, Allison D (eds) (1997) *Diagnostic Radiology: a Textbook of Organ Imaging*, 3rd edn. Edinburgh: Churchill Livingstone.

Sutton D (ed) (1998) *A Textbook of Radiology and Imaging*, 6th edn. Edinburgh: Churchill Livingstone.

SPECIALIST MONOGRAPHS

Dalinka MK (ed) (1990) Orthopedics. *Radiologic Clinics of North America* **28** (2) (includes chapters on MRI, densitometry and metastatic bone disease).

Klenerman L (ed) (1991) *The Foot and Its Disorders*, 3rd edn. Oxford: Blackwell Scientific Publications.

Weiss L, Gilbert HA (eds) (1981) *Bone Metastasis*. Boston: GK Hall Medical Publishers.

RHEUMATOLOGY

Forrester DM, Brown JC (1987) *The Radiology of Joint Disease*, 3rd edn. Philadelphia: WB Saunders.

Maddison PJ, Isenberg D, Woo P, Glass DN (eds) (1998) *Oxford Textbook of Rheumatology*, 2nd edn. Oxford: Oxford University Press.

Weissman BN (ed) (1991) Imaging of rheumatic diseases. *Rheumatic Diseases Clinics of North America* **17**, 457–816.

INHERITED DISORDERS

Taybi H, Lachman RF (1990) *The Radiology of Syndromes, Metabolic Disorders and Skeletal Dysplasias*, 3rd edn. Chicago: Year Book Medical Publishers.

Wynne-Davies R, Hall CM, Apley AG (1985) *Atlas of Skeletal Dysplasias*. Edinburgh: Churchill Livingstone.

NORMAL VARIANTS

Keats TE (1996) *Atlas of Radiological Variants*, 6th edn. Chicago: Year Book Medical Publishers.

Kohler A, Zimmer F (1968) *Borderlands of the Normal and Early Pathologic in Skeletal Roentgenology*, 3rd American edn (arranged by Stefan P Wilk). New York: Grune & Stratton.

NUCLEAR MEDICINE

Fogelman I, Maisey M, Clark S (1994) *An Atlas of Clinical Nuclear Medicine*, 2nd edn. London: Martin Dunitz.

COMPUTED TOMOGRAPHY

Scott WW, Magid D, Fishman EK (1987) *CT of the Musculoskeletal System*. Edinburgh: Churchill Livingstone.

MAGNETIC RESONANCE IMAGING

Berquist T (1995) *MRI of the Musculoskeletal System*, 3rd edn. Philadelphia: Lippincott-Raven.

Chan W, Lang P, Genant H (1994) *MRI of the Musculoskeletal System*. Philadelphia: WB Saunders.

Deutsch AL, Mink JH (eds) (1997) *MRI of the Musculoskeletal System*, 2nd edn. Philadelphia: Raven.

Mink JH, Reicher M, Crues J, Deutsch AL (1993) *MRI of the Knee*, 2nd edn. New York: Raven.

Munk PL, Helms CA (1996) *MRI of the Knee*. Philadelphia: Raven.

Steinbach LS, Tirman PFJ, Peterfy CG, Feller JF (1997) *MRI of the Shoulder*. Philadelphia: Raven.

ULTRASOUND

Fornage BD (ed) (1995) *Musculoskeletal Ultrasound*. Edinburgh: Churchill Livingstone.

Van Holsbeeck M, Introcaso JH (1991) *Musculoskeletal Ultrasound*. St Louis: Mosby.

GROWTH AND DEVELOPMENT

Greulich WW, Pyle SI (1959) *Radiographic Atlas of Skeletal Development of the Hand and Wrist*, 2nd edn. Stamford: Stamford University Press.

Tanner JM, Whitehouse RH, Cameron N et al (1983) *Assessment of Skeletal Maturity and Prediction of Adult Height*. London: Academic Press.

Index

Page numbers in *italics* refer to figures, where they occur on pages without accompanying text. The use of *vs* in sub-entries indicates differential diagnosis. The alphabetical order of the index is letter-by-letter.

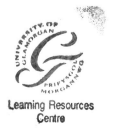